Big Data Management and the Internet of Things for Improved Health Systems

Brojo Kishore Mishra
C. V. Raman College of Engineering, India

Raghvendra Kumar
LNCT Group of Colleges, India

I0868988

A volume in the Advances in Healthcare Information Systems and Administration (AHISA) Book Series

IGI Global
DISSEMINATOR OF KNOWLEDGE

Published in the United States of America by
IGI Global
Medical Information Science Reference (an imprint of IGI Global)
701 E. Chocolate Avenue
Hershey PA, USA 17033
Tel: 717-533-8845
Fax: 717-533-8661
E-mail: cust@igi-global.com
Web site: http://www.igi-global.com

Copyright © 2018 by IGI Global. All rights reserved. No part of this publication may be reproduced, stored or distributed in any form or by any means, electronic or mechanical, including photocopying, without written permission from the publisher. Product or company names used in this set are for identification purposes only. Inclusion of the names of the products or companies does not indicate a claim of ownership by IGI Global of the trademark or registered trademark.

Library of Congress Cataloging-in-Publication Data

Names: Mishra, Brojo Kishore, 1979- editor. | Kumar, Raghvendra, 1987- editor.
Title: Big data management and the internet of things for improved health systems / Brojo Kishore Mishra and Raghvendra Kumar, editors.
Description: Hershey PA : Medical Information Science Reference, [2018] | Includes bibliographical references.
Identifiers: LCCN 2017037992| ISBN 9781522552222 (hardcover) | ISBN 9781522552239 (ebook)
Subjects: | MESH: Data Mining | Medical Informatics | Telemedicine | Cloud Computing | Telemetry | Internet
Classification: LCC R119.95 | NLM W 26.55.I4 | DDC 610.285--dc23 LC record available at https://lccn.loc.gov/2017037992

This book is published in the IGI Global book series Advances in Healthcare Information Systems and Administration (AHISA) (ISSN: 2328-1243; eISSN: 2328-126X)

British Cataloguing in Publication Data
A Cataloguing in Publication record for this book is available from the British Library.

All work contributed to this book is new, previously-unpublished material. The views expressed in this book are those of the authors, but not necessarily of the publisher.

For electronic access to this publication, please contact: eresources@igi-global.com.

Advances in Healthcare Information Systems and Administration (AHISA) Book Series

Anastasius Moumtzoglou
Hellenic Society for Quality & Safety in Healthcare and
P. & A. Kyriakou Children's Hospital, Greece

ISSN:2328-1243
EISSN:2328-126X

Mission

The **Advances in Healthcare Information Systems and Administration (AHISA) Book Series** aims to provide a channel for international researchers to progress the field of study on technology and its implications on healthcare and health information systems. With the growing focus on healthcare and the importance of enhancing this industry to tend to the expanding population, the book series seeks to accelerate the awareness of technological advancements of health information systems and expand awareness and implementation.

Driven by advancing technologies and their clinical applications, the emerging field of health information systems and informatics is still searching for coherent directing frameworks to advance health care and clinical practices and research. Conducting research in these areas is both promising and challenging due to a host of factors, including rapidly evolving technologies and their application complexity. At the same time, organizational issues, including technology adoption, diffusion and acceptance as well as cost benefits and cost effectiveness of advancing health information systems and informatics applications as innovative forms of investment in healthcare are gaining attention as well. **AHISA** addresses these concepts and critical issues.

Coverage

- Medical informatics
- Decision Support Systems
- Measurements and Impact of HISA on Public and Social Policy
- Management of Emerging Health Care Technologies
- Pharmaceutical and Home Healthcare Informatics
- Nursing Expert Systems
- Telemedicine
- Clinical Decision Support Design, Development and Implementation
- IT Applications in Physical Therapeutic Treatments
- E-Health and M-Health

IGI Global is currently accepting manuscripts for publication within this series. To submit a proposal for a volume in this series, please contact our Acquisition Editors at Acquisitions@igi-global.com or visit: http://www.igi-global.com/publish/.

The Advances in Healthcare Information Systems and Administration (AHISA) Book Series (ISSN 2328-1243) is published by IGI Global, 701 E. Chocolate Avenue, Hershey, PA 17033-1240, USA, www.igi-global.com. This series is composed of titles available for purchase individually; each title is edited to be contextually exclusive from any other title within the series. For pricing and ordering information please visit http://www.igi-global.com/book-series/advances-healthcare-information-systems-administration/37156. Postmaster: Send all address changes to above address. Copyright © 2018 IGI Global. All rights, including translation in other languages reserved by the publisher. No part of this series may be reproduced or used in any form or by any means – graphics, electronic, or mechanical, including photocopying, recording, taping, or information and retrieval systems – without written permission from the publisher, except for non commercial, educational use, including classroom teaching purposes. The views expressed in this series are those of the authors, but not necessarily of IGI Global.

Titles in this Series

For a list of additional titles in this series, please visit: www.igi-global.com/book-series

Handbook of Research on Data Science for Effective Healthcare Practice and Administration
Elham Akhond Zadeh Noughabi (University of Calgary, Canada) Bijan Raahemi (University of Ottawa, Canada) Amir Albadvi (Tarbiat Modares University, Iran) and Behrouz H. Far (University of Calgary, Canada)
Medical Information Science Reference • copyright 2017 • 545pp • H/C (ISBN: 9781522525158) • US $255.00 (our price)

Patent Law and Intellectual Property in the Medical Field
Rashmi Aggarwal (Institute of Management Technology Ghaziabad, India) and Rajinder Kaur (Panjab University, India)
Medical Information Science Reference • copyright 2017 • 257pp • H/C (ISBN: 9781522524144) • US $200.00 (our price)

Design, Development, and Integration of Reliable Electronic Healthcare Platforms
Anastasius Moumtzoglou (P&A Kyriakou Children's Hospital, Greece)
Medical Information Science Reference • copyright 2017 • 357pp • H/C (ISBN: 9781522517245) • US $205.00 (our price)

Cloud Computing Systems and Applications in Healthcare
Chintan M. Bhatt (Charotar University of Science & Technology, India) and S. K. Peddoju (Indian Institute of Technology Roorkee, India)
Medical Information Science Reference • copyright 2017 • 282pp • H/C (ISBN: 9781522510024) • US $205.00 (our price)

Handbook of Research on Healthcare Administration and Management
Nilmini Wickramasinghe (Epworth HealthCare, Australia & Deakin University, Australia)
Medical Information Science Reference • copyright 2017 • 825pp • H/C (ISBN: 9781522509202) • US $345.00 (our price)

Reshaping Medical Practice and Care with Health Information Systems
Ashish Dwivedi (University of Hull, UK)
Medical Information Science Reference • copyright 2016 • 399pp • H/C (ISBN: 9781466698703) • US $150.00 (our price)

M-Health Innovations for Patient-Centered Care
Anastasius Moumtzoglou (P&A Kyriakou Children's Hospital, Greece)
Medical Information Science Reference • copyright 2016 • 438pp • H/C (ISBN: 9781466698611) • US $235.00 (our price)

IGI Global
DISSEMINATOR OF KNOWLEDGE

701 East Chocolate Avenue, Hershey, PA 17033, USA
Tel: 717-533-8845 x100 • Fax: 717-533-8661
E-Mail: cust@igi-global.com • www.igi-global.com

Table of Contents

Detailed Table of Contents

In the process of Internet evolution, the transition from IPv4 to IPv6 has become inevitable and fairly urgent. IANA (Internet Assigned Numbers Authority) has finally exhausted the global IPv4 address space, which leaves the community no choice but pushes forward the IPv6 transition process. IPv4 and IPv6 networks both will exist during the transition period, while the two are not compatible in nature. Therefore, it is indispensable to maintain the availability, as well as to provide the inter-communication ability of IPv4 and IPv6. Years ago, a series of transition techniques were actually proposed. However, because of their technical immatureness, they failed to cover the solution space well. Some of these techniques were even obsoleted by IETF due to their flaws.

To study state-of-the art associated to Twitter mining replica as well as prognostic analytic by means of Agile Software Engineering. To recognize sentiment analysis by means of agile knowledge. To obtain as well as analysis given repository for classifying sentiments into positive, negative and neutral emotions. Analysing of all the tweets obtained from the twitter keywords as positive, negative or neutral opinions and comparing all the keywords to judge which keyword is better, there is a requirement to improve from the conventional ways of sentiment analysis. This paper emphasizes on the implementation of an algorithm for automatic classification of text into positive, negative or neutral by fetching the live tweets from twitter server by using twitter API. Graphical representation of the sentiment for the purpose of comparison in the form of pie chart and bar graph. Scan the twitter and fetching the Live Tweets from Twitter server using Twitter4J Advance Java Interface and implementing the Stanford NLP Library (Natural Language Parsing) using Advance Java for classifying the tweets into positive, negative and neutral tweets.

Cloud computing has become a revolution in the field of computing, which enables flexible, on-demand, usage of computing resources in pay-as-per-use model. However, data and computation go to some third-party cloud server beyond the physical control of client escalates various privacy and security concern. This paper proposes an improved outsourcing algorithm for system of linear equation (SLE). The improvements are first, the existing work uses expensive cryptographic computation such as Paillier encryption for security arrangement, the proposed solution does not use such cryptographic primitives rather uses efficient linear transformation method. Secondly, the previous work uses an iterative process, which required L rounds of communication between the client and cloud server, at the same time each iteration causes burden of a decryption followed by a matrix vector multiplication. However, the proposed solution required an optimal one round of communication and one-time transformation and retransformation service. Third, the previous work gives result verification method with (1/2l) error probability, the value of l is a trade-off between security and efficiency. However, the proposed solution gives an error checking with an optimal probability of one. Moreover, a security analysis has been performed on the previous method, which proves marginal security arrangement due to inappropriate use of the Paillier encryption scheme. The proposal has been verified through theoretical and experimental analysis, which demonstrate the superiority of the proposed algorithm as compared to the existing algorithm.

Unintentional falls are a frequent cause of hospitalization that mostly increases health service costs due to injuries. Fall prediction systems strive to reduce injuries and provide fast help to the users. Typically, such systems collect data continuously at a high speed through a device directly attached to the user. Whereas such systems are implemented in devices with limited resources, data volume is significantly important. In this chapter, a real-time data analyzer and reducer is proposed in order to manage the data volume of fall prediction systems.

Population aging is the most significant social transformations of our century. In this context, affordable senior housing with supportive services is a key component to the world's long-term care continuum. One of the main issues is how to cost-efficiently provide adapted (and increasingly complex) care services in senior residences to an exponentially growing number of people considering staff shortage. The rise in operating costs (energy, food, etc.) forces companies to find new ways to stay competitive. In that context, this chapter tries to propose avenues of solutions by giving some answers to a simple question: how to optimize the work of the staff to meet the growing demand considering the context of staff shortage. More precisely, this chapter studies methods and strategies to exploit Ambient Intelligence and Big Data to increase the number of residents an employee can support by automating a part of his daily work.

Availability of huge amount of data has opened up a new area and challenge to analyze these data. Analysis of these data become essential for each organization and these analyses may yield some useful information for their future prospectus. To store, manage and analyze such huge amount of data traditional database systems are not adequate and not capable also, so new data term is introduced – "Big Data". This term refers to huge amount of data which are used for analytical purpose and future prediction or forecasting. Big Data may consist of combination of structured, semi structured or unstructured data and managing such data is a big challenge in current time. Such heterogeneous data is required to maintained in very secured and specific way. In this chapter, we have tried to identify such challenges and issues and also tried to resolve it with specific tools.

In the healthcare field, plenty of clinical data is generated every day from patient records, surveys, research papers, medical devices, among others sources. These data can be exploited to discover new insights about health issues. For helping decision makers and healthcare data managers, a survey of research works and tools covering the process of handling big data in the healthcare field is included. A methodology for CVD prevention, detection and management through the use of tools for big data analysis is proposed. Also, it is important to maintain privacy of patients when handling healthcare data; therefore, a list of recommendations for maintaining privacy when handling healthcare data is presented. Specific clinical analysis are recommended on those regions where the incidence rate of CVD is high, but a weak relation with the common risk factors is observed according to historical data. Finally, challenges which need to be addressed are presented.

In this chapter, the authors have introduced the use of Internet of Things (IoT) applications and services in Indian Railway Transportation System (IRTS). Railway transportation infrastructure is one of the most important factors for the development of any country. India is a developing country and we have a vision to transform India into a developed nation by 2020 using different technologies and tools. Therefore, we need to adopt smart and secure technology for advancement in each area especially in railway transportation for growth and betterment of the country. Further, authors has introduced Vehicular Ad-Hoc Network (VANET) concept for automatic railway gate controlling system to reduce number of accidents over railway premises and enhance the system components for the Indian railway transportation system to provide the comfort, security, safety and infotainment services to the passengers.

The phrase Internet of Things (IoT) heralds a vision of the future Internet where connecting physical things, from banknotes to bicycles, through a network will let them take an active part in the Internet, exchanging information about themselves and their surroundings. This will give immediate access to information about the physical world and the objects in it leading to innovative services and increase in efficiency and productivity. In general, it may be beneficial to incorporate a number of the technologies of IoT with the use of services that can act as the bridge between each technology and the applications that developers wish to implement in IoT. This chapter studies the state-of-the-art of IoT and presents the key potential applications, challenges and future research areas in the domain of IoT. This chapter presents four main categories of services according to technical features. Some major issues of future research in IoT are identified and discussed briefly.

This chapter proposes an optimal cost security approach for the current and emerging trends in the Engineering centric IoT applications that offer an optimized infrastructure and human safety through bimodal deep face recognition. Human face determines the person identity that reveals information like age, gender, emotions, attractiveness and others. Face recognition attracted researchers to enhance its performance because of its potential usage in several commercial, law enforcement, government and video surveillance applications in which individuals perceive each other. In this chapter, authors propose a new secured optimal cost approach for deep face recognition based on feature level fusion of bi-features extracted through unsupervised deep learner, Autoencoder and Local Binary Patterns (LBP) respectively. The dimensionality of fused feature map is reduced and protected through Forward Error Correction (FEC) technique. An efficient optimal cost region matcher (OCRM) is accomplished with Canny edge detector to maximize the face recognition accuracy. OCRM uses north-west corner rule of the transportation problem that fulfills the Monge property. The experimental results demonstrate the superiority of the proposed face recognition system over unimodal systems (Autoencoder and LBP alone) when tested on ORL and Real face datasets with OCRM matcher which is interfaced through diverse IoT applications.

Lifestyle and eating habits with the special focus on young university grads are considered to design and develop a Knowledge Management System (KMS). An appropriate ice cream is suggested via KMS to university grads, which keeps blood glucose level in control and acts as a diabetes preventive KMS. Designed KMS is based on effective Data Science (DS), Big Data techniques considering standalone and proposed distributed versions of Analytical Hierarchy Process (AHP), Monte Carlo AHP (MC-AHP), Goal Programming (GP), K-Means and Artificial Neural Network (ANN) Clustering and Collaborative Filtering (CF). Incremental-learning gains and updates knowledge at each level of applied DS techniques. Developed KMS analyzed ice cream consumption pattern, lifestyle & health condition attributes of university students to promote a novel KM strategy in terms of ice cream recommendation and can give altogether novel trigger to health-conscious students. The confluence of health, students, ice creams and DS is achieved and discussed in this chapter.

This research will identify different patient's online behaviours and similarities that can help patient-clinician communications to improve to discover the future or additional threats to raise awareness of causes and consequences. To scale the model, the prototype will rely on the High Performance Computing (HPC) platform running Hadoop file system for storing patient data at distributed locations and Map-reduce paradigm with machine learning algorithms will be deployed to detect the symptoms. In this approach the authors protect online data of patients from privacy issues. In this, the author's effort this difficulty by means of a new advance utilising new similarity measures between patients. The authors are also providing a research investigation on grouping behavior which is affecting by diverse series demonstration, diverse distance similarity measures, the number of genuine patients, and the number of online doctors obtainable, similarity among patient symptoms, minimizing the feasibility, the number of patients for sittings, and the number of clusters to form.

Big data analytics is a growth area with the potential to provide useful insight in healthcare. Big Data can unify all patient related data to get a 360-degree view of the patient to analyze and predict outcomes. It can improve clinical practices, new drug development and health care financing process. It offers a lot of benefits such as early disease detection, fraud detection and better healthcare quality and efficiency. This chapter introduces the Big Data concept and characteristics, health care data and some major issues of Big Data. These issues include Big Data benefits, its applications and opportunities in medical areas and health care. Methods and technology progress about Big Data are presented in this study. Big Data challenges in medical applications and health care are also discussed. While many dimensions of big data still present issues in its use and adoption, such as managing the volume, variety, velocity, veracity, and value, the accuracy, integrity, and semantic interpretation are of greater concern in clinical application.

Huge amount of data is generated from Healthcare transactions where data are complex, voluminous and heterogeneous in nature. This large dataset can be used as an ideal store which can be analyzed for knowledge discovery as well as various future predictions. So, Data mining is becoming increasingly popular as it offers set of innovative tools and techniques to handle this kind of data set whereas traditional methods have limitations for that. In summary, providing the better patient care and reduction in healthcare cost are two major goals of application of data mining in healthcare. Initially, this chapter explores on the various types of eHealth data and its characteristics. Subsequently it explores various domains in healthcare sector and shows how data mining plays a major role in those domains. Finally, it describes few common data mining techniques and their applications in eHealth domain.

Health care is considered as the fundamental right of every citizen and it is principle duty of every country to provide good health care facilities. Many developed countries spend substantial amount of gross domestic product (GDP) on healthcare. In this chapter, we discuss kernel based machine learning techniques, i.e., k-PCA (Kernel principal component analysis) and its related properties with a aim to prescribe cost effective treatments and easy diagnosis of diseases. This objective could be met only by the serious collaboration between physician and data scientist. We discussed that how we could construct a kernel and exact features based on the given dataset. Also, we compared the proposed method with the other methods. For the sake of easy understanding, applications of the proposed method are included in the text.

Preface

Big data storage and processing is considered as one of the main applications for cloud computing systems. Moreover, the development of the Internet of Things (IoT) paradigm has advanced the research on Machine to Machine (M2M) communications and also has enabled novel tele-monitoring architectures for E-health applications. E-health is an emergent topic that poses several challenges to multiple disciplines, such as Computer Science, Engineering, Health and Social Sciences. Cloud computing, Big data and Internet of Things (IoT) are the prevalent Information and Communication Technology (ICT) paradigms, whose attributes can collaborate to structure the future of E-health systems. Big data in E-health enables the metamorphosis of hypothesis driven research to data-driven research by processing large volumes of hypothetical medical data. Furthermore, by using a search based routine, it is probable to realize feeble signals in Big data.

The Internet of Things (IoT) is a network of physical devices and other items, embedded with electronics, software, sensors, and network connectivity, which enables these objects to collect and exchange data. Its impact on medicine will be perhaps the most important, and personal, effect. By 2020, 40% of IoT-related technology will be health-related, more than any other category, making up a $117 billion market. The convergence of medicine and information technologies, such as medical informatics, will transform healthcare as we know it, curbing costs, reducing inefficiencies, and saving lives. This revolution in medicine will look in a typical IoT hospital, in practice. A patient with diabetes will have an ID card that, when scanned, links to a secure cloud which stores their electronic health record vitals and lab results, medical and prescription histories. Physicians and nurses can easily access this record on a tablet or desktop computer.

The book is organized into 15 chapters. Chapter 1 discussed about IPv4 and IPv6 networks both will exist during the transition period, while the two are not compatible in nature. Therefore, it is indispensable to maintain the availability, as well as to provide the inter-communication ability of IPv4 and IPv6. Years ago, a series of transition techniques were actually proposed. However, because of their technical immatureness, they failed to cover the solution space well. Some of these techniques were even obsolete by IETF due to their flaws.

Chapter 2 emphasized on the implementation of an algorithm for automatic classification of text into positive, negative or neutral by fetching the live tweets from twitter server by using twitter API. Graphical representation of the sentiment for the purpose of comparison in the form of pie chart and bar graph. Scan the twitter and fetching the Live Tweets from Twitter server using Twitter4J Advance Java Interface and implementing the Stanford NLP Library (Natural Language Parsing) using Advance Java for classifying the tweets into positive, negative and neutral tweets.

In Chapter 3, the proposed solution gives an error checking with an optimal probability of one. Moreover, a security analysis has been performed on the previous method, which proves marginal security arrangement due to inappropriate use of the Paillier encryption scheme. The proposal has been verified through theoretical and experimental analyses, which demonstrate the superiority of the proposed algorithm as compared to the existing algorithm.

In Chapter 4, a real-time data analyzer and reducer is proposed in order to manage the data volume of fall prediction systems, and Chapter 5 studies methods and strategies to exploit Ambient Intelligence and Big Data to increase the number of residents an employee can support by automating a part of his daily work. In Chapter 6, we have tried to identify such challenges and issues and also tried to resolve it with specific tools.

Chapter 7 surveyed research works, and tools covering the process of handling big data in the healthcare field is included. A methodology for CVD prevention, detection and management through the use of tools for big data analysis is proposed. Also, it is important to maintain privacy of patients when handling healthcare data; therefore, a list of recommendations for maintaining privacy when handling healthcare data is presented. Specific clinical analysis are recommended on those regions where the incidence rate of CVD is high, but a weak relation with the common risk factors is observed according to historical data. Finally, challenges which need to be addressed are presented, and Chapter 8 introduced Vehicular Ad-Hoc Network (VANET) concept for automatic railway gate controlling system to reduce number of accidents over railway premises and enhance the system components for the Indian railway transportation system to provide the comfort, security, safety and infotainment services to the passengers.

Chapter 9 studies the state-of-the-art of IoT and presents the key potential applications, challenges and future research areas in the domain of IoT. This chapter presents four main categories of services according to technical features. Some major issues of future research in IoT are identified and discussed briefly. Chapter 10 proposed a new secured optimal cost approach for deep face recognition based on feature level fusion of bi-features extracted through unsupervised deep learner, Auto encoder and Local Binary Patterns (LBP) respectively. The dimensionality of fused feature map is reduced and protected through Forward Error Correction (FEC) technique. An efficient optimal cost region matcher (OCRM) is accomplished with Canny edge detector to maximize the face recognition accuracy. OCRM uses north-west corner rule of the transportation problem that fulfills the Monge property. The experimental results demonstrate the superiority of the proposed face recognition system over unimodal systems (Auto encoder and LBP alone) when tested on ORL and Real face datasets with OCRM matcher which is interfaced through diverse IoT applications.

The confluence of health, students, ice-creams and DS is achieved and discussed in Chapter 11. Developed KMS analyzed ice-cream consumption pattern, lifestyle and health condition attributes of university students to promote a novel KM strategy in terms of ice-cream recommendation and can give altogether novel trigger to health-conscious students.

In Chapter 12, the author's effort this difficulty by means of a new advance utilizing new similarity measures between patients. The authors are also providing a research investigation on grouping behavior which is affecting by diverse series demonstration, diverse distance similarity measures, the number of genuine patients, and the number of online doctors obtainable, similarity among patient symptoms, minimizing the feasibility, the number of patients for sittings, and the number of clusters to form. This drives the need to investigate healthcare information to control and reduce the burgeoning cost of healthcare, as well as to seek evidence to improve patient outcomes. It identifies massive shortage of proper health care facilities and addresses how to provide greater access to primary health care services in rural India. It presents the reforms in the health care sector and boosts the discussions on how government can harness innovations in the big data analytics to improve the rural health care system are discussed in Chapter 13.

Chapter 14 explores the various types of eHealth data and its characteristics. Subsequently it explores various domains in healthcare sector and shows how data mining plays a major role in those domains. Finally, it describes few common data mining techniques and their applications in eHealth domain, and Chapter 15 discussed kernel-based machine learning techniques, i.e., k-PCA (Kernel principal component analysis) and its related properties with a aim to prescribe cost effective treatments and easy diagnosis of diseases. This objective could be met only by the serious collaboration between physician and data scientist. We discussed that how we could construct a kernel and exact features based on the given dataset. Also, we compared the proposed method with the other methods. For the sake of easy understanding, applications of the proposed method are included in the text.

There have been several influences from our family and friends who have sacrificed lot of their time and attention to ensure that we are kept motivated to complete this crucial project.

The editors are thankful to all the members of IGI Global especially Jan Travers and Maria Rohde for the given opportunities to edit this book.

Brojo Kishore Mishra
C. V. Raman College of Engineering, India

Raghvendra Kumar
LNCT Group of Colleges, India

Chapter 1
IPv6-Based IoT Smart Cities

Aashish Gadgil
KLS Gogte Institute of Technology, India

ABSTRACT

In the process of Internet evolution, the transition from IPv4 to IPv6 has become inevitable and fairly urgent. IANA (Internet Assigned Numbers Authority) has finally exhausted the global IPv4 address space, which leaves the community no choice but pushes forward the IPv6 transition process. IPv4 and IPv6 networks both will exist during the transition period, while the two are not compatible in nature. Therefore, it is indispensable to maintain the availability, as well as to provide the inter-communication ability of IPv4 and IPv6. Years ago, a series of transition techniques were actually proposed. However, because of their technical immatureness, they failed to cover the solution space well. Some of these techniques were even obsoleted by IETF due to their flaws.

INTRODUCTION

The Internet has been remarkably successful in scaling from a small community of users to a global network of networks serving more than a billion users. Over a short period it has also become a fundamental infrastructure for economies and societies around the world. Along the way, what was being interconnected expanded from one mainframe per university or company, to a one computer per person paradigm, to a multi-device environment, including greater use and all forms of access. In the future, vast numbers of objects may be connected to the Internet.

Growth in the use of the Internet has meant greater demand for Internet addresses. IP addresses combine "WHO", "WHERE" and "HOW" roles in the Internet's architecture. Internet addresses uniquely identify devices on the network i.e. "endpoints", enabling the identification of the parties to a communication transaction ("WHO" role). In addition, addresses are used by the network to transfer data as they determine the network location of the identified endpoint ("WHERE" role). Addresses are also used to support routing decisions ("HOW" role). Therefore, IP addresses enable connection to the Internet, both through identification of the endpoints to a conversation and enabling the carriage of the data of the conversation through the network.

DOI: 10.4018/978-1-5225-5222-2.ch001

Copyright © 2018, IGI Global. Copying or distributing in print or electronic forms without written permission of IGI Global is prohibited.

IPv6 is a new version of the Internet layer protocol (IP) in the TCP/IP suite of protocols. It replaces the current Internet protocol layer commonly referred to as IPv4. IPv6 is not new. RFC 2460 (IPv6) was released in December 1998. It has been more than a decade, so where are we with IPv6?

The transition between today's IPv4 Internet and the future IPv6-based one will be a long process during which both protocol versions will coexist. Moving from IPv4 to IPv6 is not straightforward and guidelines to simplify transition between the two versions have to be standardized. Network transition has been discussed in detail; however applications should be reviewed to complete the porting process.

Existing applications are written assuming IPv4. Only very recently IPv6 has been taken into account. Unless most of basic distributed applications are available now; there is too much work to do yet. The aim of this paper is to provide general recommendations to be taken into account during the porting process of applications and services to IPv6. This will allow developers to move smoothly their applications into the new environment.

IPv4 has been the network layer protocol since the very early stage of the Internet. The scale of IPv4 Internet has become far larger than one could ever imagine when designing the protocol. Currently IPv4 Internet is facing a series of problems including address exhaustion, routing scalability, and broken end-to-end property. IANA (Internet Assigned Numbers Authority) had run out of global IPv4 address pool in Feb 2011, while simulations show that within 3 years all the RIRs (Rigional Internet Registries) will exhaust their IPv4 address space. On the other hand, the scale of Internet is still growing fast, especially on the user side where the number of Internet-enabled mobile devices increases rapidly. This leads to continuous demands for new IP address allocation, which seems impossible to satisfy with IPv4. ChinaTelecom, one of the largest telecom ISPs (Internet Service Providers) in the world claims that by the end of 2012, they will use up all the IPv4 addresses they have acquired or can acquire. Besides, the prefix de-aggregation caused by address block subdivision, multihoming and traffic engineering has caused a burst in Global IPv4 RIB (Routing Information Base) and FIB (Forwarding Information Base). The Internet is suffering from this routing scalability problem. Moreover, the wide use of NAT has broken down the fundamental end-to-end property all over the Internet.

The objective of this chapter is divided in three parts. The first analyzes in which conditions is possible the transition to IPv6 without changing applications. This chapter includes recommendations on how to proceed when source code is not available and explains which mechanisms can be used. The second is the main part. It starts describing IPv6 transition scenarios from the application point of view. The focus is on analyzing existing applications looking for characteristics, which usually should be reviewed during transition to IPv6. It includes a brief description of basic socket interface extensions for IPv6, fully described in RFC2553. The chapter concludes providing general recommendations for new IPv6 applications. In the future all IPv4 networks will be IPv6 however during a long period mixed scenarios with both IPv4 and IPv6 will be the real environments. Therefore, new applications should be designed to work only in a pure IPv6 environment, but a design to allow mixed IPv4 and IPv6 environment is better now.

TRANSITION TO IPV6 WITHOUT CHANGING APPLICATIONS

Many methodologies have been studied to support transition to IPv6 depending on initial network architectures. To make IPv6 network available to the user it's necessary to provide a great number of IPv6 applications. Although, existing applications are written assuming IPv4, it isn't desirable to wait until all necessary applications will be ready to start network transition.

The simple approach during initial transition stages is to use IPv4 applications over the new IPv6 network environment. Unfortunately, this is not a simple task. A pure IPv6 node provides only the IPv6 socket interface but old applications only work over IPv4 socket interface. Both interfaces are similar, but there are some incompatible differences related with:

- Name (DNS) and IP addresses management,
- Communication constants and data structures or
- Functions names and parameters

Therefore, the IPv4 stack should be available to continue using IPv4 applications. The network is IPv6, so to operate with the network the stack which should be used is the IPv6 one. Then dual stack is required.

But dual stack is not enough. If both IPv4 and IPv6 network interfaces are available but only there are IPv4 applications, IPv6 will not be used. A real IPv6 scenery implies removing IPv4 network and operating only through IPv6 one. The solution is to provide a translator from the IPv6 network interface into the IPv4 programming interface required by applications; see Figure 1.

A translator intercepts data flowing between application and the link layer modules and translates all IPv4 related issues into IPv6 and vice versa. When IPv4 application communicates with an IPv6 node, the translator changes addresses into IPv6, changes the call into the new environment and outputs an IPv6 packet. The reception is similar. All input packets are examined, translated and emitted to the upper layer in the IPv4 format. Thus it seems as if it was dual stack host with both IPv4 and IPv6 or dual applications. Translation can be made at three different levels: link, socket or application.

Figure 1. Application interface translators

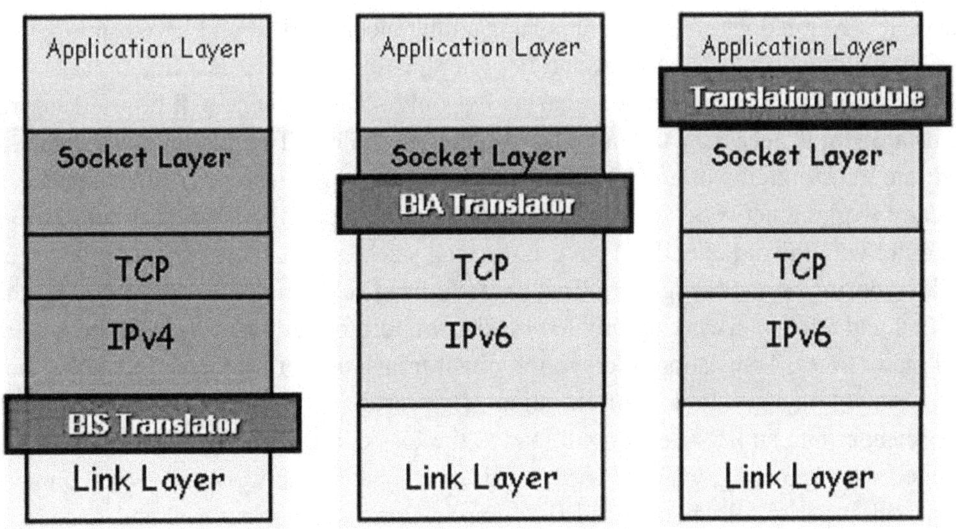

Link translation [BIS] takes place between IP level and network driver modules (the link layer). At this level the translator intercepts all input and output IP packets. If correspondent node is IPv4 the packet is emitted without changes. If correspondent node is an IPv6 one, it is revised and translated into an IPv4 packet. If it is an output packet, the translator obtains the IPv6 address of the correspondent node and outputs an IPv6 packet. When the node receives an IPv6 packet, it obtains the correspondent node IPv4 address (or builds it) and translates the original IPv6 packet into the IPv4 one.

Socket interface translation [BIA] takes place between socket API module and the TCP/IP module. Now translation is at interface programming level, so translation is simplified without translating IP packet headers. To communicate with an IPv6 node, the translator intercepts all IPv4 sockets calls and translates them into IPv6 sockets functions. The returns from IPv6 calls (packets reception) are translated into the correspondent IPv4 returns. The mechanism is complemented with translations of addresses and names, similar to the previous one.

Finally, sometimes applications use user level communications library, for example when a prototype or an interpreted programming language is used. In such a case, it is possible to introduce the translator at application level. The communications API module remains unchanged but it is rewritten in order to transform part of the IPv4 connections into IPv6 ones. Translation of names and addresses are also required to provide only IPv4 information to the application when it connects with an IPv6 node.

Unfortunately, there are many applications without a clear modularization or have addresses dependencies, in such cases application code should be revised to integrate the application in the new IPv6 environment.

The most important requirement in IPv6 transition is that existing services should work in the new environment but also continue to work with IPv4 nodes. The simplest approach to introduce IPv6 without changing applications is to use dual-stack: supporting IPv4 and IPv6 simultaneously, maintaining old IPv4 applications and adding new ones to communicate with IPv6 nodes. This largely increases the complexity of network administration and maintains the address space scarce resource.

There is a pressure to start up new networks in the new IPv6 environment without IPv4 support. However, there is no a single global IPv6 network on the same scale as the actual IPv4 and it will take some time to get it. Therefore, new applications should be designed to work in all environments: single IPv4, single IPv6 or mixed environment connecting IPv6 with IPv4 nodes. That is, dual protocol stack is necessary. However, it does not mean supporting simultaneously IPv4 and IPv6 routing. It is possible to use IPv6 applications on IPv4 network and IPv4 applications on IPv6 network.

Therefore, there are many possible scenarios but only some of them will be used in practice. To select the best one it is necessary to know the initial environment. Two possible environments can be considered: the transition of working IPv4 network and the setup of new network or service.

For already working networks the better solution is to maintain the IPv4 stack and introduce IPv6 stack in parallel with the old one; that is to use the dual stack environment [DSTM]. It is the principal building block during transitioning from IPv4 to IPv6. Dual stack mechanisms do not, by themselves, solve the IPv4 and IPv6 interworking problems; other important building block, addresses translation, is required many times. Translation refers to the direct translation of protocols, including headers and sometimes protocol payload. Protocol translation often results in features loss. For instance, translation of IPv6 header into an IPv4 header will lead to the loss of the IPv6 flow label. Translation can be complemented with tunneling; which is used to bridge compatible networks across incompatible ones.

After transition period, IPv4 stack and IPv4 applications will be removed and result a pure IPv6 environment.

The organizations transition from IPv4 to IPv6 follows more or less the same steps. Each step defines one transition scenario; see Figure 2. The systems manager should provide applications to work in all of them. We can consider various scenarios in application porting process using dual-stack:

Start Point: Applications have been designed on IPv4 and the network is working with IPv4 only.
Step 1: The network remains unchanged. Some IPv6 applications are available but IPv6 communication is only possible through IPv6 over IPv4 tunnels.
Step 2: IPv6 is available at network level unless applications remain unchanged and only support IPv4. Only IPv6 applications can use the IPv6 network.
Step 3: Applications are ready to work simultaneously on IPv4 and IPv6.
Step 4: IPv4 network has been removed. Communication with IPv4 nodes is only possible with the help of an IPv4 over IPv6 tunnel.
End Point: Finally all IPv4 networks and applications use IPv6.

The application porting process takes place between steps II and III. This chapter is devoted to describe how to make such application adaptations. There are two probable scenarios during the transition. The first is based on maintaining two application versions and the second with only one dual version.

We can forget old IPv4 applications and maintain them only to communicate with IPv4 nodes during transition period. The transition methodology consists in developing a complete set of applications designed to work only over IPv6 transport layer. The main advantage is to be ready with new applications after transition period. To finish IPv6 transition it is necessary only to removed IPv4 applications and dual stack network. However, the selection of suitable applications during transition period it's a user responsibility. When tests, configuration or management of applications are considered, the application selection is not a problem because their users normally have technical knowledge. However, with most of end-user applications, the user hasn't enough knowledge or doesn't want to know, which is the proper

Figure 2. Transition scenarios

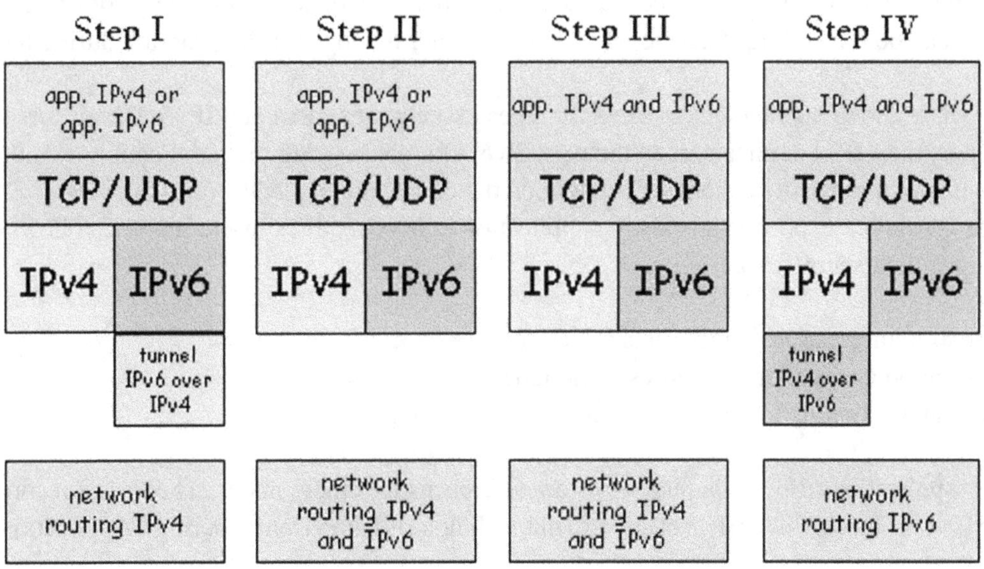

application version that should be used in each connection. Moreover, during transition period it will be necessary to provide data servers working both IPv4 and IPv6 to accept connections not only from new but also from old nodes.

The second transition scenario looks for changing existing applications, not developing new ones. The porting process takes the original IPv4 application, review source code and produces a new version adapted to work over both IPv4 and IPv6 environments. The porting process is a little bit more complex than IPv6 only support, but the result is more flexible to be used during transition period. Transition period will be probably a long period during which there will be islands, not only IPv6 but also IPv4, interested for users in the new environments. This is because during a long period most of data servers will be maintained in the IPv4 only environment.

However, for new network or services an only IPv6 stack environment is better. It is not sense to define an IPv4 network so dual stack is not allowed. However, during transition period native IPv6 networks will need to maintain connectivity with applications, which can only be reached through IPv4. In such cases, one standard network transition mechanism should be provided [6to4]. Depending on the application, sometimes it is possible to use special dual-stack edge servers at the IPv4 and IPv6 border as application level proxies, removing the need for network-level transition.

PORTING APPLICATIONS

Unless there are many proposed solutions to accelerate transition from IPv4 to IPv6, ultimately, applications should be modified to simplify protocol stacks configurations and support all IPv4 and IPv6 communication types.

Most existing applications are written assuming IPv4. In general, most of them can be converted without too much effort. Many changes could be done automatically and there are some scripts to do it. However, there are applications, which make special use of IPv4 or include advanced features, such as multicasting, raw sockets or other IP options. In such cases, an exhaustive code revision should be done.

Besides, there are applications that are not only affected by modification of function calls but also by the logic behind their usage. Such code is the hardest to deal with and cannot be automatically ported. This code can be misleading if developers do not consider the logic of the program during the porting process.

Dual stack allows applications to use both types of addresses, IPv4 and IPv6. Developers will only need to port their IPv4 applications to the new IPv6 API, considering that applications could communicate using both protocol versions, depending on the destination node.

In the general case, porting an existing application to IPv6 requires to examine the following issues in the application source code:

- Network information storage: data structures.
- Resolution and conversion address functions.
- Communication API functions and pre-defined constants.

Many applications use IP addresses to store references to remote nodes. This is not recommended because IPv6 lets addresses change over time (this technique is named renumbering). Applications should use stable identifiers for other nodes, for instance, host names. If applications store IP addresses they should redo the mapping from host names to IP addresses in order to solve inconsistencies.

Client applications should be prepared to connect to multi-homed severs, nodes that have more than one IP address. Hence, when a communication channel to a multi-homed server fails, client applications should try another IP address in the multi-homed server list of IP addresses until they find one that is working.

IPv4/IPv6 Interoperability

The mechanism to select the appropriate IP address is decided by the name service. When a network node wants to reach another, it asks the name service for its IP address. If the answer is an IPv4 address, it is assumed that there is a path through Internet to link with the remote node and that this remote node is capable of receiving IPv4 connections from the source node. The same applies for a node that has only IPv6 address. It is assumed that it understands IPv6 packets. If both source and destination nodes have dual stack, the communication will use the type of address returned by the name service.

During first step of transition phase there is no IPv6 network. This document is not devoted to study how to solve other communication aspects, which are not visible to the application layer. If IPv6 addresses should be used during connection but IPv6 routers are not part of the network infrastructure, a basic IPv4 framework should be used. This is achieved by building IPv6 tunnels. They encapsulate IPv6 packets inside IPv4 header and send them through the IPv4 network.

However, dual-stack should be used during most of the transition periods, because not all IPv6-only implementations allow the interaction with any kind of network node. As such there is necessity to check the interoperability between IPv4-only nodes, IPv6-only nodes and dual stack nodes using the client/server model.

GUIDELINES ON DEVELOPING NEW APPLICATIONS

In the design of applications to use IPv6 some characteristics must be taken into account. First of all it is necessary to separate the transport module from the rest of application functional modules. This separation makes the application independent on the network system used. Then, if the network protocol is changed, only the transport module should be modified. Transport module should provide the communication channel abstraction with basic channel operations and generic data structures to represent the addresses. These abstractions could be instantiated as different implementations depending on the network protocol required at any moment. The application will deal with this generic communication channel interface without knowing the network protocol used. Using this design if a new network protocol is added, application developers only need to implement a new instance of the channel abstraction, which manages the features of this new protocol.

Once the transport module has been designed, there are some implementations details related to the type of the nodes which will run the application: IPv4-only nodes, IPv6-only nodes or both, dual stack. Within the transport module the use of the new API with extensions for IPv6 is mandatory, but it is strongly recommended to make the program protocol independent. The new IPv6 functions are only valid if this protocol is supported by all installed systems. IPv6 is now reaching maturity and most popular systems provide it as default in their standard distributions. However, IPv6 support does not force to use it, only after the complete network configuration is defined, applications will use IPv4 or IPv6. Protocol independent code is feasible if the design is based on the principal building block for transitioning, the dual stack. Dual stacks maintain two protocol stacks that operate in parallel and thus it is allowed to operate via either protocol. The operating system running dual stack translates IPv4 addresses to IPv4-mapped IPv6 ones when communicating to IPv4 remote applications. Although applications are written following program protocol independent rules, other points have to be considered such as the movement of binary code between IPv4-only nodes, dual stacks nodes or IPv6-only nodes.

Compilation options (#ifdefs in C language) can be provided throughout the code to select the proper use environment. If IPv6 is not supported the IPv4-only code will be selected for compilation during installation process. However, if IPv6 is supported (Kernel level support) by installed systems, the code for IPv6 or the IPv4 could be selected for compilation, depending on the requirements of applications. Notice that if the kernel supports IPv6, it only means the IPv6 option could be activated and while this option is disabled the node will be only use IPv4 stack. During the transition period nodes are usually running dual stack, both IPv4 and IPv6 stacks. The problem with the conditional compilation approach is that the code becomes littered with compilation options very quickly and harder to follow and maintain.

If an application is compiled on a system, which supports dual stack and move the binary code to an IPv4-only node without IPv6 kernel support, the source code must be recompiled to use the original IPv4 API. The binary code generated on the dual stack uses the new system functions, which are not supported in the IPv4-only node.

If the binary code is moved, which has been compiled on a dual stack, to an IPv4-only node with IPv6 kernel support and IPv6 stack not activated, recompilation is not required. Since the IPv6 stack is not activated, the node cannot establish IPv6 connections. However, the resolver system could return an IPv6 address to an application query and the application should be prepared to discard this IPv6 address and select the IPv4 one to open connections.

All these alternatives are summarized in Table 1.

Table 1. IPv4 or IPv6 activation

NODE		APPLICATION		CONNECTIONS	
IPv6 kernel support	**Dual stack activated**	**Network API used**	**Application type**	**IPv4 connection**	**IPv6 connection**
Yes	Yes	IPv6 extensions (portable code)	IPv6-enabled	IPv4 stack	IPv6 stack
	No	IPv6 extensions (portable code)	IPv6-enabled	IPv4 stack	IPv6 address resolution Connection error.
No		Without IPv6 extensions (old API)	IPv4-only (compiled with IPv4 options)	IPv4 stack	Error

In summary, if applications follow the recommendations explained above, using a separated protocol independent transport module, which provides a generic communication API, it is easy to adapt them to new network protocols. Besides, the generic communication API could be implemented as a communication library to be used for many applications. This solution encourages the code reusability and makes communication modules of applications easy to maintain.

Finally, if the new application is designed only for the new IPv6 environment, the code is simpler than dual stack implementation. The new application will work only with other IPv6 nodes. When the local IPv6 node wants to use IPv6 application to communicate with a remote IPv4 node, one standard network transition mechanism should be provided [6to4]. Depending on the application, sometimes it is possible to use special dual-stack edge servers at the IPv4 and IPv6 border as application level proxies, removing the need for network-level transition.

Future of IPv6

IPv6 enabled Internet version 2 will replace todays IPv4 enabled Internet. When Internet was launched with IPv4, developed countries like U.S. and Europe took the larger space of IPv4 for deployment of Internet in their respective countries keeping future need in mind. But Internet exploded everywhere reaching and connecting every country of the world increasing the requirement of IPv4 address space. As a result, till this day U.S. and Europe have many IPv4 address space left with them and countries like India and China are bound to address their IP space requirement by means of deployment of IPv6. Most of the IPv6 deployment is being done outside U.S., and Europe. India and China are moving forward to change their entire space to IPv6. China has announced a five year deployment plan named China Next Generation Internet. After June 06, 2012 all major ISPs were shifted to IPv6 and rest of them are still moving. IPv6 provides ample of address space and is designed to expand today's Internet services. Feature-rich IPv6 enabled Internet version 2 may deliver more than expected.

CONCLUSION

Given that IANA has eventually run out IPv4 address space, the Internet is bound to enter the IPv6 era. Nevertheless, IPv4 networks will coexist with IPv6 networks for a long time during the transition. The IPv6 transition process should be steady and smooth. Therefore, the IPv4-IPv6 coexisting networks should sustain the availability of both IPv4 and IPv6, and support IPv4-IPv6 interconnection as well.

The transition techniques are still facing challenges and require further research efforts. For translation techniques, the most critical issue is the lack of feasible, stateful IPv4→IPv6 translation mechanisms. Unfortunately, based on the current understanding of IPv4-IPv6 translation, this problem seems unlikely to be solved. We need to find a new angle to develop a solution. As for the existing translation mechanisms, there are still the issues of scalability, heterogeneous addressing and application layer translation. IPv6 is the only technology currently available that is mature enough to provide a viable, long term solution. It is not perfect as it is not backwards compatible and does not work with IPv4. But it does work alongside IPv4 and can integrate via a number of methods providing co-existence and transition.

REFERENCES

de Miguel, T. P., & Castro, E. M. (2012). *Programming guidelines on transition to IPv6*. LONG (Laboratories Over Next Generation networks) project, IST-1999-20393.

de Miguel & Castro. (2001). *Requirements and guidelines for distributed laboratorios applications migration*. LONG Project IST-1999-20393, D3.1.

Gilligan. (2002). *Basic Socket Interface Extensions for IPv6*. Obsoletes RFC 2553.

Huston, G. (2010). *IPv4 Address Report*. Tech. Rep. Available: http://www.potaroo.net/tools/ipv4

I. S. I. at University of Southern California. (1981). *Internet Protocol, DARPA Internet Program, Protocol Specification*. Author.

IETF RFC 791. (2011). *Internet Usage Statistics*. Miniwatts Marketing Group, Tech. Rep. Available: http://www.internetworldstats.com

Nordmark, E. (2000). *Stateless IP/ICMP Translator (SIIT)*. RFC 2765.

Shin et al. (2002). *Application Aspects of IPv6 Transition*. Academic Press.

Srisuresh & Egevang. (2001). *Traditional IP Network Address Translator (Traditional NAT)*. RFC 3022.

Tsirtsis & Srisuresh. (2000). *Network Address Translation – Protocol Translation (NAT-PT)*. RFC 2766.

Tsuchiya, Higuchi, & Atarashi. (2000). *Dual Stack Hosts using the Bump-In-The-Stack technique (BIS)*. RFC 2767.

Wu, Cui, & Wu, Liu, & Metz. (n.d.). Transition from IPv4 to IPv6: A State-of-the-Art Survey. *IEEE Communications Surveys and Tutorials*.

Chapter 2
Agile-Model-Based Sentiment Analysis From Social Media

Tarandeep Kaur Bhatia
Chandigarh Group of Colleges, India

ABSTRACT

To study state-of-the art associated to Twitter mining replica as well as prognostic analytic by means of Agile Software Engineering. To recognize sentiment analysis by means of agile knowledge. To obtain as well as analysis given repository for classifying sentiments into positive, negative and neutral emotions. Analysing of all the tweets obtained from the twitter keywords as positive, negative or neutral opinions and comparing all the keywords to judge which keyword is better, there is a requirement to improve from the conventional ways of sentiment analysis. This paper emphasizes on the implementation of an algorithm for automatic classification of text into positive, negative or neutral by fetching the live tweets from twitter server by using twitter API. Graphical representation of the sentiment for the purpose of comparison in the form of pie chart and bar graph. Scan the twitter and fetching the Live Tweets from Twitter server using Twitter4J Advance Java Interface and implementing the Stanford NLP Library (Natural Language Parsing) using Advance Java for classifying the tweets into positive, negative and neutral tweets.

INTRODUCTION

The difficulty in sentimental_analysis is categorizing the polarity of a specified manuscript at a sentence, document or feature/aspect level whether the uttered belief in a sentence, document and feature/aspect is positive, negative or neutral. (Ågerfalk, Pär, Fitzgerald, 2006). Twitter is a public networking as well as micro_blogging examination that permit clients to post real_time message, known as tweets. Tweets are tiny posts, limited to 140 lettering in extent. (Charalabidis, Yannis, Triantafillou, Karkletsis, Loukis, 2012). Due to the natural world of this micro_blogging examination, public apply acronyms; create spelling_mistakes, make use of emoticons as well as extra fonts that state extraordinary significance. Subsequent is a concise vocabulary linked by means of tweets. (Colbaugh, Richard and Galss, 2011).

DOI: 10.4018/978-1-5225-5222-2.ch002

Copyright © 2018, IGI Global. Copying or distributing in print or electronic forms without written permission of IGI Global is prohibited.

- **Emoticons:** They are facial_expressions, diagrammatically signifying by means of punctuation as well as letters; they state the consumer's humor. (Hogenboom, Alexander, Bal, Fransincar, Bal, Joung and Kaymak, 2013).
- **Target:** Consumers of Twitter make use of the @ sign to refer to further consumers on the micro_blog. Referring to further consumers in this way robotically aware them. (Yi, Jeonghee, Nasukawa, Bunescu, Niblack, 2003).
- **Hash_Tags:** Consumers frequently make use of hash_tags to spot subject. This is first and foremost prepared to enlarge the visibility of their tweets. (Naveed, Nasir, Gottron, Kunegis, Alhadi, 2011).

PROPOSED SYSTEM AND SYSTEM DESIGN

Methodology

1. To study state-of-the art associated to Twitter mining replica as well as prognostic analytics by means of Agile Software Engineering.
2. To recognize sentiment analysis by means of agile knowledge.
3. To obtain as well as analysis given repository for classifying sentiments into positive, negative and neutral emotions.

Procedure

This study job is paying attention on the prognostic investigation as well as alliance of consumer account through their timeline. (Rosenthal, Sara, Nakov, Kiritchenko, Mohamad, Ritter, Stoyanov, 2015). There are numerous parts of planned job as well as execution by which the withdrawal of live social_media as well as particular characteristic are interconnected for the connection in addition to bond (Prabowo, Rudy, Thelwall, 2009). By means of this strategy, the outline of whichever consumer can be straightforwardly obtained from numerous social_media as well as after that the chance or connection features through additional functions can be completed. (Whitworth, Biddle, 2007).

In this study job, the sentiment facts investigation as well as forecast is prepared on the large data obtained during live tweets. By means of forecasting tools in addition to algorithms, the successful as well as correct outcomes shall be calculated. (Hao, Ming, Rohrdantz, Janetzko, Dayal, Keim, Haug, Hsu, 2011).

Work Objective

Scan the twitter and fetching the Live Tweets from Twitter server using Twitter4J Advance Java Interface and implementing the Stanford NLP Library (Natural Language Parsing) using Advance Java for classifying the tweets into positive, negative and neutral tweets. Sentiment Analysis aims to determine the attitude of the mass as positive, negative or neutral towards the subject of interest. Graphical representation of the sentiment for the purpose of comparison in the form of pie chart and bar graph.

Research Methodology

1. Input the keyword for which the sentiment need to be analysed.
2. Scan the twitter and fetching the Live Tweets from Twitter server using Twitter4J Advance Java Interface.
3. Real time dataset creation is done with the help of twitter server tokens or secured key.
4. Set of tweets has been created.
5. Fragmentation of each tweet as line wise as well as word wise.
6. Extraction of the Interesting / Feature Points from the Tweets that represent emotions or sentiment. This collection will be match with repository of positive, negative and neutral words.
7. Analysis of each tweet is done.
8. Sentiment Score is assigned.
9. If all the tweets are over then plotting is done for comparison.
10. If all tweets are not over then again go to step 6 and continue the same process. This all the iterations will be followed by agile model.

Process

See Figure 1.

Common Tools of Sentiment Analysis (Cambria, Hussain, 2015)

1. Meltwater
2. Google Alerts
3. People Browser
4. Tweet stats
5. Pagelever
6. Social Mention
7. Twitter Sentiment
8. TweetFeel

Technologies Used in Sentiment Analysis (Feldman, 2015)

1. Advance Java
2. Eclipse IDE
3. Twitter4J
4. Dia - The Diagram Editor
5. Stanford NLP API
6. JFreeCharts JAVA APIs for Plotting of Graphs

Figure 1. Process of sentiment analysis

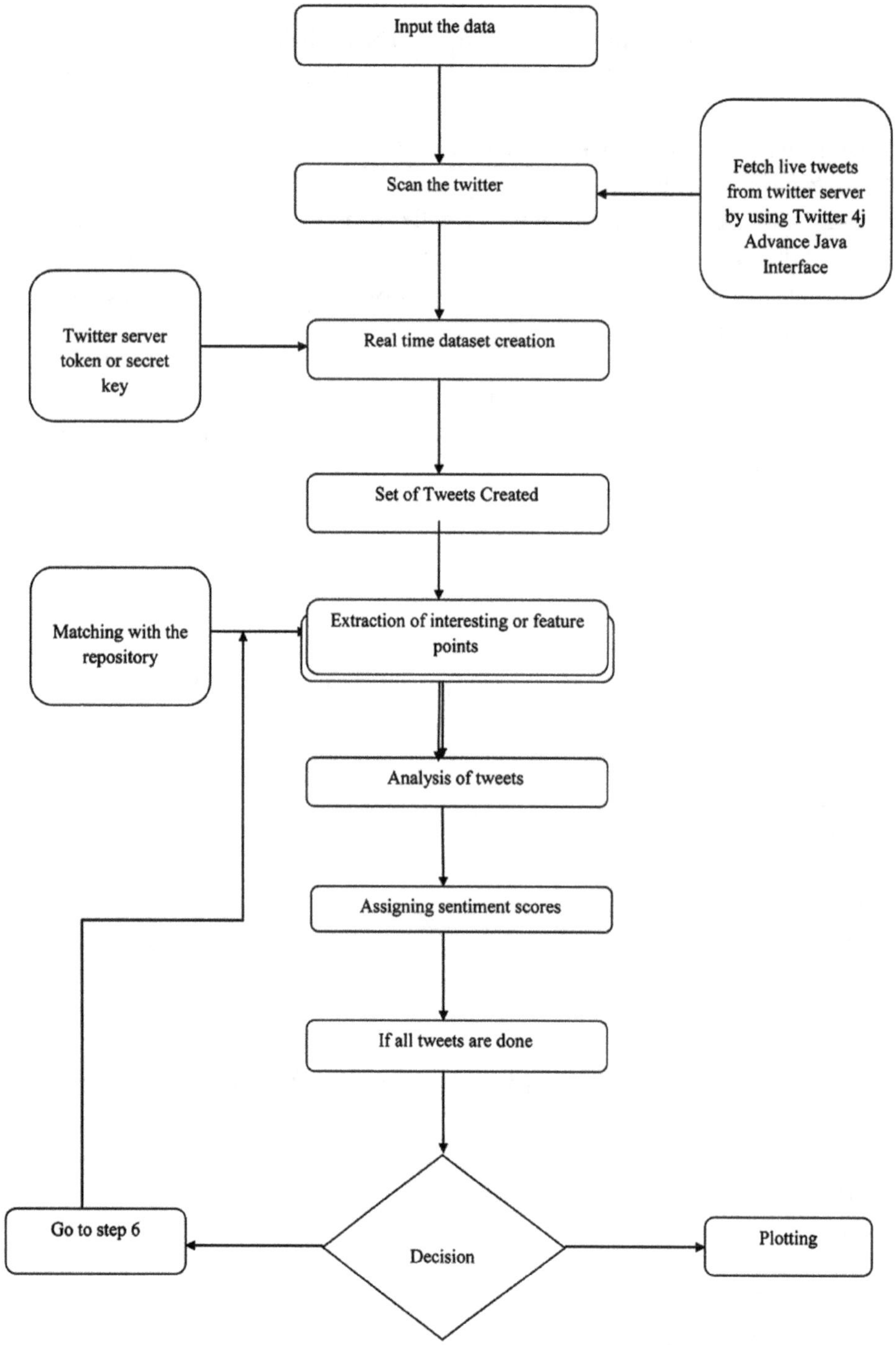

Applications of Sentiment Analysis (Goncalves, Pollyanna, Araujo, Benevenuto, Cha, 2013)

1. It is being used in purchasing products.
2. Improving the quality of products.
3. Recommendation system.
4. Decision Making.
5. Policy Making.
6. Customer Satisfaction.
7. Used in Surveys.
8. Business purposes.
9. Key role in Politics.
10. Promotions of movies.

Challenges of Sentiment Analysis (Saif, 2016)

1. Detection of spam and fake reviews.
2. Limitation of classification filtering.
3. Domain – Dependence.
4. Natural Language processing overheads.
5. People express opinions in a complex way

EXPERIMENTAL RESULTS AND DISCUSSION

See Figures 2-13.

Figure 2. Sign in the Twitter account (https://apps.twitter.com)

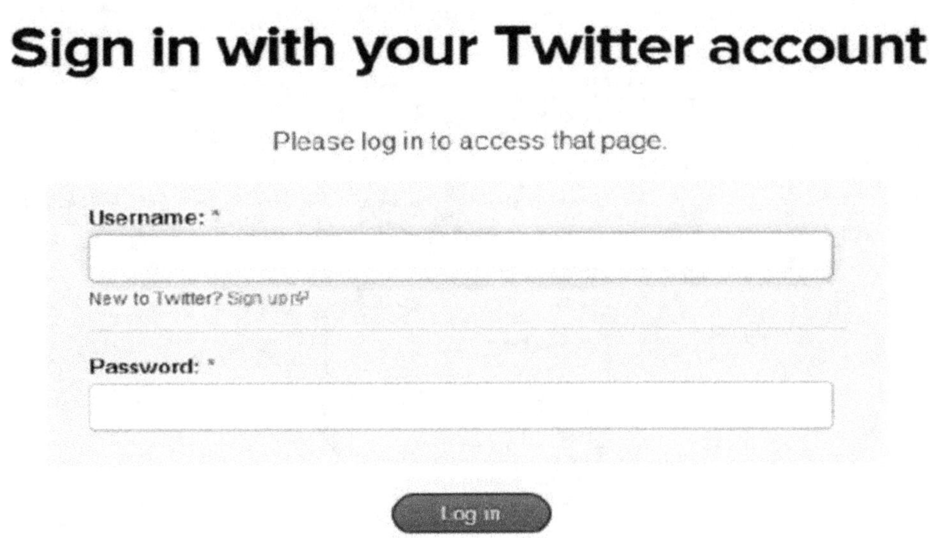

Figure 3. Assignment of the twitter tokens

OAuth settings

Your application's OAuth settings. Keep the "Consumer secret" a secret. This key should never be human-readable in your application.

Access level	Read-only About the application permission model
Consumer key	
Consumer secret	
Request token URL	https://api.twitter.com/oauth/request_token
Authorize URL	https://api.twitter.com/oauth/authorize
Access token URL	https://api.twitter.com/oauth/access_token
Callback URL	None
Sign in with Twitter	No

Your access token

Use the access token string as your "oauth_token" and the access token secret as your "oauth_token_secret" to sign requests with your own Twitter account. Do not share your oauth_token_secret with anyone.

Access token	
Access token secret	
Access level	Read-only

Figure 4. Selection of domain

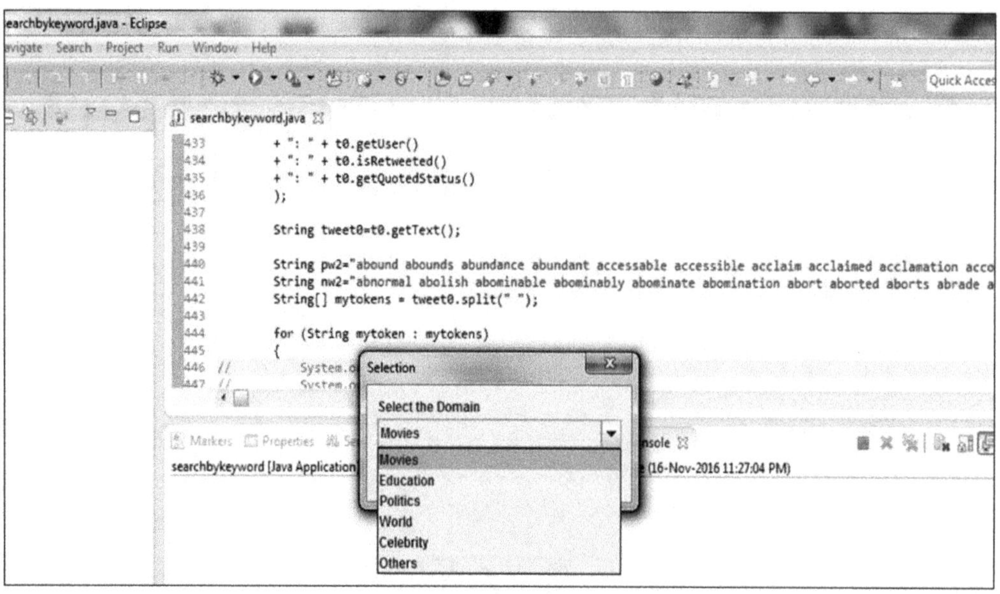

Figure 5. Enter the first keyword for Twitter mining

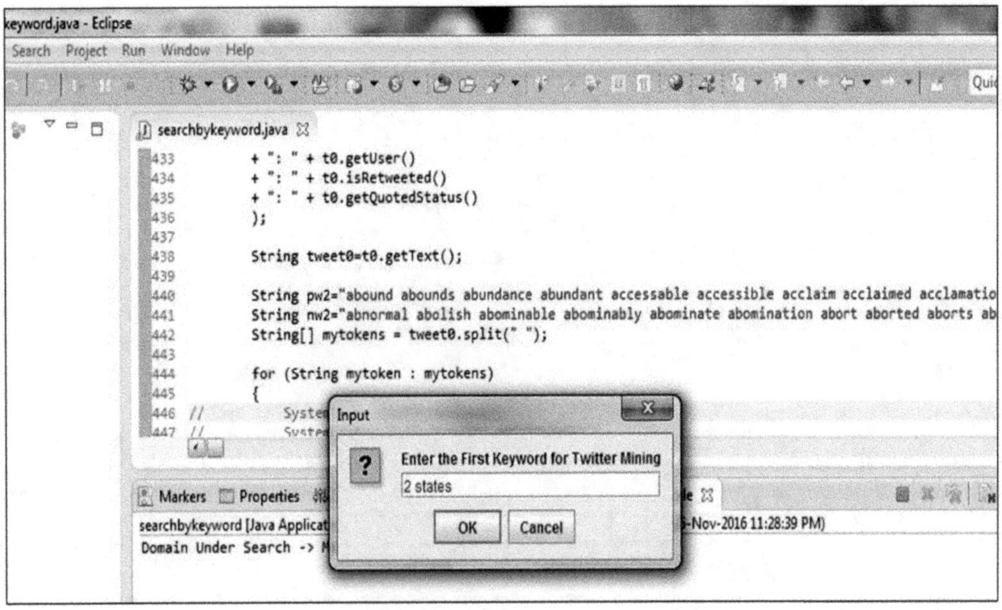

Figure 6. Enter the second keyword for Twitter mining

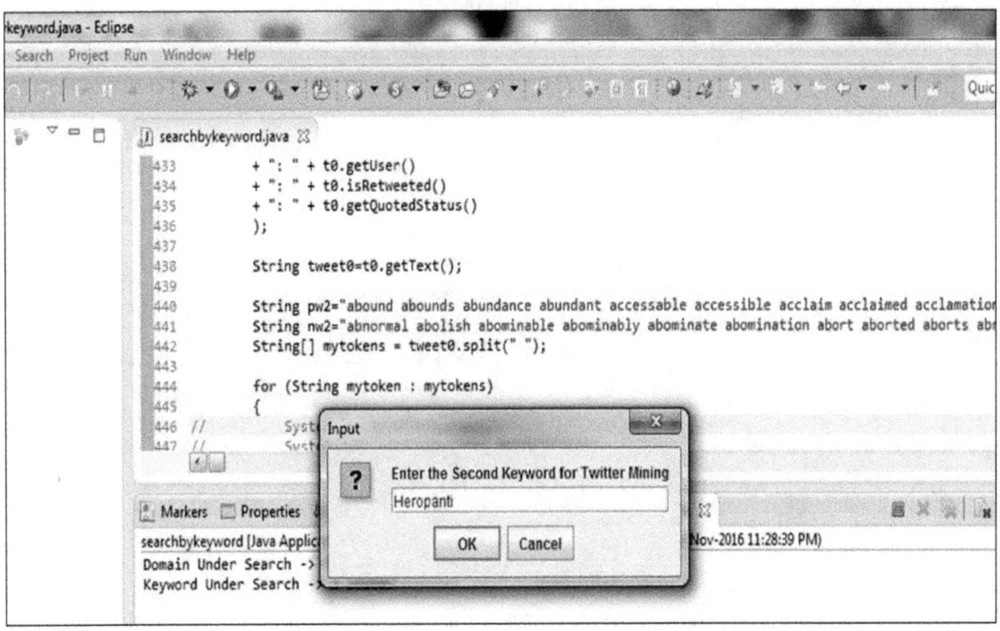

Figure 7. Fetching of live tweets from Twitter

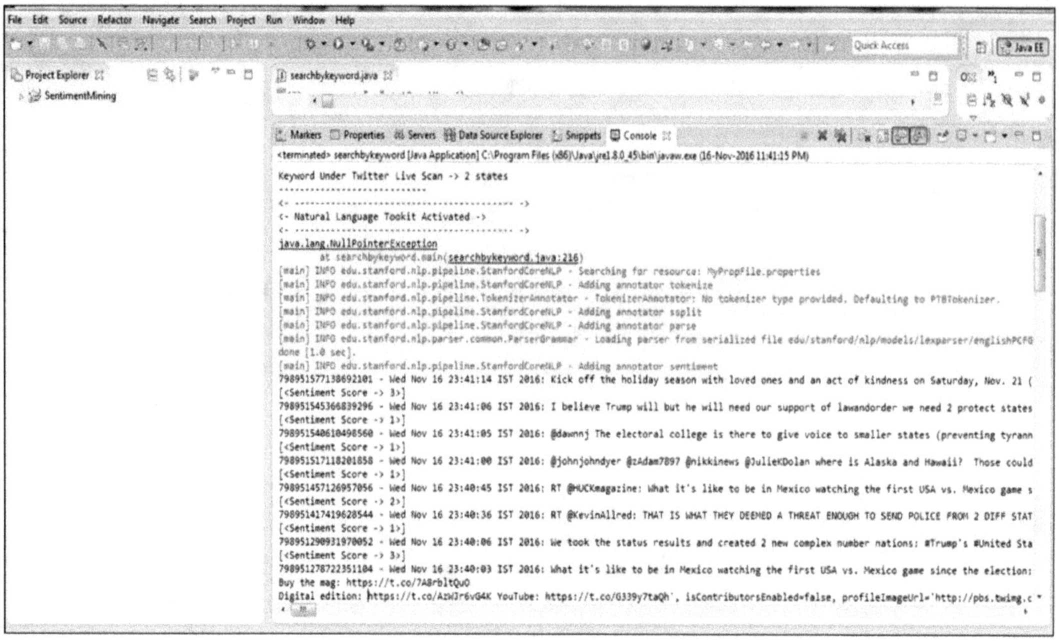

Figure 8. Assignment of sentiment score to the keywords

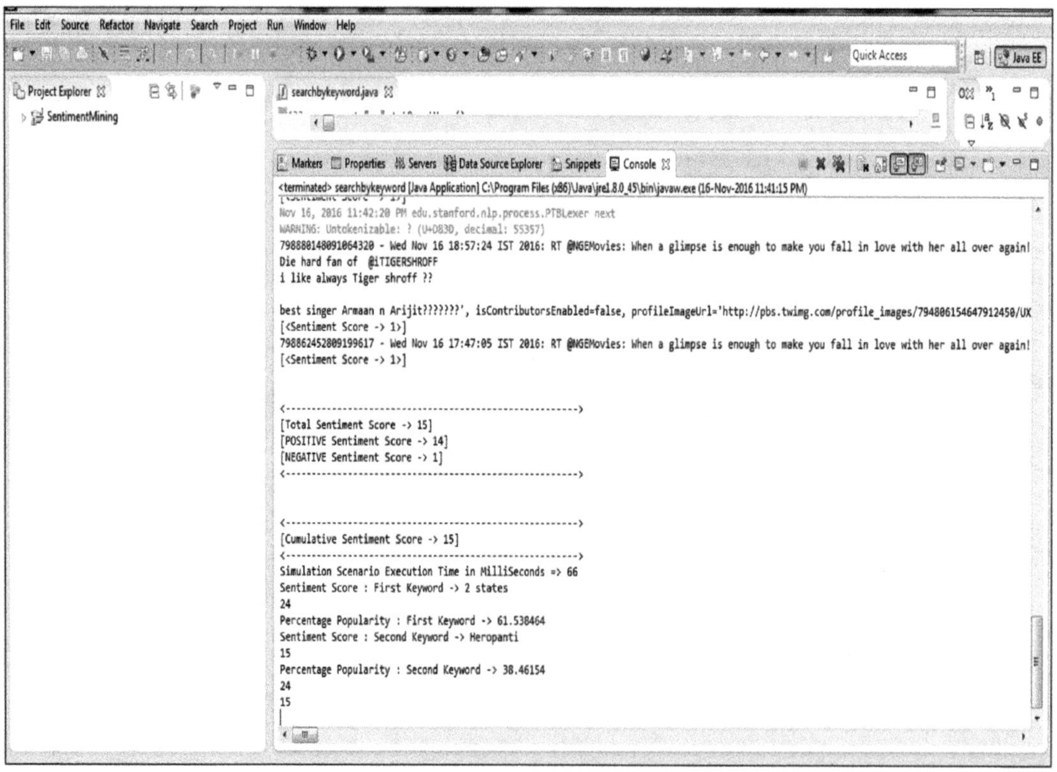

Figure 9. Execution time in milliseconds

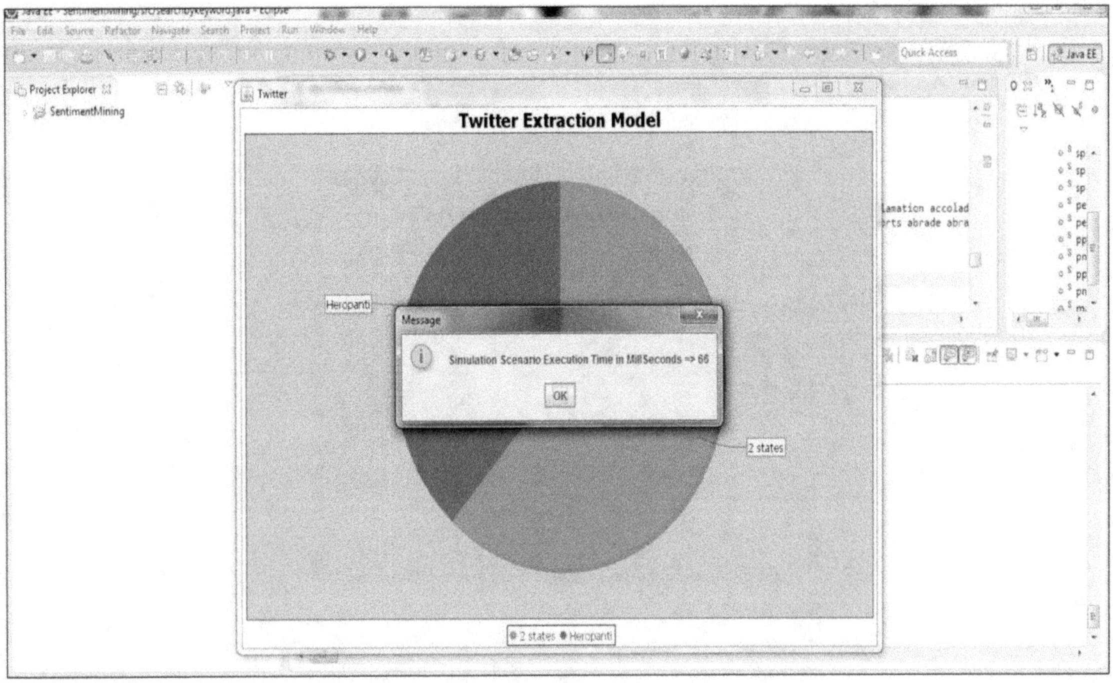

Figure 10. Pie chart of twitter extraction model

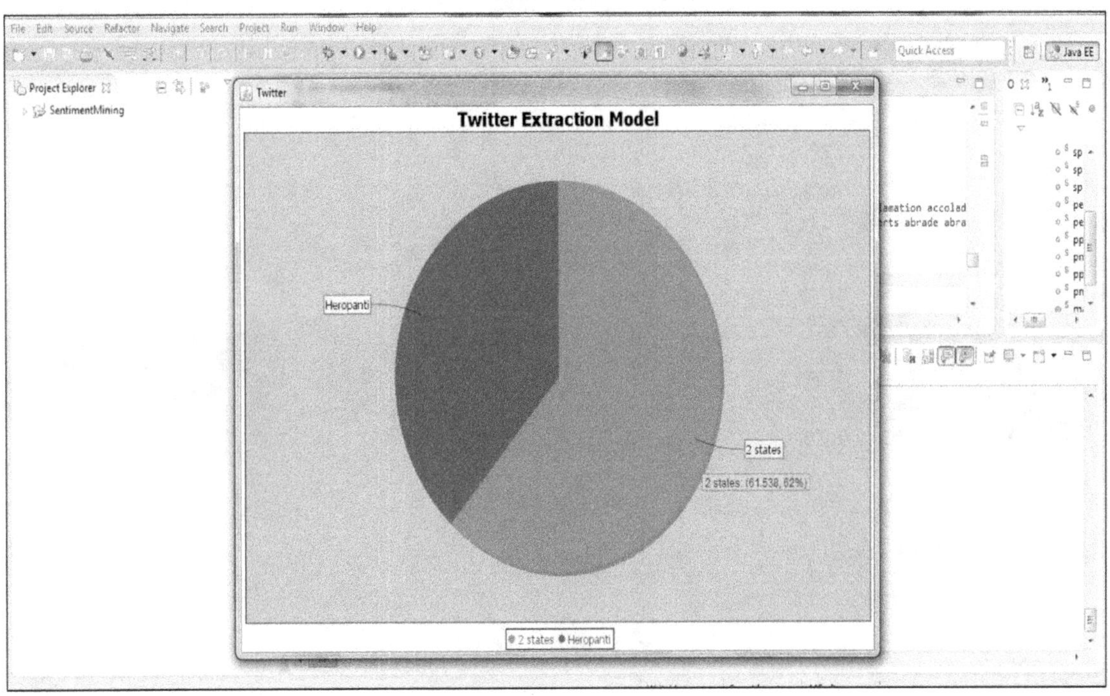

Figure 11. Bar graph of twitter extraction model

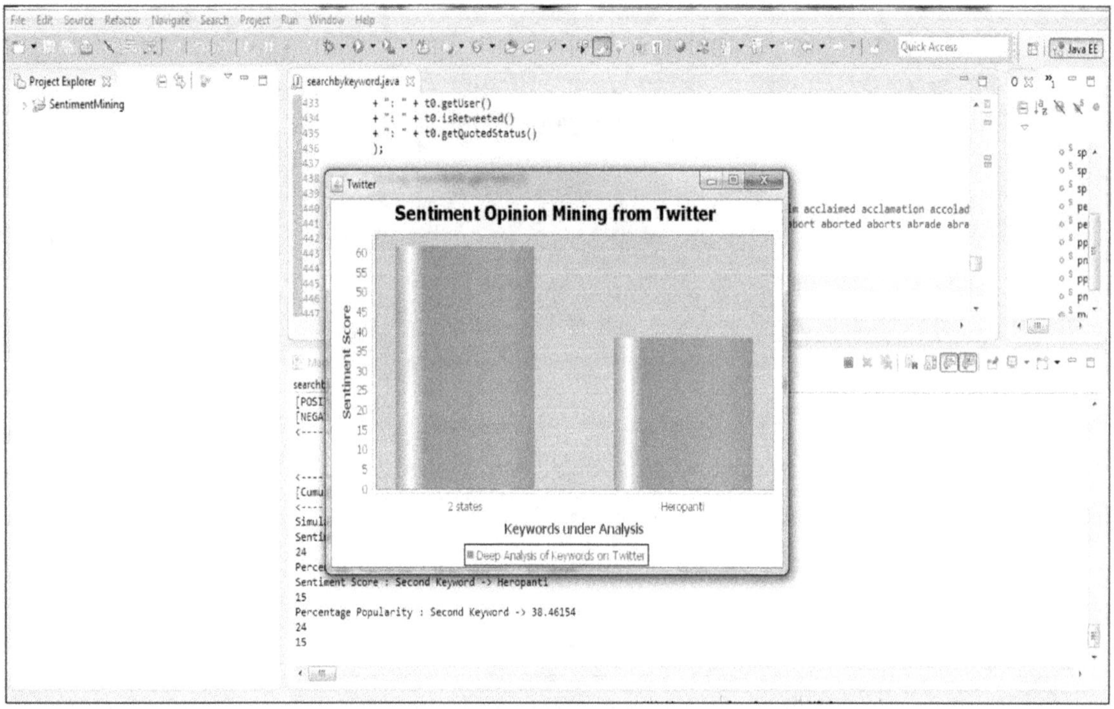

Figure 12. Code for setting the tokens of Twitter account

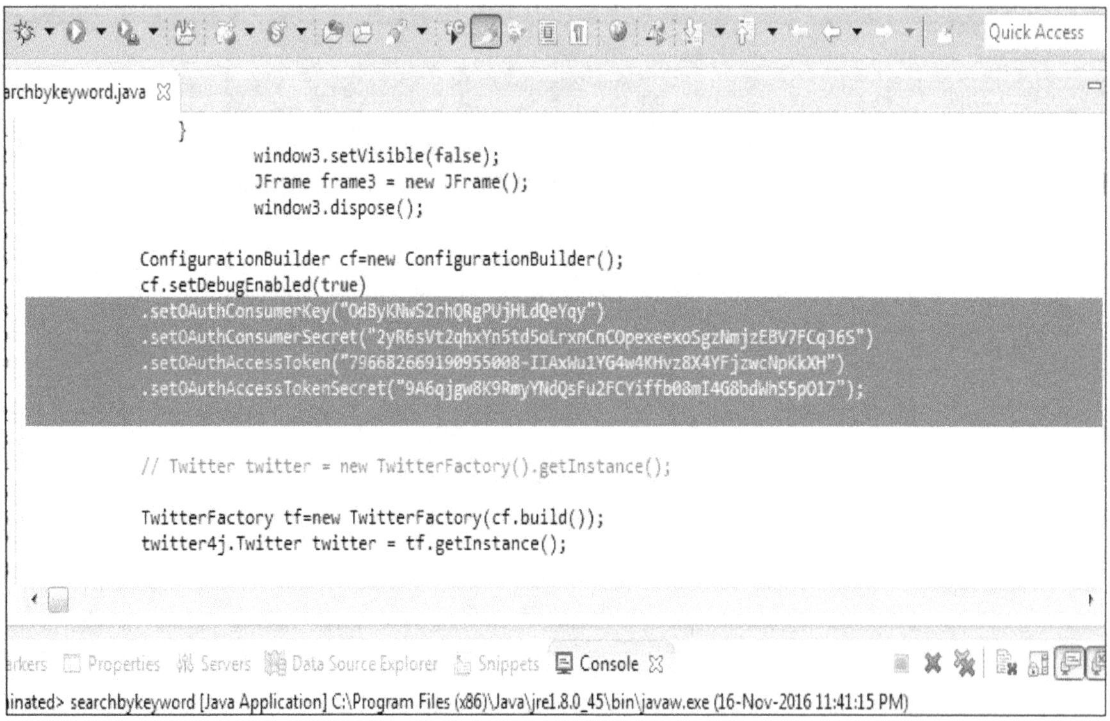

Figure 13. Repository of positive and negative words

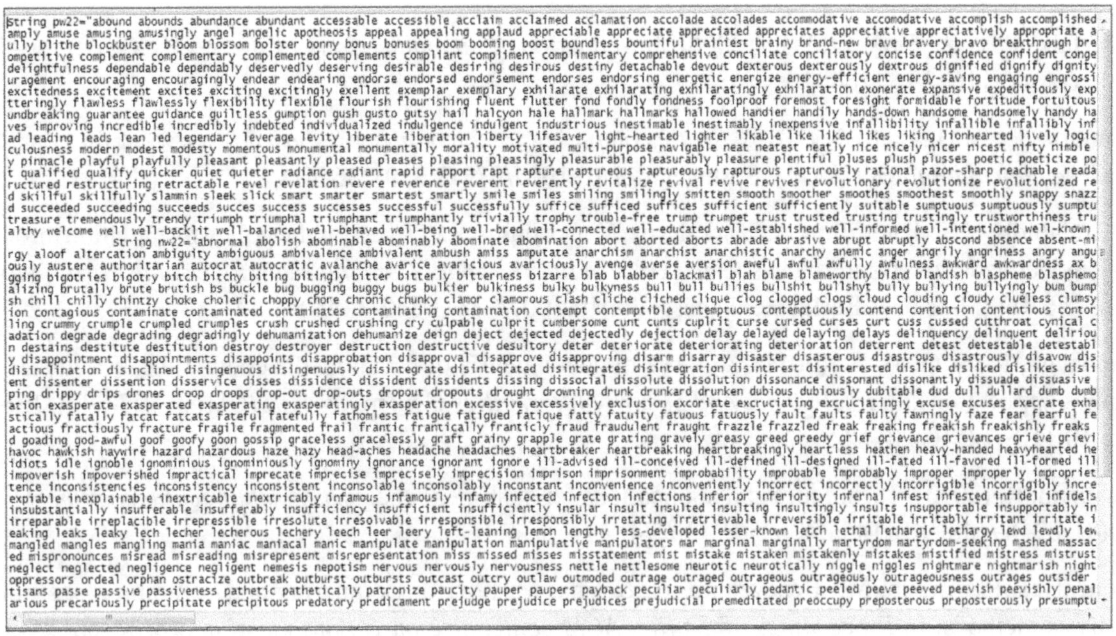

FUTURE RESEARCH DIRECTIONS

For future scope of the work, following techniques can be used in hybrid approach to better and efficient results:

1. Spam Detection Sentiment Analysis.
2. Sentiment Analysis on Short Sentence like abbreviations.
3. Successful handling of bi polar sentiments.
4. ANN and hybrid approaches are used to improve the accuracy by decreasing the execution time and increasing the speed.
5. Enhancing the repository.
6. Dynamic Authentication can be imposed to enrich the security.

CONCLUSION

- Enter the two keywords for any of the following domains: Movies, Education, Politics, World, Celebrity and Others. Then Fetch the Live Tweets for the entered keywords from Twitter server using Twitter4J Advance Java Interface.
- Also classify the live tweets fetched from twitter into Positive, Negative or Neutral opinions and assigning the sentiment scores to them. Also plot the pie chart and bar graph as the result of the two keywords showing the comparison between them.

REFERENCES

Ågerfalk, P. J., & Fitzgerald, B. (2006). Introduction. *Communications of the ACM*, *49*(10), 26–34. doi:10.1145/1164394.1164416

Cambria, E., & Hussain, A. (2015). *Sentic computing: a common-sense-based framework for concept-level sentiment analysis* (Vol. 1). Springer. doi:10.1007/978-3-319-23654-4

Charalabidis, Y., Triantafillou, A., Karkaletsis, V., & Loukis, E. (2012). Public policy formulation through non moderated crowdsourcing in social media. In *International Conference on Electronic Participation* (pp. 156-169). Springer Berlin Heidelberg. doi:10.1007/978-3-642-33250-0_14

Colbaugh, R., & Glass, K. (2011). Agile sentiment analysis of social media content for security informatics applications. In *Intelligence and Security Informatics Conference (EISIC)* (pp. 327-331). IEEE. doi:10.1109/EISIC.2011.65

Feldman, R. (2013). Techniques and applications for sentiment analysis. *Communications of the ACM*, *56*(4), 82–89. doi:10.1145/2436256.2436274

Gonçalves, P., Araújo, M., Benevenuto, F., & Cha, M. (2013). Comparing and combining sentiment analysis methods. In *Proceedings of the first ACM conference on Online social networks* (pp. 27-38). ACM. doi:10.1145/2512938.2512951

Hao, M., Rohrdantz, C., Janetzko, H., Dayal, U., Keim, D. A., Haug, L.-E., & Hsu, M.-C. (2011). Visual sentiment analysis on twitter data streams. In *Visual Analytics Science and Technology (VAST)* (pp. 277-278). IEEE. doi:10.1109/VAST.2011.6102472

Hogenboom, A., Bal, D., Frasincar, F., Bal, M., de Jong, F., & Kaymak, U. (2013). Exploiting emoticons in sentiment analysis. In *Proceedings of the 28th Annual ACM Symposium on Applied Computing* (pp. 703-710). ACM. doi:10.1145/2480362.2480498

Mohammad, S. M. (2016). Challenges in sentiment analysis. In A Practical Guide to Sentiment Analysis. Springer.

Naveed, N., Gottron, T., Kunegis, J., & Alhadi, A. C. (2011). Bad news travel fast: A content-based analysis of interestingness on twitter. In *Proceedings of the 3rd International Web Science Conference* (p. 8). ACM. doi:10.1145/2527031.2527052

Prabowo & Thelwall. (2009). Sentiment analysis: A combined approach. *Journal of Informetrics, 3*(2), 143-157. doi.org/10.1016/j.joi.2009.01.003

Rosenthal, S., Nakov, P., Kiritchenko, S., Mohammad, S. M., Ritter, A., & Stoyanov, V. (2015). Semeval-2015 task 10: Sentiment analysis in twitter. In *Proceedings of the 9th international workshop on semantic evaluation (SemEval 2015)* (pp. 451-463). doi:10.18653/v1/S15-2078

Whitworth, E., & Biddle, R. (2007). The social nature of agile teams. In Agile conference (AGILE), 2007 (pp. 26-36). IEEE. doi:10.1109/AGILE.2007.60

Yi, J., Nasukawa, T., Bunescu, R., & Niblack, W. (2003). Sentiment analyzer: Extracting sentiments about a given topic using natural language processing techniques. In *Data Mining, 2003. ICDM 2003. Third IEEE International Conference on* (pp. 427-434). IEEE. doi:10.1109/ICDM.2003.1250949

Chapter 3
Data Confidentiality and Integrity Preserving Outsourcing Algorithm for System of Linear Equation to a Malicious Cloud Server

Malay Kumar
National Institute of Technology Raipur, India

Manu Vardhan
National Institute of Technology Raipur, India

ABSTRACT

Cloud computing has become a revolution in the field of computing, which enables flexible, on-demand, usage of computing resources in pay-as-per-use model. However, data and computation go to some third-party cloud server beyond the physical control of client escalates various privacy and security concern. This paper proposes an improved outsourcing algorithm for system of linear equation (SLE). The improvements are first, the existing work uses expensive cryptographic computation such as Paillier encryption for security arrangement, the proposed solution does not use such cryptographic primitives rather uses efficient linear transformation method. Secondly, the previous work uses an iterative process, which required L rounds of communication between the client and cloud server, at the same time each iteration causes burden of a decryption followed by a matrix vector multiplication. However, the proposed solution required an optimal one round of communication and one-time transformation and retransformation service. Third, the previous work gives result verification method with ($1/2l^l$ error probability, the value of l is a trade-off between security and efficiency. However, the proposed solution gives an error checking with an optimal probability of one. Moreover, a security analysis has been performed on the previous method, which proves marginal security arrangement due to inappropriate use of the Paillier encryption scheme. The proposal has been verified through theoretical and experimental analysis, which demonstrate the superiority of the proposed algorithm as compared to the existing algorithm.

DOI: 10.4018/978-1-5225-5222-2.ch003

Copyright © 2018, IGI Global. Copying or distributing in print or electronic forms without written permission of IGI Global is prohibited.

INTRODUCTION

Cloud computing has become increasingly important in both business and academia due to strong financial viability. It reduces both the capital and operational investment spend on the procurement and maintenance of IT infrastructure. Cloud computing enables ubiquitous, convenient, on-demand network access to a shared pool of configurable computing resources (e.g., networks, servers, storage, applications, and services) that can be rapidly provisioned and released with minimal management effort or service provider interaction (NIST, Mell, & Grance, 2011). A resource-constrained client usually has relatively limited CPU, storage and battery. If a client connected to cloud server over internet is no longer restricted to limited CPU, storage, and bandwidth else it leverages the abundance of computing resources due to seamless access to the data centers (Shiraz, Gani, Khokhar, & Buyya, 2013). The cloud computing paradigm empowers them to execute massive computations by outsourcing their computation load to the cloud server. Despite the tremendous benefits, this promising paradigm brings many security and privacy concerns, which makes a client reluctant to outsource their sensitive and classified data to the cloud server. The first security concern is the privacy of confidential data. The input data have been often sensitive, it may be personal identifiable information, financial records, and trends of stock prices, scientific research data and many more. Therefore, the input data needs to be encrypted to maintain the confidentiality and integrity of data before transferring to the cloud server. One method to address such security concern is to apply some encryption scheme, but the tradition encryption scheme would not work out here, because it changes the input into the cipher and performing computation on cipher is very difficult. The second concern is the correctness of the result. The client has no information about how the cloud server performs the computation inside their data centers. The cloud server may return invalid result due to a flaw, bug in the logic or may be intentionally deviated from the algorithm instruction (behave maliciously), means there is no guaranty on the integrity of the result. Therefore, an outsourcing algorithm must be capable of providing privacy to the confidential data (input and output) and proficiently in verification of the result. The other challenges are efficiency and correctness of algorithm. To outsource the computation on the cloud server, it is required to do some preprocessing such as input transformation for privacy, result verification, computation of the problem and ultimately the re-transformation. Therefore, the computation perform on the client system (viz., transformation, verification, and retransformation) must be substantially lesser than executing the SLE else the outsourcing has no mean (F. Chen, Xiang, & Yang, 2014; Lin & Chen, 2010; Mohassel, 2011).

In summary an outsourcing algorithm must satisfy the following four design goals: correctness, security, verifiability, and efficiency (Xiaofeng Chen et al., 2015).

1. **Correctness:** The client and the cloud server should follow the outsourcing algorithm instructions then only the outsourcing algorithm will produce correct result.
2. **Security:** There are two goals of the transformation operation. The first is to provide security to the confidential data and the second is to allow the cloud server to carry out meaningful operation on the transformed data (Lei, Liao, Huang, & Heriniaina, 2014; Wang, Ren, & Wang, 2011; Wang, Ren, Wang, & Urs, 2011; Zhang & Blanton, 2014).
3. **Verification:** The verification algorithm of the outsourced computation should be design in such a way that the client will able to detect cheating and server misbehavior. However, the verification algorithm should be efficient and not involved in expensive computation. Moreover the cost of verification should strictly be less than executing the problem itself.

4. **Efficiency:** The client-side computation (transformation, verification and re-transformation) time must be substantially lesser than executing the outsourcing problem itself (F. Chen, Xiang, & Yang, 2014; Lin & Chen, 2010; Mohassel, 2011).

System of linear equation (SLE) plays an important role in various analysis and optimization problem of engineering and scientific discipline. For example, the system of linear equation solve to fit a polynomial function to a set of data points in a plane. The SLE could be modeled to represent network of electricity and Kirchhoff's Laws for electricity, other application of SLE are also seen in astronomy, traffic management, and electromagnetics. Therefore a variety of clients needed an efficient and secure solution of SLE.

There are many algorithms are available in literature for various core problems of linear algebra, which includes system of linear equations (Cramer & Damgård, 2001; W. Du & Atallah, 2001; Kiltz, Mohassel, Weinreb, & Franklin, 2007; Mohassel & Weinreb, 2008; Nissim & Weinreb, 2006; Ram & Comesa, n.d.; Saad, 2001). These algorithm were not suitable in the context of secure outsourcing of large system of linear equation in cloud computing environment. Recently, an algorithm for secure outsourcing of system of linear equation on cloud server has been proposed by wang et al., (Wang, Ren, Wang, et al., 2011; Wang, Ren, Wang, & Wang, 2013). However, the algorithm has few shortcomings, which makes it far from practical usage in real-world application. First, the algorithm is insufficient in providing privacy to client's data. There is a possibility that an adversary could recover meaningful information from the client's dataset. Second, the algorithm requires many rounds of interactive communication between the client and the cloud server, and overhead due to Pilliaer encryption system. Third, the result verification technique verifies the result with an error probability of $(\frac{1}{2^l})$, in order to reduce the error probability the verification needed to execute (l) times, which is an additional overhed for the SLE algorithm. Interested with the fact that system linear equation is an important problem in many domains, and there exist gap in the current state of the art algorithm. The authors are motivated to design an improved algorithm for system of linear equation.

In this paper, we proposed a new secure outsourcing algorithm for the system of linear equation $Ax=b$ in a fully malicious environment, i.e., the cloud server could be deceitful, lazy, and inquisitive. The proposed outsourcing algorithm for SLE provides better security, verifiability, and efficiency than the wang et al. (Wang et al., 2013).

The main contribution of this paper summarized in following points.

1. A new outsourcing algorithm has been proposed, which is based on efficient linear transformation unlike the previous algorithm, which is based on Paillier encryption system. The proposed algorithm is suitable for any non-singular dense matrix A, where A is a coefficient matrix. However, the existing algorithm (Wang et al., 2013) work only with the diagonally dominant matrix.
2. The proposed algorithm requires only one round of communication between client and the cloud server, while the previous algorithm required L round of communication before convergence and each interaction increase burden on client for a decryption followed by matrix vector multiplication that significantly reduces the performance gain of client. However, if $(L \geq n)$ the privacy will be compromised.

3. The previous work gives a result verification method with $(\frac{1}{2^l})$ an error probability, the value of l is trade-off between security and efficiency. However, the proposed solution give an error checking with an optimal probability of one without involving in complex computation.
4. A thorough security analysis of the existing algorithm has been presented, which proves that security breach is possible in the existing approach and the cloud server could retrieve meaningful client information (Wang et al., 2013). Further, a security analysis of proposed algorithm has presented, which proves that the malicious cloud will unable to retrieve any meaning full information.
5. The proposed algorithm is developed without using any complex cryptographic method. The asymptotic running time complexity of the client system at any point of time is $O(n2)$. A comparison of complexities of the proposed algorithm with the existing algorithm reveals that the proposed algorithm is much more efficient.
6. The experimental evaluation validates the proposal. The result analysis shows that the algorithm is highly efficient and endorses the practical usability of the algorithm. All the experimental results can be reproduced.

The rest of the paper is organized as follows: Section 2, discusses the related work done in the area of secure computation. Section 3, provides detail discussion on the system of linear equation problem, its mathematical elements, and system model to solve them. Section 4, formulates the proposed SLE outsourcing algorithm and provide detail discussion on the improvement of the outsourcing algorithm. Section 5, provides analytical analysis of the proposed algorithm on correctness, security, verifiability and efficiency parameter. This section also provides the security analysis of existing algorithm. Section 6, presents the experimental analysis of the proposed algorithm. Finally, concluding remark and future direction is incorporated in Section 7.

RELATED WORK

In literature, there are various algorithms available for secure outsourcing of various core problems of linear algebra. However, these algorithms are providing cryptographic solutions of the problems. Moreover, secure outsourcing is divided into two parts i.e., semi-trusted computing model and un-trusted computing model. In the semi-trusted computing model, the cloud server follows the algorithm instructions and produces the correct result, but the cloud server secretly records the accessible data and attempt to retrieve meaningful information from those records. A taxonomy is presented in figure. 1. In the semi-trusted model, the first one is audit based model (Belenkiy et al., 2008; Monrose, Wyckoff, & Rubin, 1999; Seshadri et al., 2005), the client or the trusted workers in audit-based approach re-computes some part of the computation performed by the un-trusted workers. This approach is unfeasible for a computationally weak client because if the client is capable of performing the computation, then there is no need to outsource the computation to the cloud server. This method also required that some workers must be honest or at least non-colluding in nature. The second one is secure-co-processors (Bajikar, 2002; Smith & Weingart, 1999; Yee, 1994), or Trusted Platform Modules (TPMs) method, which required to deploy trusted hardware on the server to provide an isolated execution environment. This model is also impractical, since it is not possible to install TPM on third party cloud server. The last one is secure multiparty computation, the computation is divide among two or more workers without allowing any participated worker to view another secret data. The resultant of computation is union of the output of all workers (Dreier & Kerschbaum, 2011; Wenliang Du, Chen, & Han, 2004; Lindell & Pinkas, 2009; López-Alt, Tromer, & Vaikuntanathan, 2012). This model is not feasible for cloud environment since this model required that the participating workers must have comparable computing capability. However, in the outsourcing paradigm, the client transfers the entire computation load to the massive cloud servers.

In untrusted computing model, the server can deviate from the algorithmic instructions and behave arbitrarily. The solution of this problem applies some encryption techniques to perform a secure computation and handle the result verification to verify the correctness of the result. There exist two types of verifiable outsourcing i.e., interactive proof and non-interactive proof. In interactive proof, a weak verifier actively challenges a server (prover). The prover replies a probabilistic proof to the client (verifier) to convince him (verifier) about the truth of the statement that he is unable to compute (Fortnow & Lund, 1993; Goldwasser, Kalai, & Rothblum, 2008; Goldwasser, Micali, & Rackoff, 1989). The second one is the non-interactive proof, where a weak client outsources the computation to a powerful server, the server returns the result along with the proof of verification [22]–[33].

Our solution applies non-interactive proof to provide verifiability of computation. Therefore, the attention is more on non-interactive verifiable algorithms. Gentry's provides a novel Fully Homomorphic Encryption (FHE) scheme (Gentry, 2009). This scheme allows the server to perform arbitrary computation on encrypted input, but the solution suffers from the complexity and efficiency of FHE that makes it far from practical use for outsourcing (Gennaro et al., 2010; Gentry, 2010; Mohassel, 2011; Van Dijk, Gentry, Halevi, & Vaikuntanathan, 2010). Moreover, FHE does not guarantees that the server performs correct computation. Gennaro et al., (Gennaro et al., 2010) has proposed a non-interactive solution for the secure outsourcing of polynomial function. First, they model the polynomial function into Yao's grabbled circuit (A. C.-C. Yao, 1986; A. C. Yao, 1982). Then homomorphically (Gentry, 2009) encrypt the circuit and send to the server for the execution of the polynomial function. The cloud server performs the execution & returns a computationally sound non-interactive proof that can verify in $O(m)$ time. Another elegant solution is proposed by Chung et al. (Chung, Kalai, & Vadhan, 2010). The client performs pre-processing and create hundreds of problem instances mostly of same type. Then apply homomorphic encryption for privacy on problem instances. The server computes these functions without knowing the actual inputs. Finally, the client verifies the solution of the same type of problem for ensuring their correctness. The main drawback of these two algorithms that they are incurring huge computation load on

Figure 1. Taxonomy of secure computation outsourcing

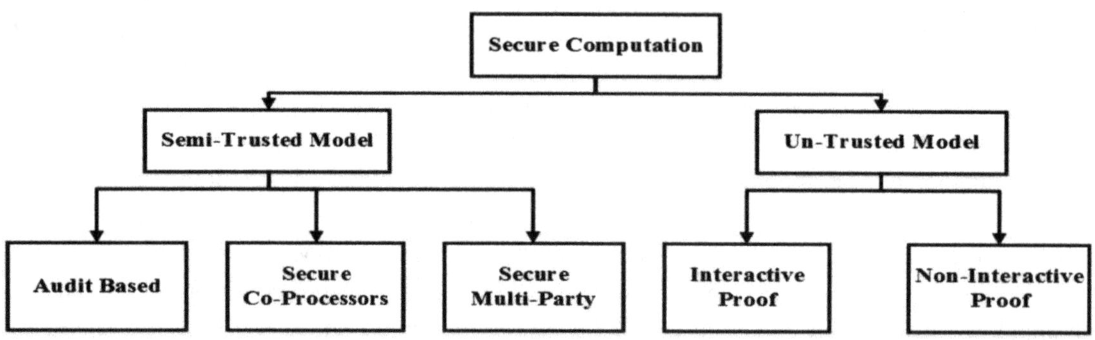

both client and server due to the complex homomorphic encryption. These algorithms are also require modeling of problem into circuit, which needed to dealing with large amount of parameters. However, one main advantage of these methods that they took constant time for verification.

Furthermore, there are many algorithms available, which address some specific type of problems. (Atallah, Pantazopoulos, Rice, & Spafford, 2002) have carried out an investigation for many problems such as matrix multiplication, quadrature, a solution of the differential equation, the system of linear equations. Their solution explicitly leaking private information. Besides, the proposed work do not handle the result verification. Further, (Benjamin & Atallah, 2008) gave an outsourcing algorithm for matrix multiplication. The algorithm developed on the assumption of two non-colluding servers. They assumed that servers would not share secret information between them. However, this method is vulnerable to colluding attack. Later on (Atallah & Frikken, 2010) proposed a secure matrix multiplication outsourcing algorithm based on the theory of secret sharing. This algorithm is an improvement of their previous work in (Benjamin & Atallah, 2008), regarding single server and computational efficiency. However, this algorithm also suffers from computational overhead due to Shamir's secret sharing technique. The scalar multiplication complexity expands up to polynomial time. (Blanton, Zhang, & Frikken, 2013) addressed the large scale computation of biometric computation. The implementation leverages individual structures of distance computation and random sampling. The result verification method can verify the result with modest overhead and high probability. In (Lei et al., 2014; Xinyu Lei et al., 2013) presented matrix inversion outsourcing algorithm. They uses monomial matrix for the privacy of input/output matrix. The algorithm efficiently outsources the matrix inversion to the cloud server, while maintaining the correctness, privacy of the input-output, and verifies the result efficiently. Next, an algorithm addresses linear programming (LP) in (Wang, Ren, & Wang, 2011). This method split the LP solver into two parts; those are the LP solver on cloud and the LP parameters on client-side. The client transforms the input data using a transformation technique and outsources to the LP solver on a cloud server. Then cloud server solves the linear programming problem with the help of LP solver and returns the result. The client verifies the result using the fundamental theorem of duality. Further, another algorithm is presented for LP problem, which reduces the computation and communication time significantly (Hong et al., 2012). The algorithm proposed by (Wang, Ren, Wang, et al., 2011) requires (***L***) round of communication between the client and cloud before the client get the convergent solution. The algorithm encrypts the input in ***O*(*n*2)** i^{n} setup phase and verify the output in ***O*(*n*2)**. The ^{L} round of communication between the client and the cloud is the main drawback of this method which increses the communication overhead and also add security vulnerability to the algorithm.

SECURITY DEFINITIONS AND SYSTEM MODEL

Security Definition

The client C securely outsources their computation load to the cloud server CS , (C, CS) is said to be a correct implementation of a secure outsourcing algorithm for SLE, if a pair of algorithm (C, CS) produces a correct solution for SLE. The client C has given an oracle access to the server CS that records all of the computation and the data came into possession and tries to act maliciously. However, due to efficient and rigorous implementation of security mechanism, the server CS unable to retrieve any meaningful information from the input and output.

- **Definition 1 Correctness:** A pair of algorithm $\left(C, CS\right)$ is said to be a correct implementation of SLE, if $A\lg = C^{CS}$ correctly implements the SLE and it produces a correct solution for the system of linear equation problem.
- **Definition 2 Privacy:** Given on the input of security parameter $\left(\lambda\right)$, The SLE algorithm $A\lg = C^{CS}$ is said to be secure, if the cloud server CS unable retrieve the original information from the transformed input and output.

Let the vectors of input a' & b', the encryption of two vectors are said to be computationally indistinguishable only if for every probabilistic polynomial time adversary there exist a negligible function $negl(\cdot)$ such that,

$$(\Pr\left(a'\right) = 1) - \left(\Pr\left(b'\right) = 1\right) \leq negl\left(\cdot\right)$$

Moreover, this security definition can be extended to the case where the cloud server *CS* has access to the input matrices $\left(A', b'\right)$ & the result matrices x', i.e.,

The client performed the key generation and the problem transformation procedures on his premise and kept the secret keys $\left(k\right)$ secret from the cloud server, only public information after the transformation of coefficient matrix $\left(A'\right)$ and solution vector $\left(b'\right)$ shared with the cloud server.

$$\Rightarrow KeyGen\left(\lambda\right) \rightarrow \left(k\right)$$

$$\Rightarrow ProbTrans\left(\varphi\left(A, b\right), k\right) \rightarrow (A', b')$$

$$\Rightarrow Compute\left(\varphi\left(A', b'\right)\right) \rightarrow x'$$

The cloud server CS has the oracle access to the transformed input dataset and the computed result (x'), the probabilistic polynomial time adversary Å get negligible information about $\left(A, b, x\right)$. The malicious cloud server get only the public information $\left(A', b', x'\right)$.

$$\Rightarrow Pr\left[KeyGen\left(\lambda\right)\right] \leq negl\left(\cdot\right)$$

$$\Rightarrow Pr\left[ProbTrans\left(\varphi\left(A, b\right), k\right)\right] \leq negl\left(\cdot\right)$$

$$\Rightarrow Pr_{A}\left[Compute\left(\varphi\left(A', b'\right)\right)\right]) \leq negl\left(\cdot\right)$$

$$\Rightarrow CS^{Pr_A\left[Compute\left(\varphi\left(A',b'\right)\right)\right]\to x')PPTA\left(\varphi\left(A',b'\right)\right)} \leq negl\left(\cdot\right)$$

Since, the cloud server has access to the transformed input $\left(A',b'\right)$ & the solution of SLE $\left(x'\right)$, the adversary attempt to retrieve information from $Pr_A\left[Compute\left(\varphi\left(A',b'\right)\right)\right]$, but this function only returns the public information about the solution x'.

- **Definition 3 Efficiency:** A pair of algorithms $\left(C,CS\right)$ for the implementation of SLE is said to be efficient if the running time of algorithms at C is always be less than the running of SLE itself.
- **Definition 4 Verifiability:** A pair of algorithms $\left(C,CS\right)$ in the implementation of SLE is said to be verifiable, if the $\left(C,CS\right)$ correctly implement the SLE algorithm and if the cloud server CS deviates from the algorithm instructions or perform maliciously client C will verify the correctness of result $\forall x \in \mathbb{R}$.

SYSTEM MODEL

The system model for secure computation outsourcing algorithm for system of linear equation is depicted in Figure 2. The resource-constrained client C wants to compute the solution for the system of linear equation, but due to lack of computing resources, the client is unable to perform the analysis, therefore, the client outsources the computation to the massive cloud servers. The client C first performs a linear transformation on the input problem $\varphi\left(A,b\right)$ using a secret key $\left(k\right)$ to protect the input. Then the client C outsources $\left(Alg = C^{CS} = \varphi_k\left(A',b'\right)\right)$ to the system of linear equation to the cloud server CS to harness the computing power of massive cloud servers. The cloud server is expected to compute

Figure 2. Proposed system model for SLE algorithm

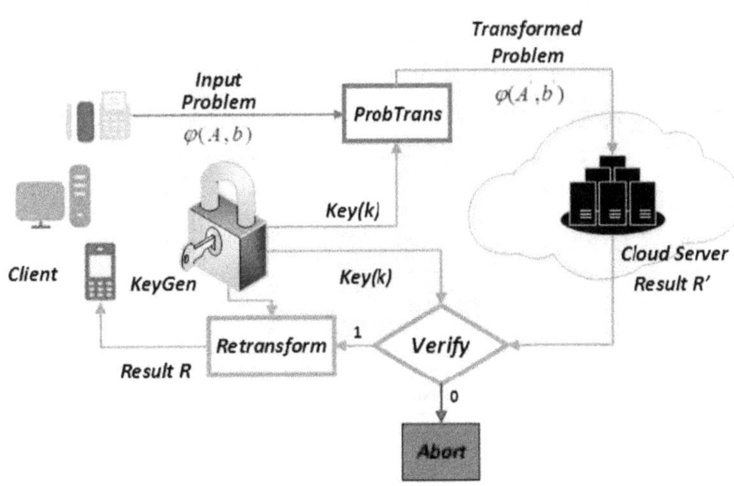

the correct result for the outsourced SLE problem(φ_k). But for the assurance, the client verifies the result received from the cloud server. The client first verifies the result received from the cloud server. If the client found that the result received from the cloud server is correct, then only the client performs a retransformation to obtain decrypted result. Table 1, listed the common notations used in the paper.

Threat Model

The security threat in outsourcing system model comes from the suspicious behavior of the cloud server. The previous work for the secure outsourcing computation defines three threat model that are "Trusted Model", "Semi-Trusted Model", and "Un-trusted Model" (Xiaofeng Chen et al., 2015; Lei et al., 2014; Xinyu Lei et al., 2013).

1. **Trusted Model:** The cloud server follows the algorithm instructions correctly and it does not attempt to unauthorized access to the client information. Therefore, no need of encryption and verification.
2. **Semi-Trusted Model:** In this model, the cloud behaves as "honest but curious" or "lazy but honest" or even both. Goldreich et al. (Goldreich, O.; Micali S., Goldreich, Micali, & Wigderson, 1987) first introduces the honest but curious model. The server follows the algorithm instructions and produces the correct result, but the cloud server tries to secretly record the accessible data and attempt to retrieve meaningful information. However, the proposed algorithm has been design to handle such threat model. The cloud server is not able to extract the original information from the transformed input or the result. The *lazy but honest* model behaves honestly; it does not record any such information or computation but behave lazily, that the cloud server might not perform on the agreed service level. It might send some invalid result to save computing resources. To, share the

Table 1. List of common notations and symbols

Notations and Symbols	Description
$D(A:b)$	Input Data Set (A Coefficient Matrix, b Solution Vector)
Key	k (The key Matrices k_1, k_2)
$\varphi(A,b)$	System of Linear Equation Problem
$\varphi_k(A',b')$	Transformed Outsourcing Problem
(π)	Permutation Function
(γ,δ)	Non-Zero Random Numbers
(D)	Diagonal Matrix

remaining resources with other clients to increase the financial gain. The proposed system model for SLE successfully addresses this security threat. The client can detect the correctness of result with an optimal probability.

3. **Un-Trusted Model:** The third threat model comes from the *malicious* behavior of cloud server, which is the strongest adversarial model. In this model, the server could be "lazy", "curious", and "dishonest". The proposed algorithm is developed in completely malicious cloud environment, where the cloud server attempt to retrieve information from the computation and the data that came into its possession during the execution of the SLE. The malicious cloud server also performs randomly, it may deviate from the actual algorithm instructions and produce random indistinguishable result. The proposed algorithm proficient and able to manage such malicious behavior of the cloud server.

Outsourcing Algorithm Framework

A secure and verifiable outsourcing algorithm framework has five sub-steps in the following order: *KeyGen, ProbTrans, Compute, Verify, and Retransform.*

1. $KeyGen(\lambda)$: The algorithm takes input security parameter λ and generates the key matrices, which is used for transformation step. The key generation step runs for every new problem submission.
2. $ProbTrans(\varphi,k)$: The client first encrypts the input data set $\varphi(A,b)$ with key $(k = k_1 \;\&\; k_2)$ and generates the transformed problem $\varphi_k(A',b')$.
3. $Compute\ \varphi_k(A',b')$: The client outsources the transformed dataset to the cloud server. Then the cloud server computes the solution of the system of linear equation (x') on the transformed dataset.
4. $Verify\ (x',k)$: The client verifies the solution (x') obtained from the cloud server.
5. $Retransform\ (x',k)$: The client retransform/decrypts SLE solution (x) (if verification step is successfully passed), to obtain the original SLE solution (x).

Basic Idea of System of Linear Equation Outsourcing Algorithm

The system of linear equation is presented as

$$Ax = b \qquad (1)$$

where

$$A \in \mathbb{R}^{n*n} b \in \mathbb{R}^{n}$$

The Matrix A is called the coefficient matrix, where $A \in \mathbb{R}^{n*n}$, x is the column vector of unknowns and $b \in \mathbb{R}^{n}$ is the column vector of solutions. Further, if the matrix A is a non-singular square matrix the system of linear equation of (n) variables produces unique solution. The basic idea of SLE outsourcing algorithm follows: Let the resource constrained client want to evaluate solution of system of linear equation large input size, but due to lack of computing resources the client outsources this problem to the cloud server. The SLE problem is denoted as $\varphi = (A, b)$ and its solution as x. Further, the client applies a transformation on input data. Then this transformed input is send to the cloud. Thus, from the viewpoint of cloud server, this transformed problem is same as any other SLE problem. Although, the cloud server read the input, but unable to recover the original input data values. In this way, the input is protected from the cloud server. Then, the cloud server evaluates the system of linear equation on the transformed input and produces the encrypted result (x'). Then, the client verifies the integrity of result (x'), once the result passes the verification step, client retransform/decrypts and accepts the result.

Mathematical Details

The proposed outsourcing algorithm uses some basic functions for the transformation operation such as Cauchy's permutation function, Kronecker delta function. The Cauchy's two-line notation has two rows. The first row has list of elements and the second row list the permutation of each element respectively.

The Cauchy's Permutation function is written as

$$\pi = \begin{pmatrix} 1 \ldots\ldots\ldots\ldots\ldots\ldots n \\ \mu_1 \ldots\ldots\ldots\ldots\ldots \mu_n \end{pmatrix} \tag{2}$$

Cauchy's permutation function generates random permutations, which applies on matrix to shuffle the matrix values row-wise and column-wise.

The Kronecker delta function is written as

$$\delta_{i,j} = \begin{Bmatrix} 1 \; if\, i = j \\ 0\, if\, i \neq j \end{Bmatrix} \tag{3}$$

Further, these functions are helpful in the construction of key matrices. First the Kronecker delta function uses to generate an identity matrix. Let the identity matrix $I_{(i,j)} = \begin{bmatrix} 100 \\ 010 \\ 001 \end{bmatrix}$

Further, applying the Cauchy's two-line permutation function on the identity matrix $I_{(i,j)}$.. Since, the matrix dimension is $(3 * 3)$ i.e. $(i = 3), (j = 3)$, Let the $random\, \pi(i) = (3, 1, 2)$ that randomizes the row indices of identity matrix.

$$I_{(\pi(i),j)} = \begin{bmatrix} 010 \\ 001 \\ 100 \end{bmatrix} \tag{4}$$

Let the value of input data matrix $X = \begin{bmatrix} 893 \\ 965 \\ 219 \end{bmatrix}$, the identity matrix $I_{(\pi(i),j)} = \begin{bmatrix} 010 \\ 001 \\ 100 \end{bmatrix}$ when multiplies the input matrix it randomly permutes the row values that is $tempX = \begin{bmatrix} 010 \\ 001 \\ 100 \end{bmatrix} * \begin{bmatrix} 893 \\ 965 \\ 219 \end{bmatrix} = \begin{bmatrix} 965 \\ 219 \\ 893 \end{bmatrix}$.

The values of identity matrix $I_{(\pi(i),j)}$ are further multiplied by the positive random numbers such that $\gamma \to \{\gamma_1, \gamma_2, \dots\dots\dots\gamma_n\}$ here $0 \notin \gamma$ multiplies in each row. This process generates the key matrices, which are used in the transformation operation. Let the transformation matrices are denoted as k_1, and k_2. There is only one non-zero element in each row and each column. Thus, the key matric generated from this process is square non-singular matrix, therefore also called invertible matrix.

The matrix $k_{(\pi(i),j)} = \begin{bmatrix} 0\gamma_2 0 \\ 00\gamma_3 \\ \gamma_1 00 \end{bmatrix}$ So, in this way we find the matrix.

$$k_{(\pi(i),j)} * X = \begin{bmatrix} 0\ 40 \\ 005 \\ 200 \end{bmatrix} * \begin{bmatrix} 893 \\ 965 \\ 219 \end{bmatrix}$$

$$k * X = \begin{bmatrix} 362420 \\ 10545 \\ 16186 \end{bmatrix}$$

Similarly, when the permutation matrix is multiplied from the right-side, it permutes the column values of the input matrix (X). These key matrices are also known as monomial matrix. The special arrangement of the key matrix, that is one element in each row causes only linear time in key generation and problem transformation phase.

DATA CONFIDENTIALITY AND INTEGRITY PRESERVING SYSTEM OF LINEAR EQUATION

This section discusses the design details of privacy preserving SLE. The section discusses the privacy of input data-set (A, b), and the output of linear equation (x). A secure outsourcing algorithm required to construct the following sub-algorithms $KeyGen(\lambda)$, $ProbTrans(\varphi,k)$, $Compute\ \varphi_k(A',b')$, $Verify\ (x',k)$, $Retransform\ (x',k)$. Further, the development of each sub-algorithm is discussed in the below sections.

Key Generation

The client invokes this algorithm with an input security parameter λ, this algorithm first generates two sets of non-zero random numbers $\gamma \rightarrow \{\gamma_1, \gamma_2, ...\gamma_n\}, \delta \rightarrow \{\delta_1, \delta_2, ...\delta_n\}$, where $\{0 \notin (\gamma, \delta)\}$ and random permutations $\{\pi_1, \pi_2\}$. The client generates two identity matrices (I_1, I_2); then the random permutations $\{\pi_1, \pi_2\}$ are applied to these diagonal matrices that will generate random permutation matrix $\left(I_{1(\pi_1(i),j)}, I_{2(\pi_2(i),j)}\right)$. These matrices are further masked with the non-zero random numbers $\gamma \rightarrow \{\gamma_1, \gamma_2, ...\gamma_n\}, \delta \rightarrow \{\delta_1, \delta_2, ...\delta_n\}$ and then the key matrices are generated (k_1, k_2). These matrices are square and non-singular, so they could be easily invertible in (k_1^{-1}, k_2^{-1}). Therefore, in this way the key matrices are generated, which are $\{key = k_1, k_2, k_1^{-1}, k_2^{-1}\}$. This implementation is very efficient and takes only $O(n)$ time complexity. The key generation algorithm has got inspiration form algorithm (Xinyu Lei et al., 2013), which was developed for secure outsourcing of matrix inversion algorithm.

Problem Transformation

This section explains the transformation operation $ProbTrans(\varphi, k)$ applied on the client's dataset to preserve the confidentiality. The transformation operation has two aim. First, the transformation operation satisfies the privacy & confidentiality concern of the client. Second, it should be efficient because the transformation operation is executed on client's system. The client first generates two random monomial key matrices $\{k_1, k_2\}$, where $\{ \{k_1, k_2\} \in \mathbb{R}^n$. The special arrangement of these key matrices allows them to invertible. Interestingly, the key generation, and the inversion of keys, that is $\{k_1^{-1}, k_2^{-1}$ only requires $O(n)$ complexity. Further, the client performs the transformation on the input data set (A, b) using the key matrices $\{k_1, k_2^{-1}\}$, the transformation operation of coefficient matrix A generates $A\, A' = k_1 * A * k_2^{-1}$ and $b' = k_1 * b$. Putting these values in the equation (1), the SLE in equation (1) transformed to $A'x' = b'$. Then, the client outsources this transformed to cloud server.

System of Linear Equation Function Computation on Cloud Server

This section explains the $Compute\ \varphi_k(A', b')$ operation executed on the cloud server. The client generates (A', b') from the transformation, then this transformed matrices send to the cloud server. The cloud server executes the system of linear equation function $Compute\ \varphi_k(A', b')$. The details of cloud server execution explain below

$$A'x' = b' \tag{5}$$

Further, the cloud server will compute the values of x'.

$$x' = (k_1 * A * k_2^{-1})^{-1} * b'$$

Further, the property of invertible matrix that it reverses the order of multiplication that is $((k_1) * (k_2))^{-1} = (k_2)^{-1}(k_1)^{-1}$. Applying the matrix property on equation (2)

$$x' = k_2 * A^{-1} * k_1^{-1} * k_1 * b$$

Since, the invertible matrix $k_1^{-1} * k_1 = I$ the values in the equation (2) reduce to

$$x' = k_2 * A^{-1} * b \tag{6}$$

The cloud server produces the values of output variable x'. Besides, preserving the privacy of the input and the output dataset, an important aim of transformation techniques is that the client could establish a relation between the original result and the transformed result produced by the cloud server. The retransformation operation should be efficient and not involve in any complex computation.

Result Verification

The result verification process is a critical step in the design of outsourcing algorithm since the SLE algorithm is developed in completely malicious environment. The malicious cloud server may return a random result, or may converse early to save computation cycle and return random indistinguishable result. Therefore, there is no integrity on the result received from the cloud server. Thus, an outsourcing algorithm should be proficient in verify the correctness of the result computed by the cloud server.

The cloud server solves the system of linear equation for the transformed input (A', b') and returned the result (x'). To, verify the result obtained from the cloud server. The client establishes a relation $D = A' * x' - b'$, if the cloud produces correct result the value of $D = 0.$. The effectiveness of result relation lies that, the client able to verify the result without decryption and not involved in complex computation and the client only have to perform $O(n^2)$ work. Further, we provide a mathematical proof of the result verification process, which proves our claim in the next section.

Retransformation

The client verifies the result obtained from the cloud server, If the result obtained from the cloud server successfully passed the verification step then only the client retransforms the result (x') to obtained the original result of SLE (x). The steps of retransformation explained further,

$$x' = k_2 * A^{-1} * b$$

From equation (1), $Ax = b$, this equation could be written as $x = A^{-1} * b$ substituting the value of (x) into equation (6)

⇨ $x' = k_2 * x$

⇨ $x = k_2^{-1} x'$

Thus, we can easily retransform the result obtained from the cloud server without involving into any complex computation this retransformation process requires only $O(n)$ time complexity.

ANALYSIS OF PROPOSED SLE OUTSOURCING ALGORITHM

This section provides theoretical analysis of the proposed system of linear equation outsourcing algorithm. The proposed outsourcing algorithm meeting all the design goals such as correctness, privacy, verifiability, and efficiency.

Correctness Analysis

The system of linear equation outsourcing algorithm will perform correctly, only if the client and the cloud server follow the algorithm instructions and produces correct results.

Theorem 1: The proposed SLE algorithm is correct if both the client and cloud follow the algorithm properly.

Proof: The client first transforms the input (A, b) into $A' = \left(k_1 * A * k_2^{-1}\right)$, and $b' = k_1 * b$, Next the cloud server will solve the system of linear equation function for the transformed input (A', b').

⇨ $A'x' = b'$

⇨ $x' = A'^{-1} * b'$, substituting the value of (A', b')

⇨ $x' = \left(k_1 * A * k_2^{-1}\right)^{-1} * k_1 * b$, applying the matrix property $((k_1) * (k_2))^{-1} = (k_2)^{-1}(k_1)^{-1}$

⇨ $x' = k_2 * A^{-1} * k_1^{-1} * k_1 * b$, applying the matrix property $k_1 * k_1^{-1} = I$

⇨ $x' = k_2 * A^{-1} * b$, multiplying the value of x', with k_2^{-1}

⇨ $k_2^{-1} * x' = x$

Thus, the client will get the solution of original system of linear equation problem, which implies the correctness of the outsourcing algorithm.

Privacy Analysis

In the malicious cloud environment, the cloud server behaves as curious cloud. Therefore, the server may record all the client input and output data, which came into its control during the execution of SLE algorithm. Then the server tries to retrieve the original information from the recorded information. However, the cloud server never succeeded to recover the original information. Further, a security analysis is presented, which justify our claim. The security analysis follows the previous work on secure outsourcing on cloud computing (F. Chen, Xiang, Lei, et al., 2014; Wang et al., 2013).

Theorem 2: In the fully malicious model the proposed algorithm for SLE able to provide privacy to the input dataset *A*, *b* and the output *x*.

Proof: The cloud server may behave as lazy, curious and dishonest. Here the cloud server is considered as a malicious cloud, which is a strongest adversarial model. However, the cloud server will never able to recover the original client information (input and output) due to the proposed security arrangement. Further, a mathematical discussion has been presented to justify the claim.

The original input dataset is (A,b), where (A) is an $(n*n)$ matrix in $\mathbb{R}^{n*n}$ and (b) is an $(n*1)$ vector in $\mathbb{R}^n$, has been transformed to $\varphi(A',b')$ in following steps:

Step 1: First each entry in original matrix is randomly permuted row-wise & then column-wise using permutation function $\{\pi_1,\pi_2\}$ *where* $\pi_i \in \{1,\ldots\ldots\ldots,n\}$ and $i \in \{1,2\}$ ie.,

$$A'_{(i,j)} = A_{(\pi_1(i),\pi_2(j))}$$

similarly, for $b'_{(i,1)} = b_{(\pi_1(i),1)}$

Step 2: Each entry in matrix (A,b) is further masked by multiplicative factor $\gamma \rightarrow \{\gamma_1,\gamma_2,\ldots\ldots\ldots\gamma_n\}$, $\delta \rightarrow \{\delta_{1,}\delta_{2,}\ldots\ldots\ldots\ldots\delta_n\}$ *where* $\{0 \notin \gamma \cup \delta\}$, i.e.,

$$X'(i,j) = \left(\gamma_i \big/ \delta_j\right) X_{(\pi_1(i),\pi_2(j))} \quad (7)$$

similarly, for

$$b'_{(i,1)} = \gamma_i \left(b_{(\pi_1(i),1}\right) \quad (8)$$

In step 1, each entry is randomly permuted by two permutation functions $\{\pi_1,\pi_2\}$, so there are $(n)!*(n)!$ cases for each entry in the matrix where each case occurs with the probability of $1/((n)!)^2$. The estimated time of brute-force attack on the key space to recover the original matrix (A) is $(n)!^2/2$, which is a non-polynomial bound quantity in terms of (n).

In step 2, the matrix produced in step (1) is further multiply by the multiplying factor γ & δ, *where* $\{0 \notin \gamma \cup \delta\}$. The approximate time for brute-force attack to recover the key space γ & δ) is $\left(|K_\gamma|^n * |K_\delta|^n\right)/2$. A large choice of (γ & δ) will sufficiently reduce the chance of guessing the value of (γ & δ).

Similarly, the output result is also protected in the same way as the input data is protected. Therefore, resultant matrix is also not leaking any information to thc cloud. Thus, a malicious cloud server even if record the input and the output data, it never able to recover the original input and output data. Besides, the client generates a pair of new securities keys for every new problem submission to the cloud server. Thus, our encryption system is similar to one-time-pad encryption system. Therefore, there is no chance of known-plain-text attack or chosen-plain-text attack. Thus, the SLE outsourcing algorithm is secure and not leaking any information to cloud servers.

Verifiability Analysis

In the malicious threat model, the cloud server may deviate from the actual instruction of the SLE outsourcing algorithm and return a random arbitrary result. Thus, the SLE outsourcing algorithm must be equipped with the result verification process, which is able to verify the correctness of the result.

Theorem 3: In result verification step if $Ax \neq b$ the verification fails with the probability of 1.

Proof: In the malicious threat model the cloud server may deviate from the actual algorithmic instructions and return random arbitrary results. Thus, the proposed algorithm must be equipped with the rigorous result verification process, which verifies the correctness of the result. The client receives the solution of system of linear equation (x') from the cloud server. The client already has the transformed input (A',b'). If the solution vector (x') is correctly computed by the cloud server then only the equation $(A'x' = b')$ holds true. If the equation $(A'x' = b')$ holds true then,

$$D = A'x' - b' = (0,0,0.................0)^T \tag{9}$$

The client in the algorithm verifies the correctness of the result produces by the cloud server. To, perform such task, the client verifies the equation $(A'x' = b')$ must holds true. The verification process is yet efficient since it required only a matrix-vector multiplication that cost only $O(n^2)$ to the client. If $(A'x' - b' \neq 0)$ there must be at least one row that is not equal to zero.

$$\Rightarrow D = A'x' - b'$$

$$\Rightarrow D = (d_1, \ldots, d_k, \ldots, d_n)^T$$

Let, some $d_i \neq 0$, then

$$\Rightarrow d_i = (a'_{i1} * x'_1 + a'_{i2} * x'_2 + \ldots + \ldots + a'_{in} * x'_n) - b'_i$$

$$\Rightarrow d_i = \sum_{j=1}^{n} a'_{ij} * x'_j - b'_i$$

$$\Rightarrow d_i = a'_{i1} * x'_1 + \sum_{j=2}^{n} a'_{ij} * x'_j - b'_i$$

$$\Rightarrow a'_{i1} * x'_1 = d_i + b'_i - \sum_{j=2}^{n} a'_{ij} * x'_j$$

$$\Rightarrow x'_1 = \frac{d_i + b'_i - \sum_{j=2}^{n} a'_{ij} * x'_j}{a'_{i1}} \tag{10}$$

The value of (x'_1) could be any real number, but if the server correctly computes the values of (x'_1), there should be only one value which satisfies equation (7). So, (x'_1) has only one value, so the probability ($Pr = 1 / n$, where $n \in \mathbb{R}$ so $Pr \cong 0$. So, the server misconduct detected with the probability of $\left(Pr = 1 - 1 / n\right) \cong 1$. Thus, the result verification step verifies the result with the probability of (1).

Efficiency Analysis

The outsourcing algorithm for SLE has two parts, the client-side computation, and the cloud-side computation. The client performs the following sub-operations: the *KeyGen*, *ProbTrans*, *Verify*, and *Retransform*. However, cloud server runs the complex computation of solution to the SLE on the transformed input *Compute*.

Theorem 4: The proposed secure outsourcing algorithm is $O(n)$ times efficient implementation of SLE.

Proof: In order to execute the proposed SLE outsourcing algorithm the client needs to carry out matrix multiplication in $ProbTrans(\varphi,k)$, $Verify\ (x',k)$, and $Retransform\ (x',k)$. The problem transformation operation requires to perform the following matrix multiplication such that $A' = k_1 * A * k_2^{-1}$, $b' = k_1 * b$. Due to the special arrangement of key matrices k_1 and k_2 that is one element in each row and column, the matrix multiplication operation causes only the complexity of matrix-vector multiplication because the cost of addition operation is omitted during the matrix multiplication. So, the upper bound asymptotic requirement of this operation is only $O(n^2)$. In the result verification, the client needed to perform $(A'x' = b')$, where A' is a general $(n \times n)$ matrix and x' is a column matrix $(n \times 1)$. So, a single matrix-vector multiplication only causes $O(n^2)$. Finally, the retransformation operation, which requires to carry out $k_2^{-1} * x' = x$. The multiplication of the key matrix k_2^{-1} with a column vector only causes $O(n)$. Thus, the client side computation never cross the asymptotic upper bound of $O(n^2)$ during the entire course of execution of SLE outsourcing algorithm. However, in order to solve a system of linear equation causes $O(n^3)$. Therefore, the client system has the computer saving of $O(n)$. Thus, the SLE outsourcing algorithm is $O(n)$ times efficient implementation.

Comparision Analysis

In the section, the proposed algorithm for SLE has been compared against the existing work. A privacy analysis has also been performed for the (Wang et al., 2013) algorithm to point out marginal security arrangement due to inappropriate use of the Paillier encryption system.

Privacy Comparison

The prime objective of outsourcing algorithm is offload the large computation without revealing the input and output to the cloud server. However, the security analysis for (Wang et al., 2013) has reached to a conclusion that the cloud server could recover partial information about the coefficient matrix A.

Proof: The authors have proposed an interactive solution for the system of linear equation $Ay = b$. First the SLE convert to an iterative form that is $y^{(k+1)} = T * y^{(k)} + c'$ where $T = -D^{-1} * R$ and $c' = D^{-1}(b + A * r)$. In each round of computation, the client provides the decryption service for $Enc(T * y^k)$. The client first decrypts $(T * y^k)$, then the client computes $y^{(k+1)} = T * y^k + c'$ and send it to the cloud server for the next round of computation of $y^{(k+1)}$ and here the trapdoor lies. Let the cloud server returns the $(T * y^k)$ with an adversary for gaining information about T that is $Enc(T_{ij} * z)$, where T_{ij} is the element of the matrix T, and z is a random number. The client is not able to verify the correctness of the result obtained from cloud server at this stage. Thus, provide decryption service. The cloud server could recover partial information about (T). The client provide decryption service for $Enc(T_{ij} * z)$, the client find $z * T_j$. For the next round the client computes $z * T_j + c'$ and send to the cloud server in this way the cloud server gets information about the $T_{j(th)}$ column of T. Similarly, this process will repeat several times until the problem conveses, after L round of interaction. Therefore the cloud server could access information about up to L column of matrix T. Further, the matrix T came into the form of Diophantine approximation problem.

The Diophantine approximation problem approximates a real number α by rational number a / b. A rational number a / b is a good approximation of a real number α, if the absolute difference of $\left|\alpha - \frac{a}{b}\right|$ is not decreases and the rational number is replaced by some other rational number a'/b' with smaller denominator. Further, we show that, if the cloud server has information about matrix T. The cloud server could recover partial information about the coefficient matrix A by using Diophantine approximation. This problem is similar to Diophantine Approximation problem, where the real number α could be obtained from the good approximation of rational number. These columns are the good approximations of real number of the coefficient matrix A. Therefore, the cloud server could recover several columns of coefficient matrix A. The number of columns that the cloud server will able to recover depends upon the number of interactions between the client and the cloud server, which is L. The value of $L < n$ (n is the size of the problem). So, the cloud server would not able to recover entire coefficient matrix A. However, if the algorithm is submitted multiple times for the same set of problem then it possible that the cloud server will able to recover entire coefficient matrix A.

Finally, the point, which rises from the above discussion that the decryption service along with simultaneous multiple round of interaction between client and the cloud server causes security breach for the client's input data. This makes the algorithm vulnerable for security threat. Interested readers may read (Cao & Liu, 2016) for more information.

Efficiency Comparison

The secure outsourcing algorithm proposed by (Wang et al., 2013), first it generates the Paillier encryption key and secure vector for encryption. Then it takes three matrix-vector multiplications for problem transformation. The client C interact with the cloud server SC in the multiple round communications L, where each round of communication required a vector decryption and one matrix-vector computation until the problem reaches to a result. The result verification algorithm takes another matrix-vector multiplication to verify the correctness of the result for l times where $\left(l \leq L \leq n\right)$ causes additional burden on client. The summary of the running time of the sub-algorithms of existing and proposed SLE outsourcing algorithms are shown in Table 2.

Verifiability Comparison

In the (Wang et al., 2013) algorithm result verification provides probabilistic verification of result with an error probability of $\left(\frac{1}{2^l}\right)$, the result verification is efficient causes only matrix-vector multiplication but to reduce the error probability the verification process required to run l time where $\left(l \leq L \leq n\right)$. The size of l is trade-off between security and efficiency.

The comparison analysis reveals that the existing algorithm is lagging in all the three parameters of security, efficiency and verifiability parameters. First, an adversary might get access to dataset due to inappropriate decryption service in each round of interaction. Second, the L round interaction between the client and the cloud server not only open opportunity for the adversary to gain access of dataset but it also adds overhead of one decryption and matrix-vector multiplication in each round of communication that also make the algorithm inefficient. Third, the verification service is also probabilistic, for rigorous checking the verification algorithm should be execute l times. The size of $\left(l\right)$ is a trade-off between security and efficiency.

Table 2. Theoretical analysis of complexities

Algorithm Primitives	(Wang et al., 2013)	Proposed Algorithm
$ProbTrans$	$O\left(2n^2\right)$	$O\left(3n^2\right)$
$Compute$	$O\left(n^3 + Ln^2\right)$	$O\left(n^3\right)$
$Retransform$	$O\left(Ln * dec\right)$	$O\left(n\right)$
$Verify$	$O\left(l * n^2\right), \left(l \leq L \leq n\right)$	$O\left(n^2\right)$
$Encryption\,System$	*Paillier Encryption*	*Linear Transformation*
$Interaction$	$L\left(dec + n^2\right)$	NA
$Data\,Set$	$\left(T', b'\right) + 2L\,Vector$	$\left(A', b'\right)$
$Communication$	*L-Round*	1

EXPERIMENTAL ANALYSIS

The experimental analysis has been performed to validate the correctness and effectiveness of the proposed algorithm. The proposed SLE algorithm is implemented in Matlab version 2014a. The client & the cloud server both implemented on a system having same computing capacity. The CPU is Intel® Xenon® CPU E5-2620 v2 @ 2.10 GHz ~ 8GB RAM. The reason for implementing client and server on the same node is to show the outsourcing algorithm actual efficiency and performance gain. If there are differences between the computing performance of client and server, then the performance of algorithm will be case specific. However, in reality, the cloud server always has more computing resources than the client.

Three standard parameters the efficiency, performance gain and the relative extra are measured to present the experimental analysis of the algorithm.

$$Efficiency\left(\eta\right) = \frac{T_{original}}{T_{cloud}} \tag{11}$$

where $T_{original}$ is an original time of execution of SLE problem without encryption, T_{cloud} execution time of the encrypted problem. Ideally, the efficiency of the algorithm should be close to one. If the efficiency is nearby one. It indicates that the execution time of the original problem and the encrypted problem is almost same.

The second parameter is the Performance Gain (PG) for the client "It represents the actual speed-up the client has gained from outsourcing the problem."

$$PG = T_{original} / T_{client} \tag{12}$$

where, T_{client} is client processing time for computing. Theoretically, the performance gain for the client should always be greater than one.

The relative extra cost (REC) is define as the amount of extra work done by the client and cloud server in outsourcing paradigm as compared to direct method. Ideally, REC should be near to zero that is there should be no extra burden incur by the outsourcing paradigm.

$$REC = \frac{\left(T_{client} + T_{cloud} - T_{original}\right)}{\left(T_{original}\right)} \tag{13}$$

Further the notations use to calculate the performance of the algorithms presented in Table 3.

Table 3. Terms and description

Notations	Meaning
MD	Matrix Dimension $\left(A,b\right)$
$T_{original}$	Time to execute the SLE without Transformation/Encryption and outsourcing paradigm (Direct Method)
T_{cloud}	Time to execute transformed/encrypted SLE
T_{client_1}	Time for Key Generation + Time for Problem Transformation
T_{client_2}	Result Verification Time + Time for re-transformation
T_{client}	$T_{client} = T_{client_1} + T_{client_2}$
$\left(\eta\right)$	$Efficiency\left(\eta\right) = \frac{T_{original}}{T_{cloud}}$
PG	$PG = T_{original} / T_{client}$
REC	$REC = \frac{\left(T_{client} + T_{cloud} - T_{original}\right)}{\left(T_{original}\right)}$

We execute the SLE outsourcing algorithm multiple times for each problem instance to get a stable system performance. The experimental performance analysis of the proposed algorithm is shown in Table 4 & Figure 3. We can see in Figure 3 (a) & Table 4, that the efficiency parameter remains close to one, which means the outsourcing paradigm adds no extra burden on the cloud server for executing an encrypted problem. Further, it is shown in Table 4 that the REC parameter stays 0.2045 for a problem size of (500*500) whereas 0.01186 for (5000*5000) 94% decrease in relative extra cost. However, we have conduct the experiments for other bigger size problem too, but after certain point the rec parameter remain constant. It is evident from experimental result that the overhead reduces to great extent as the problem size increases. Further, Figure. 3(c) demonstrates the comparison of execution the times between direct algorithm and proposed algorithm for SLE. The time to execute a problem of size (5000*5000) is 11.8995 seconds. However, when the computation is outsourced by using the proposed algorithm it takes only 0.3798 seconds. This happen because the client in our algorithm work only $O\left(n^2\right)$ for SLE rather the computation burden of $O\left(n^3\right)$. A computational saving of $O\left(n\right)$ for the client, and as the size of problem $\left(n\right)$ increases the client got substantial computational saving.

Furthermore, the performance-gain parameter is in double-digit for larger size problem and able to attain more than 31.33 times, which is a very motivating factor to use SLE outsourcing algorithm in real-world scenarios. Moreover, the theoretical and experimental analysis of SLE outsourcing algorithm proves, that the resource constrained client can execute large SLE by offloading their computation load to massive cloud servers using SLE outsourcing algorithm. The proposed work is very efficient and able to maintain the privacy of data under the malicious cloud environment. Due to rising demand of outsourcing solution for more practical problem the proposed work would be very helpful for the research community to carry out further research work. It is worth noting that the experimental performance depends on problem dimension, the underlying execution platform, and algorithm for solving matrix

Table 4. Performance analysis of SLE algorithm

Problem Size	Original Time	Cloud Time	Client-Side Computation			Performance Gain	Efficiency	Relative Extra Cost
	$T_{original}$	T_{cloud}	T_{client_1}	T_{client_2}	T_{client}	$\frac{T_{original}}{T_{client}}$	$\frac{T_{original}}{T_{cloud}}$	$\frac{T_{client}+T_{cloud}}{T_{original}}-1$
500	0.0375	0.0356	0.00606	0.00354	0.0096	3.9183	1.0534	0.2045
1000	0.1098	0.1032	0.01327	0.00724	0.0205	5.3462	1.064	0.12659
1500	0.3488	0.3389	0.02436	0.01294	0.0373	9.3429	1.0294	0.0785
2000	0.8026	0.7864	0.04586	0.01925	0.0651	12.3268	1.0206	0.06094
2500	1.6946	1.6579	0.0714	0.0378	0.1106	15.3214	1.0221	0.0436
3000	2.8907	2.8261	0.10402	0.05369	0.1577	18.3287	1.0229	0.03221
3500	4.933	4.8119	0.14578	0.07492	0.2207	22.3469	1.0252	0.02019
4000	8.1	7.9246	0.19806	0.10144	0.2995	27.0485	1.0221	0.01532
4500	8.8706	8.6865	0.20008	0.10222	0.3023	29.3453	1.0212	0.01332
5000	11.8995	11.6608	0.25156	0.12824	0.3798	31.3352	1.0205	0.01186

Figure 3. The performance graphs of SLE algorithm. (a) Efficiency of SLE algorithm. (b) Relative extra cost of SLE algorithm. (c) Execution time comparison between client and cloud. (d) Performance gain of SLE algorithm.

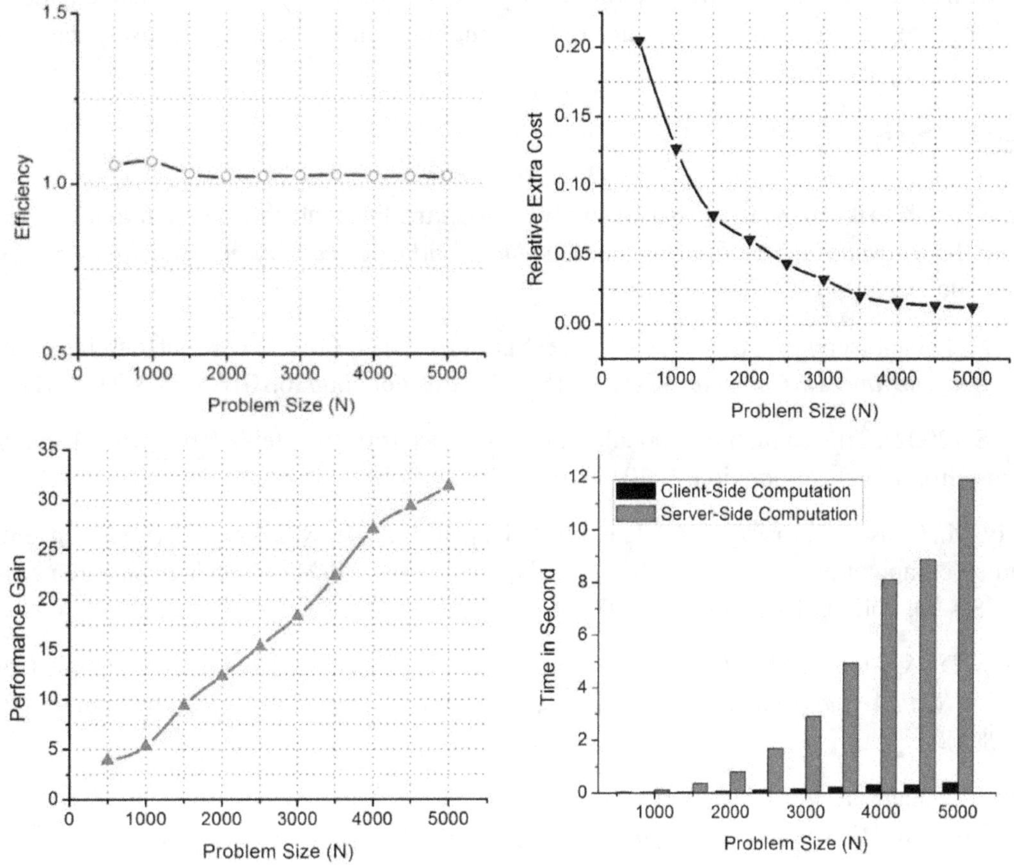

multiplication. If the cloud exploits other faster matrix operation algorithms, then client speedup will decrease to some extent. However, as long as the size of the input goes sufficiently large, the client get a significant performance-gain due to the apparent computation gap between the client-side computation and server-side computation.

CONCLUSION

In this paper, we formulated and implemented a new outsourcing algorithm for the SLE problem. Unlike the existing algorithm for SLE the proposed outsourcing algorithm is not using any such complex cryptography techniques. It is developed by utilizing the linear transformation method using the concepts of linear algebra. A comparison analysis has been performed, which shows that the proposed algorithm performs better on security, efficiency and verifiability parameter than the existing algorithm. The algorithm is able to meet the challenges of input/output privacy, correctness, verifiability, and efficiency, which is well demonstrated in the analytical analysis of the algorithm. The results of the experimental implementation demonstrate the practical usability of the algorithm. In future, it would be remarkable to see novel algorithms, which reduces the overhead cost incur by the problem transformation and verification process with greater efficiency. However, finding newer computationally expensive mathematical, scientific and engineering problem and designing outsourcing solution for them, would always be noticeable.

REFERENCES

Atallah, M. J., & Frikken, K. B. (2010). Securely outsourcing linear algebra computations. *Proceedings of the 5th ACM Symposium on Information, Computer and Communications Security - ASIACCS '10*, 48. https://doi.org/10.1145/1755688.1755695

Atallah, M. J., Pantazopoulos, K. N., Rice, J. R., & Spafford, E. E. (2002). Secure outsourcing of scientific computations. *Advances in Computers, 54*(C), 215–272. https://doi.org/10.1016/S0065-2458(01)80019-X

Bajikar, S. (2002). Trusted platform module (tpm) based security on notebook pcs-white paper. Mobile Platforms Group Intel Corporation, 1–20.

Belenkiy, M., Chase, M., Erway, C. C., Jannotti, J., Küpçü, A., & Lysyanskaya, A. (2008). Incentivizing outsourced computation. *Proceedings of the 3rd international workshop on Economics of networked systems*, 85–90. doi:10.1145/1403027.1403046

Benjamin, D., & Atallah, M. J. (2008). Private and Cheating-Free Outsourcing of Algebraic Computations. *2008 Sixth Annual Conference on Privacy, Security and Trust*, 240–245. https://doi.org/10.1109/PST.2008.12

Blanton, M., Zhang, Y., & Frikken, K. B. (2013). Secure and verifiable outsourcing of large-scale biometric computations. *ACM Transactions on Information and System Security, 16*(3), 1–33. doi:10.1145/2535523

Cao, Z., & Liu, L. (2016). Comment on harnessing the Cloud for Securely Outsourcing Large-Scale Systems of Linear Equations.. *IEEE Transactions on Parallel and Distributed Systems, 27*(5), 1551–1562. doi:10.1109/TPDS.2016.2531669

Chen, F., Xiang, T., Lei, X., & Chen, J. (2014). Highly Efficient Linear Regression Outsourcing to a Cloud. *IEEE Transactions on Cloud Computing*. https://doi.org/10.1109/TCC.2014.2378757

Chen, F., Xiang, T., Lei, X., & Chen, J. (2015). *Highly Efficient Linear Regression Outsourcing to a Cloud*. Academic Press.

Chen, F., Xiang, T., & Yang, Y. (2014). Privacy-preserving and verifiable protocols for scientific computation outsourcing to the cloud. *Journal of Parallel and Distributed Computing*, *74*(3), 2141–2151. doi:10.1016/j.jpdc.2013.11.007

Chen, X., Huang, X., Li, J., Ma, J., Lou, W., & Wong, D. S. (2015). *New Algorithms for Secure Outsourcing of Large-Scale Systems of Linear Equations*. Academic Press.

Chen, X., Li, J., & Ma, J. (2014). *New algorithms for secure outsourcing of modular exponentiations*. Academic Press.

Chung, K. M., Kalai, Y., & Vadhan, S. (2010). Improved delegation of computation using fully homomorphic encryption. *Lecture Notes in Computer Science, 6223*, 483–501. https://doi.org/10.1007/978-3-642-14623-7_26

Cramer, R., & Damgård, I. (2001). Secure Distributed Linear Algebra in a Constant Number of Rounds. *Crypto, 2139*, 119–136. https://doi.org/10.1007/3-540-44647-8_7

Dreier, J., & Kerschbaum, F. (2011). *Practical Secure and Efficient Multiparty Linear Programming Based on Problem Transformation*. Retrieved from http://eprint.iacr.org/2011/108

Du, W., & Atallah, M. J. (2001). Privacy-preserving cooperative scientific computations. *Proceedings of the Computer Security Foundations Workshop*, 273–282. https://doi.org/10.1109/CSFW.2001.930152

Du, W., Chen, S., & Han, Y. S. (2004). Privacy-Preserving Multivariate Statistical Analysis: Linear Regression and Classification. *Proceedings of the 4th SIAM International Conference on Data Mining*, 222–233. Retrieved from http://citeseerx.ist.psu.edu/viewdoc/summary?doi=10.1.1.2.423

Fortnow, L., & Lund, C. (1993, May). Interactive proof systems and alternating time—space complexity. *Theoretical Computer Science*, *113*(1), 55–73. doi:10.1016/0304-3975(93)90210-K

Gennaro, R., Gentry, C., & Parno, B. (2010). Non-interactive verifiable computing: Outsourcing computation to untrusted workers. *Lecture Notes in Computer Science, 6223*, 465–482. https://doi.org/10.1007/978-3-642-14623-7_25

Gentry, C. (2009). *A Fully Homomorphic Encryption Scheme* (PhD thesis). https://doi.org/10.1145/1536414.1536440

Gentry, C. (2010). Computing arbitrary functions of encrypted data. *Communications of the ACM*, *53*(3), 97. doi:10.1145/1666420.1666444

Goldreich, O., Micali, S. W. A., Goldreich, O., Micali, S., & Wigderson, A. (1987). How To Play Any Mental Game, or A Completeness Theorem for Protocols with Honest Majority. *Proceedings of 19th Annual ACM Symposium on Theory of Computing*. https://doi.org/10.1145/28395.28420

Goldwasser, S., Kalai, Y. T., & Rothblum, G. N. (2008). Delegating Computation: Interactive Proofs for Muggles. *Stoc, 62*(4), 113–122. https://doi.org/http://doi.acm.org/10.1145/1374376.1374396

Goldwasser, S., Micali, S., & Rackoff, C. (1989). The Knowledge Complexity of Interactive Proof Systems. *SIAM Journal on Computing*, *18*(1), 186–208. doi:10.1137/0218012

Hong, Y., Vaidya, J., & Lu, H. (2012). Secure and efficient distributed linear programming. *Journal of Computer Security*, *20*(5), 583–634. doi:10.3233/JCS-2012-0452

Hu, X., & Tang, C. (2015). Secure outsourced computation of the characteristic polynomial and eigenvalues of matrix. *Journal of Cloud Computing*, *4*(1), 4–9. https://doi.org/10.1186/s13677-015-0033-9

Kiltz, E., Mohassel, P., Weinreb, E., & Franklin, M. K. (2007). Secure Linear Algebra Using Linearly Recurrent Sequences. *Theory of Cryptography, 4th Theory of Cryptography Conference Proceedings*, *4392*, 291–310. https://doi.org/10.1007/978-3-540-70936-7_16

Laud, P., & Pankova, A. (n.d.). *Transformation-Based Outsourcing of Linear Equation Systems over Real Numbers*. Retrieved from http://eprint.iacr.org/2015/322

Lei, X., Liao, X., Huang, T., & Heriniaina, F. (2014). Achieving security, robust cheating resistance, and high-efficiency for outsourcing large matrix multiplication computation to a malicious cloud. *Information Sciences, 280*, 205–217. doi:10.1016/j.ins.2014.05.014

Lei, X., Liao, X., Huang, T., Li, H., & Hu, C. (2013). Outsourcing Large Matrix Inversion Computation to A Public Cloud. *IEEE Transactions on Cloud Computing, 1*(1), 1–1. https://doi.org/10.1109/TCC.2013.7

Lei, X., Liao, X., Member, S., Huang, T., & Li, H. (2015). Cloud Computing Service. *The Case of Large Matrix Determinant Computation, 8*(5), 688–700.

Lin, K., & Chen, M. S. (2010). Privacy-preserving outsourcing support vector machines with random transformation. *Proceedings of the 16th ACM SIGKDD International Conference on Knowledge Discovery and Data Mining*, 363–372. https://doi.org/10.1145/1835804.1835852

Lindell, Y., & Pinkas, B. (2009). Secure Multiparty Computation for Privacy-preserving Data Mining. *Journal of Privacy and Confidentiality, 1*(1), 59–98.

López-Alt, A., Tromer, E., & Vaikuntanathan, V. (2012). On-the-fly multiparty computation on the cloud via multikey fully homomorphic encryption. *Proceedings of the 44th Symposium on Theory of Computing - STOC '12*, 1219. https://doi.org/10.1145/2213977.2214086

Mell, P., & Grance, T. (2011). The NIST Definition of Cloud Computing Recommendations of the National Institute of Standards and Technology. *National Institute of Standards and Technology, Information Technology Laboratory, 145*, 7. https://doi.org/10.1136/emj.2010.096966

Mohassel, P. (2011). Efficient and Secure Delegation of Linear Algebra. *IACR Cryptology ePrint Archive*, 1–33. Retrieved from http://eprint.iacr.org/2011/605.pdf

Mohassel, P., & Weinreb, E. (2008). Efficient secure linear algebra in the presence of covert or computationally unbounded adversaries. *Lecture Notes in Computer Science, 5157*, 481–496. https://doi.org/10.1007/978-3-540-85174-5_27

Monrose, F., Wyckoff, P., & Rubin, A. (1999). Distributed execution with remote audit. *Ndss*. Retrieved from http://www.isoc.org/isoc/conferences/ndss/99/proceedings/papers/monrose.pdf

Nissim, K., & Weinreb, E. (2006). Communication efficient secure linear algebra. *Lecture Notes in Computer Science, 3876*, 522–541. https://doi.org/10.1007/11681878_27

Ram, J., & Comesa, P. (n.d.). *Secure Direct and Iterative Protocols for Solving Systems of Linear Equations. Academic Press.*

Saad, Y. (2001). Parallel iterative methods for sparse linear systems. *Studies in Computational Mathematics, 8*(C), 423–440. https://doi.org/10.1016/S1570-579X(01)80025-2

Seshadri, A., Luk, M., Shi, E., Perrig, A., Van Doorn, L., & Khosla, P. (2005). Pioneer: Verifying integrity and guaranteeing execution of code on legacy platforms. In *Proceedings of ACM Symposium on Operating Systems Principles (SOSP)* (Vol. 173). doi:10.1145/1095810.1095812

Shiraz, M., Gani, A., Khokhar, R. H., & Buyya, R. (2013). A review on distributed application processing frameworks in smart mobile devices for mobile cloud computing. *IEEE Communications Surveys and Tutorials, 15*(3), 1294–1313. doi:10.1109/SURV.2012.111412.00045

Smith, S. W., & Weingart, S. (1999). Building a high-performance, programmable secure coprocessor. *Computer Networks, 31*(8), 831–860. doi:10.1016/S1389-1286(98)00019-X

Van Dijk, M., Gentry, C., Halevi, S., & Vaikuntanathan, V. (2010). Fully homomorphic encryption over the integers. *Advances in Cryptology–EUROCRYPT '10*, 24–43. https://doi.org/10.1007/978-3-642-38348-9_20

Wang, C., Ren, K., & Wang, J. (2011). Secure and practical outsourcing of linear programming in cloud computing. *Proceedings - IEEE INFOCOM*, 820–828. https://doi.org/10.1109/INFCOM.2011.5935305

Wang, C., Ren, K., Wang, J., & Urs, K. M. (2011). Harnessing the Cloud for Securely Solving Large-Scale Systems of Linear Equations. *2011 31st International Conference on Distributed Computing Systems, 24*(6), 549–558. https://doi.org/10.1109/icdcs.2011.41

Wang, C., Ren, K., Wang, J., & Wang, Q. (2013). Harnessing the Cloud for Securely Outsourcing Large-Scale Systems of Linear Equations. *IEEE Transactions on Parallel and Distributed Systems, 24*(6), 1172–1181. doi:10.1109/TPDS.2012.206

Yao, A. C. (1982). Protocols for secure computations. *23rd Annual Symposium on Foundations of Computer Science (Sfcs 1982)*, 1–5. https://doi.org/10.1109/SFCS.1982.38

Yao, A. C.-C. (1986). How to generate and exchange secrets. *27th Annual Symposium on Foundations of Computer Science (Sfcs 1986)*, (1), 162–167. https://doi.org/10.1109/SFCS.1986.25

Yee, B. (1994). *Using secure coprocessors.* Citeseer.

Zhang, Y., & Blanton, M. (2014). *Efficient Secure and Verifiable Outsourcing of Matrix Multiplications.* https://doi.org/10.1007/978-3-319-13257-0_10

Zhou, L., Li, C., & Member, S. (2016). *Outsourcing Eigen-Decomposition and Singular Value Decomposition of Large Matrix to a Public Cloud.* Academic Press.

Chapter 4
Data Reduction Techniques for Near Real-Time Decision Making in Fall Prediction Systems

Masoud Hemmatpour
Politecnico di Torino, Italy

Renato Ferrero
Politecnico di Torino, Italy

Filippo Gandino
Politecnico di Torino, Italy

Bartolomeo Montrucchio
Politecnico di Torino, Italy

Maurizio Rebaudengo
Politecnico di Torino, Italy

ABSTRACT

Unintentional falls are a frequent cause of hospitalization that mostly increases health service costs due to injuries. Fall prediction systems strive to reduce injuries and provide fast help to the users. Typically, such systems collect data continuously at a high speed through a device directly attached to the user. Whereas such systems are implemented in devices with limited resources, data volume is significantly important. In this chapter, a real-time data analyzer and reducer is proposed in order to manage the data volume of fall prediction systems.

DOI: 10.4018/978-1-5225-5222-2.ch004

Copyright © 2018, IGI Global. Copying or distributing in print or electronic forms without written permission of IGI Global is prohibited.

1. INTRODUCTION

Hospitalized patients, people with movement-related disorders, and elderly people are high risk categories of encountering falls (Schwendimann, 2006) (Ambrose, 2013) (Canning, 2014). Currently, modern hospitals are well-equipped with monitoring and data collection devices to store and analyze patient data (Baig, 2013). Moreover, since fall is one of the negative consequences of some diseases such as Parkinson and rheumatism, which provoke disturbance in gait pattern, several gait assessment systems have been developed to measure or monitor gait parameters of patients. In addition, the risk of falling increases progressively with age, so several fall avoidance systems have been developed for elderly people in order to reduce fall injuries, in particular hip fracture.

Generally speaking, applicable fall avoidance systems can be categorized into three different types: detection, prediction, and prevention systems. Fall detection systems notify an acquaintance of the user in case of fall occurrence (Mubashir, 2013). These systems can be used to provide fast help after a fall, but they do not avoid it so, they are less effective than the other systems. Fall prediction systems strive to predict a fall before its occurrence (Staranowicz, 2013). Fall prevention systems provide solutions for preventing the fall (Majumder, 2013). Since predicting a fall is the most promising approach, the fall prediction algorithms are considered to be studied in this chapter. One category of fall prediction systems investigates balance and muscle strength through some offline tests such as Timed Up and Go (TUG), Berg Balance Scale (BBS), Sit To Stand (STS), and One Leg Stand (OLS) (Grant, 2014) (Vellas, 1997) (Muir, 2008) (Shumway-Cook, 2000). If the fall risk is high, a probable future fall can be prevented through some exercises. Typically, mentioned fall risk tests are applied by experts in clinical environments to evaluate balance and lower limb strength. The drawbacks of the mentioned tests are the demand of time and effort and they need to be conducted in a supervised environment. Therefore, they may suffer from influences such as the Hawthorne effect (McCarney, 2007), i.e., an individual modifies his/her behavior due to awareness of being observed. The other dominant category of fall prediction systems investigates real-time recognition of abnormal gait patterns to predict, or at least reduce, the injuries of a fall in real-time. Real-time fall solutions avoid a fall by alerting the user or using an external aid such as a walker or a robot (Di, 2011) (Hirata, 2006). Choosing between real-time or offline systems depends on the user circumstances. Generally speaking, if a user categorized in high risk of fall out of offline test, a real-time system can help to avoid a serious injury.

Most of the real-time fall prediction systems are based on kinematics and consider user's posture or gait variables. Kinematic-based solutions usually exploit movement sensors to investigate the parameters of a fall, i.e., the characteristics of the movement of the body. This chapter investigates real-time fall prediction systems exploiting accelerometer sensor. Real-time fall prediction systems usually have some steps in common: firstly, data are collected from sensors, and then they are analyzed to compute the appropriate feature set. Finally, the risk of a possible fall is evaluated through gait analysis techniques.

The quality of data must be guaranteed while acquiring and storing it rapidly. High-quality is a precondition attribute for analyzing and using data in order to guarantee a reliable result. The increase in data volume causes great difficulties for storage and analysis. Collected data during a walk has a quasi-periodic temporal dependence, so the time series is difficult to be modeled. Gait variables generally interact in a complex non-linear fashion, which requires high volume of data to be analyzed. Several gait models have been developed for the fall prediction systems in the literature. Most of the fall prediction systems achieve high accuracy by means of complex mathematics, which leads to high computational time. Since the data volume directly affects the performance, finding a technique with high accuracy and low data volume consumption is important for the design of a real-time application. Studying the data volume, and measuring the amount of data reduction considering its effect on the data quality can be beneficial in order to find an appropriate sampling rate, feature set, and classification model.

The analysis of quantitative gait data has traditionally been a challenging endeavor. The need for data reduction is critical due to high volume of the collected data. In terms of data reduction, there are few guiding rules for determining which variables contain useful information within a particular context. Moreover, data reduction must not harm the quality of data; otherwise the result of gait analysis is not accurate.

In the first step, a dataset with realistic parameters of abnormal and normal walks is required. Since a fall may be due to many factors such as balance and visual deficit, a flat area with different types of obstacles has been prepared. 31 users are asked to walk through obstacles without looking them. Figure 1 shows the abnormal walking test which users lose their balance due to the obstacles in the path (Weiss, 2010). Each user walks 5 times normally and 5 times abnormally. The accelerometer embedded in a smartphone is exploited in creating the dataset. Since the body Center Of Pressure (COP) reveals several information of user gait, the smartphone is placed on the lower back of trunk, near the real Center Of Mass (COM) position, assuming that this position moves parallel to the COP, and the same accelerations, velocities and positions are measured (Guimaraes, 2013).

The main contributions of this chapter are to analyze the collected gait data, then to design and implement a systematic methodology to reduce the data volume. The data generation in different stages of the fall prediction systems is investigated. Moreover, reduction techniques and their impact on data quality are experimentally evaluated.

The remainder of the chapter is organized as follows. Related works in the literature and background are reviewed in Section 2. The proposed methods are explained in Section 3. Experimental results are presented in Section 4. Finally, some conclusions are drawn in Section 5.

2. BACKGROUND

Typically, sensors generate huge raw data due to high frequency of sampling. Additionally, raw data are susceptible to include stale values. Since low-quality data will lead to low-quality results, collecting high

Figure 1. Abnormal walking simulation.

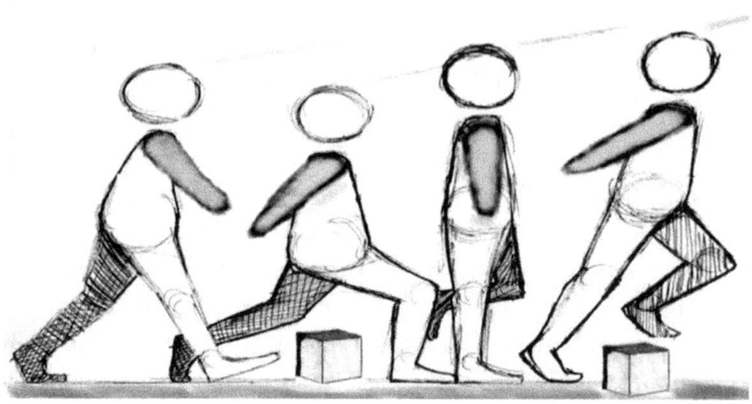

quality data is challenging for data pre-processing methods in particular with time constraint. In fact, real- time data pre-processing method is an essential component in the chain process in different context such as sensors network, intrusion detection systems, traffic control, ECG analysis, etc., (Abenstein, 1982) (Nimbalkar, 2016) (Lee, 2001) (Lopes, 2010). Basically, important data utilized by the system consists of extracted features from the output of the pre-processing unit.

In this section, the extrapolated features based on the accelerometer sensor in the kinematic analysis of user gait for real-time fall prediction systems are described (Weiss, 2010) (Majumder, 2013). In the formulas, A (t) indicates the acceleration and A_x (t), A_y (t), A_z (t) refer to its components along the 3 axes.

The *energy* of the acceleration signal specifies the amount of activity in the vertical and horizontal directions. It estimates the strength of the contact with the floor, so it can be used to recognize an abnormal walk pattern such as stumbling. The energy of the signal is computed as follows:

$$E_x = \int_{-\infty}^{+\infty} \left|A(t)\right|^2 dt\,.$$

Signal Magnitude Area (SMA) is used to classify the user activities. It is computed as:

$$SMA = \frac{1}{T}\left(\int_{-\infty}^{+\infty} \left|A(t)\right| dt\right)$$

where *T* is the monitored interval.

Signal Magnitude Vector (SMV) specifies the degree of the movement intensity and the resultant of the acceleration signal as follows:

$$SMV = \frac{1}{n}\sum_{i=1}^{n}\sqrt{A_x(t)^2 + A_y(t)^2 + A_z(t)^2}$$

where *n* is the number of samples.

The peak and peak-to-peak are useful measurements of data changing over time. The peak is the maximum value of the signal over the period of time, and the peak-to-peak is the difference between minimum and maximum values of the signal. Moreover, the derivative *A'(t)* of the acceleration can be used to indicate the vibration of a user movement.

3. DATA ANALYSIS AND REDUCTION TECHNIQUES

Healthcare is one of the most critical issues that are looking for tools to perform an automatic decision making. One of the important tools in this context is fall predictor. Such tools essentially collect data for decision making. Since data are gathered from different sensors, they may suffer from many problems such as noise, missing values and redundant features (El-Hasnony, 2015). These problems need to be carefully handled in order to improve the decision making process. Quality of the result is dependent on quality of the data, so tackling this problem is mandatory in fall prediction systems to analyze data in an efficient and an effective way.

The analytics associated with data can be described by three primary characteristics: velocity, volume (Rehman, 2016) and durability. Data will be created and accumulated continuously over time, resulting in a substantial volume. In the course of capturing and managing real-time data, some factors are important to be investigated:

- Data capturing frequency
- Data storage space
- Length of data stay
- Speed of data writing
- Speed of access to data

These factors are related to both hardware resources and to software requirements. For example, capturing data with a specific frequency might be an essential requirement of the software. However, data storage capacity, writing and reading speeds are hardware constraints. In designing a system both hardware and software characteristics should be considered. Therefore, answering to the question "which data is necessary?" is important. To do so, data processing unit of the typical fall prediction systems is investigated in more detail.

Some fall prediction systems exploit the internal processor of the embedded device to analyze the data (Guimaraes, 2013), (Majumder, 2013) whereas other systems transmit data on a remote node to analyze them (Otis, 2012), (Horta, 2013). Data volume has a big impact on the former approach due to limited resources of the embedded device and in the latter approach due to transmission latency and cost. Additionally, some fall prediction systems exploit online data and some approaches use the history of the observed data. Since the history of data is important in the latter approach a sliding window of the data are always maintained in the system. Figure 2 shows the conceptual framework of typical fall prediction systems.

Figure 2. Conceptual framework of fall prediction

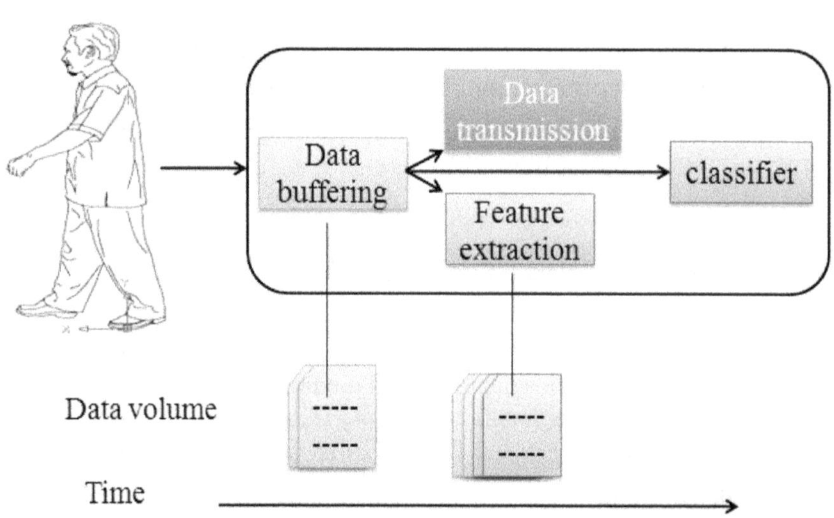

Firstly, data are captured and stored with a specific frequency in a buffering storage. Subsequently, data is transmitted either towards a central processing unit or to the feature extraction component. However, data can be exploited directly by classifier without performing any feature extraction. Two main parts that produce and consume the majority of the data are data buffering and feature extraction components.

In the mentioned framework, the data buffering completely depends on the capturing frequency that directly affects the data volume (Rehman, 2016). If the history of the observed data is required, a sliding window is always maintained in the system. Let assume f is the frequency of the capturing data and L is the size of the data in each sample. In the time period t, the maximum $(f * L * t * w)$ unit of data will be buffered where w specifies the sliding window size. Additionally, if the durability T is considered the formula can be presented as $f * L * w * g(T,t)$

$$g(T,t) = \begin{cases} t & T > t \\ T & T < t \end{cases}$$

where durability (T) specifies the life span of the data. Reducing the frequency can significantly reduce the size of the input data. Accuracy also might be sacrificed, since not all data is recorded. High frequency of data acquisition combined with the average of the observed data is a way to represent the actual data (Zakrzewska, 2009). Recording only data values that do not exceed a pre-specified band is another approach to reduce the input data size and eliminate the noises. Additionally, data compression can help but much time will be lost due to the compression and decompression algorithms.

Information about how much data is produced, how long data stays, and how data is consumed in the system can help in designing applications. This information describes fundamental issues in a supervisory control. This set of requirements leads to develop a two-tier data chronicle component to analyze and reduce the data volume. Basically, this component is proposed to be independently installed in order to dynamically analyze the data in the fall prediction application.

Figure 3 shows the proposed framework with the *data chronicle* component. The proposed component is composed of two tiers: Real-time analyzer and Reducer that work in parallel with the existing component. Data is always stored in the data buffering container. Firstly, it is passed to the real-time analyzer

Figure 3. Proposed data chronicle component

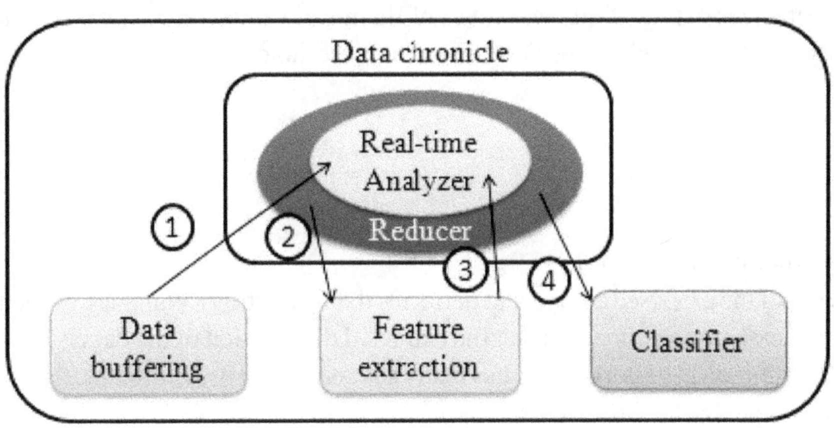

then, Reducer will clean the data out of dropping the outlier and anomaly pattern. Afterwards, the filtered data is passed to the feature extraction component. Subsequently, feature set is computed and returned back to the analyzer in order to perform the data reduction techniques. Finally, Reducer discovers the best feature set and passes it to the classifier. Basically, Reducer will reduce the data volume after two stages: once after analyzing the data buffering and once after analyzing the feature extraction. Intrinsically, Reducer uses two different approaches: data pre-processing and reduction techniques.

Pre-processing techniques strive to capture only the essential data and drop all non-essential entries. Since time is an important constraint in this context, a real-time pre-processor is required. Real-time pre-processing needs a comprehensive view of the input data. It can be done through a preliminary dataset in order to summarize the characteristics of the data. Basically, real-time techniques strive to understand the distribution of the data based on the descriptive statistics regarding both central tendency and dispersion including mean, max, and variance as measures for data dispersion. The big advantage of this method is the simplicity that leads to an easy implementation and computation, useful for real-time applications. The proposed pre-processor tier consists of filtering outliers and pattern identification.

Outliers are values that lie far from the middle of the distribution in either direction (Mendenhall, 1993). They may be due to sensor noise, acquisition and, system fails.

Firstly, pre-processor captures a sliding window of the input data. Basically, the proposed pre-processor computes the (maximum, mean, minimum) of each sliding window. In order to eliminate outliers, all samples of the sliding window must be in a feasible set. A set ∂ is said to be feasible if

$$\forall \beta \in \partial : \left(\beta - \varphi < \varepsilon\right),$$

where β is a sample in the sliding window, φ is the uncertainty set and ε is the uncertainty interval. Uncertainty interval specifies all values within [minimum, maximum]. Samples in the sliding window that do not support the mentioned property will be dropped continuously till ∂ becomes a feasible set. In this way, input data are guaranteed in the range of [minimum, maximum].

Subsequently, the proposed pre-processor identifies the input pattern in order to only accept valid patterns. A cosine similarity function based on local derivative pattern is proposed to perform the pattern identification.

In more detail, as Figure 4 shows, a large sliding windows size including *n* (e.g., *n*=4) consecutive small sliding windows are captured. Then, the derivative of mean value (m_n) is computed (r_n) and vector *R* will be created consisting of all derivatives of the mean values. Vector *R* is a valid pattern if the cosine similarity function (Singhal, 2001) is lower than threshold ε

$$\cos\theta = \frac{R.\rho}{R\rho} < \varepsilon$$

where ρ is the expected input pattern.

The second tier of the proposed component performs data reduction techniques. Basically, data reduction discovers the least number of values that the extracted distribution of the data is as close as possible to the original distribution. This techniques has many advantages in systems with central processing unit due to data transmission costs time and energy.

Figure 4. Proposed pattern identifier

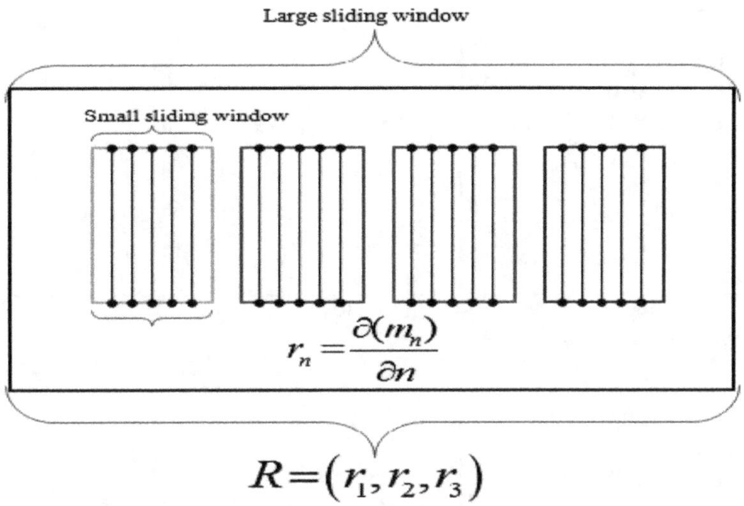

Perceptually Important Points (PIPs) is adopted as the data reduction technique in the proposed component (Chung, 2001). The PIPs is based on the importance of data points in the time series. Basically, with a given time series $T = \{T_1, ..., T_n\}$ with the fix sliding window size w, a set of time series segments can be formed which present the dominant points in the shape of time series. Firstly, all the data points are processed by the PIP identification function. The first two PIPs will be the first and last points of T. The next PIP will be the point in T with the greatest distance to the first two PIPs. The next PIP will be the one with the greatest distance to its two adjacent PIPs, either between the first and second PIPs or between the second and the last PIPs.

4. EXPERIMENTAL RESULTS

In this section, an experimental evaluation of the proposed method is performed.

An iPhone 4S equipped with the STMicro STM33DH 3-axis accelerometer is adopted in the experiments. Data are collected through MATLAB R2015b with frequency of 10Hz. The proposed model is composed of two main phases: data pre-processing and data reduction. The pre-processing handles data problems like noise and pattern identification. Data reduction aims to keep important data affecting the decision making process.

As described, the pre-processor identifies a boundary based on the maximum and lower band of each sliding window. In order to find the mentioned boundaries, an experiment on the dataset with sliding windows of 5 samples is performed. Figure 5 shows the acceleration boundaries of normal and abnormal walks on different acceleration axes. Basically, based on the identified boundaries, a sliding window consisting of samples out of the specified boundaries can be counted as outlier and removed from the sliding window.

After removing the outliers, the input pattern is compared with the valid patterns. Afterwards, the second phase shrinks the data based on the PIPs technique. Figure 6 shows the data in the original format

Figure 5. Boundaries of the input pattern

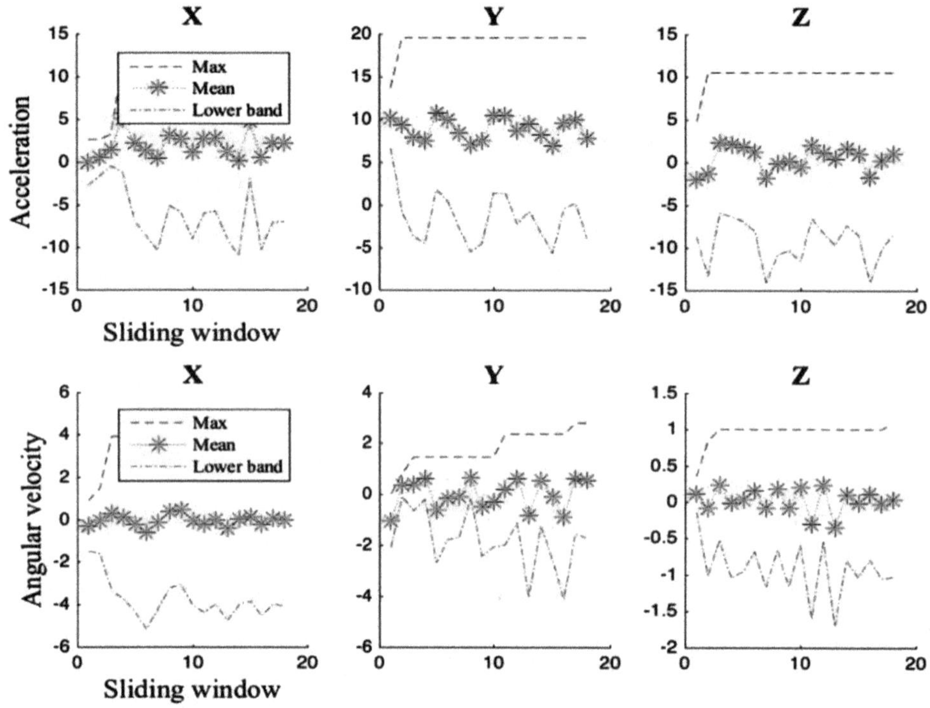

Figure 6. Original and shaped points after PIPs algorithm

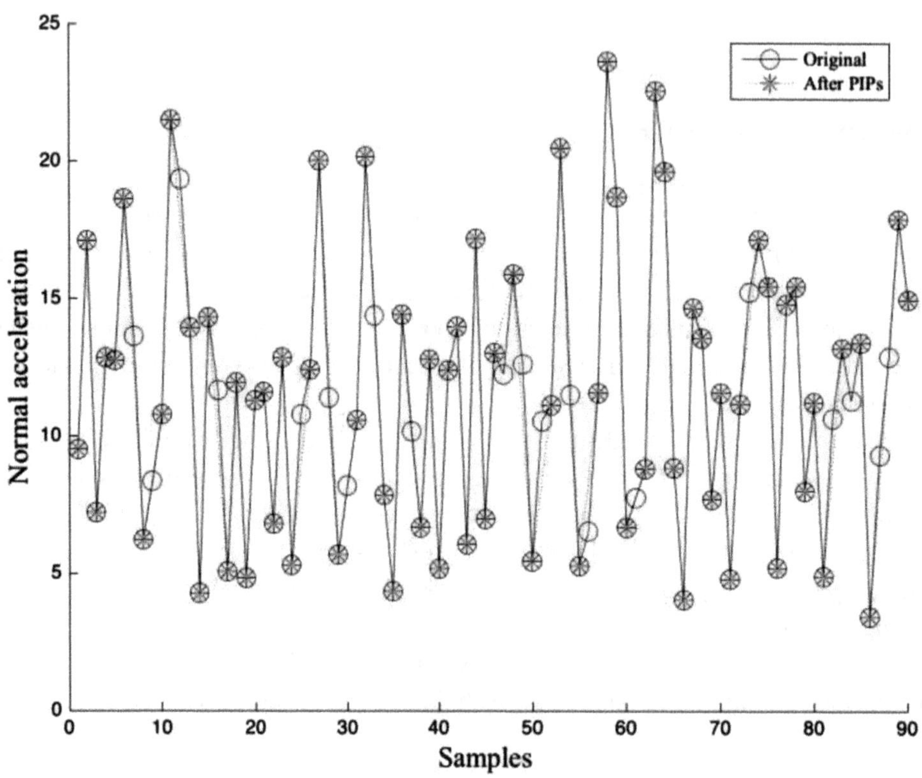

consisting of 90 samples, which are reduced to 70 samples after applying the PIPs algorithm. As can be seen, the circle points are the original points, which are reduced to the asterisk points that generate the overall shape of the input.

Basically, it is important to verify the accuracy of fall prediction algorithm after exploiting the proposed component in the system. To do so, an experiment based on the acceleration features in combination with different classifiers is performed in order to recognize the abnormal walk pattern.

The decision tree is a directed tree with a root node without incoming edges, decision nodes with one incoming edge and possible out coming edge and leaf nodes without out coming edges (Dai, 2014). At the training stage, each internal node specifies a feature of the data which splits the instance space into two or more parts with the goal to optimize the performance of the classifier. Then, every path from the root to a leaf node forms a decision rule to determine which class a new instance belongs to.

A support vector machine is used to classify separable classes of the observations. The SVM finds the best hyper plane with the maximum margin to separate two classes. The SVM can be defined as linear or non-linear according to the hyper plane function used for the classification (Cortes, 1995).

The multi-layer perceptron is a neural network with different layers between input and output. The input data flows through the layers towards the output. Each layer consists of different nodes which processes the input data and directs it towards a proper output (Haykin, 1999).

Random forest is a large collection of decision trees (Friedman, 2001). It consists of an arbitrary number of simple trees, which are used to determine the final outcome. For classification problems, the set of trees vote for the most popular class. The main idea in random forest is to reduce the correlation between the trees, without increasing the variance.

Table 1 shows the result of the experiment. The result shows that after applying the proposed component the system accuracy increases or remains the same in all cases. The increase of accuracy lies in the fact that the clean data can reveal more information, which classifiers exploit explicitly.

The important point in real-time decision making system is the time constraint. Despite the proposed component reduces the data volume without scarifying the accuracy, its computational time must be short. Basically, the heavy operation in the presented component is the PIPs algorithm. In order to experimentally evaluate the time overhead of the PIPs algorithm an experiment was performed on an Intel core i5 2.5 GHz machine. In this experiment, the computational overhead of processing 90 samples in the PIPs algorithm is measured at different intervals. Figure 7 shows the result of the experiment. As can be seen, the computational overhead is tiny and the computation time is uniformly distributed at different time instances.

Table 1. The accuracy before and after applying the component

Classifier	Before	After
Decision Tree	87.05	87.04
SVM	54.50	64.45
Multilayer perceptron	87.45	89.36
Random forest	84.31	87.37

Figure 7. Computational time overhead

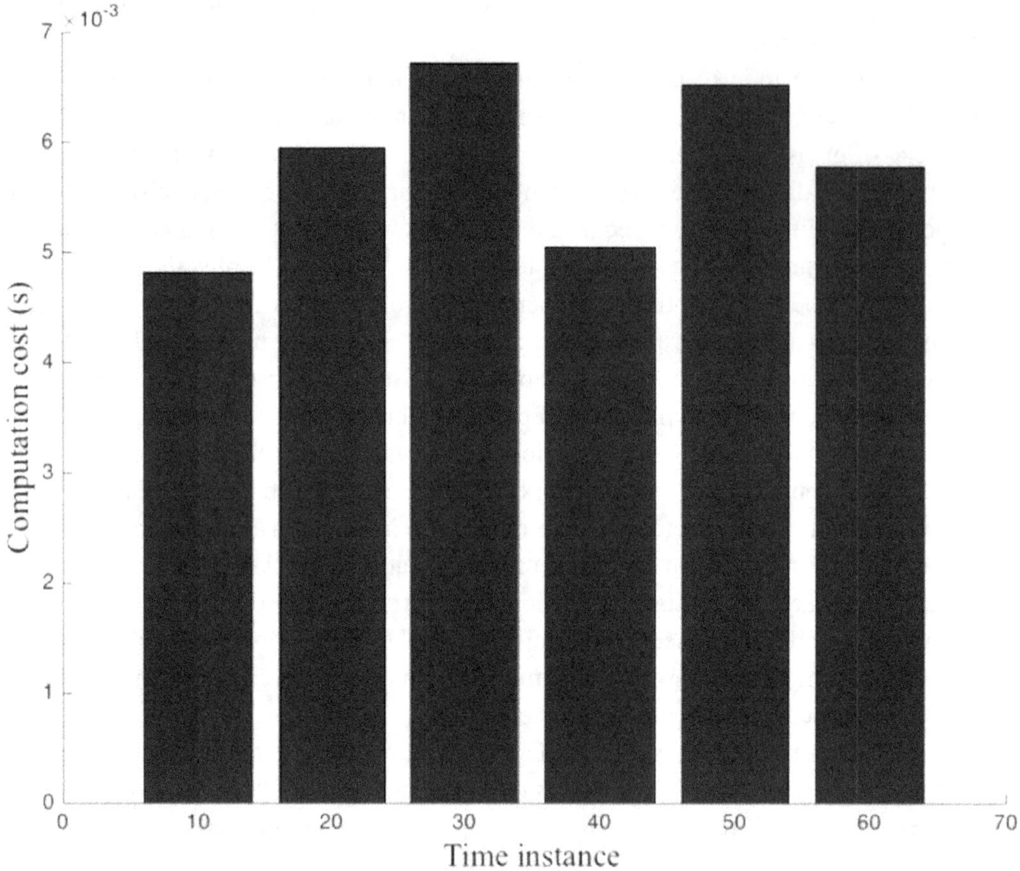

5. CONCLUSION

In this chapter, a schematic view of fall prediction systems with a chronicle component including algorithms for real-time data pre-processing in combination with PIPs reduction algorithm has been proposed. The algorithms are evaluated according to accuracy and efficiency. The result shows that the proposed component can be used with acceleration sensors and different classifiers.

REFERENCES

Abenstein, J. P., & Tompkins, W. J. (1982). A new data-reduction algorithm for real-time ECG analysis. *IEEE Transactions on Bio-Medical Engineering*, *BME-29*(1), 43–48. doi:10.1109/TBME.1982.324962 PMID:7076268

Ambrose, A. F., Paul, G., & Hausdorff, J. M. (2013). Risk factors for falls among older adults: A review of the literature. *Maturitas*, *75*(1), 51–61. doi:10.1016/j.maturitas.2013.02.009 PMID:23523272

Baig, M. M., & Gholamhosseini, H. (2013). Smart health monitoring systems: An overview of design and modeling. *Journal of Medical Systems, 37*(2), 9898. doi:10.1007/s10916-012-9898-z PMID:23321968

Canning, C. G. (2014). *Prevention of falls in Parkinson's disease: A review of fall risk factors and the role of physical interventions*. Future Medicine.

Cortes, C., & Vapnik, V. (1995). Support-vector networks. *Machine Learning, 20*(3), 273–297. doi:10.1007/BF00994018

Dai, W. (2014). A mapreduce implementation of C4. 5 decision tree algorithm. *International Journal of Database Theory and Application*, 49-60. doi:10.1007/978-3-642-02196-1

Di, P. H. (2011). *A novel fall prevention scheme for intelligent cane robot by using a motor driven universal joint. In Micro-NanoMechatronics and Human Science* (pp. 391–396). IEEE.

El-Hasnony, I. M. (2015). Comparative study among data reduction techniques over classification accuracy. *International Journal of Computer Applications*, 8-15.

Friedman, J. (2001). The elements of statistical learning (Vol. 1). New York: Springer.

Grant, T. J. (2014). *Measuring sit-to-stand timing variability over time using under mattress pressure sensor technology. In Medical Measurements and Applications*. IEEE.

Guimaraes, V. R. (2013). *A smartphone-based fall risk assessment tool: Measuring one leg standing, sit to stand and falls efficacy scale. In e-Health Networking, Applications & Services*. IEEE.

Haykin, S. (1999). *Neural Networks: A Comprehensive Foundation*. Pearson education.

Hirata, Y. M. (2006). *Motion control of intelligent passive-type walker for fall-prevention function based on estimation of user state. In Robotics and Automation* (pp. 3498–3503). IEEE.

Horta, E. T. (2013). *Real time falls prevention and detection with biofeedback monitoring solution for mobile environments. In e-Health Networking, Applications & Services*. IEEE.

Lee, W. S. (2001). *Real time data mining-based intrusion detection. In Information Survivability Conference & Exposition* (pp. 89–100). IEEE.

Lopes, J. B.-A. (2010). *Traffic and mobility data collection for real-time applications. Intelligent Transportation Systems* (pp. 216–223). IEEE.

Majumder, A. J. (2013). iPrevention: Towards a novel real-time smartphone-based fall prevention system. *Symposium on Applied Computing* (pp. 513-518). ACM. doi:10.1145/2480362.2480462

Majumder, A. J. (2013). *SmartPrediction: A real-time smartphone-based fall risk prediction and prevention system. In Research in Adaptive and Convergent Systems*. ACM. doi:10.1145/2513228.2513267

McCarney, R. W., Warner, J., Iliffe, S., van Haselen, R., Griffin, M., & Fisher, P. (2007). The Hawthorne Effect: A randomised, controlled trial. *BMC Medical Research Methodology, 7*(1), 30. doi:10.1186/1471-2288-7-30 PMID:17608932

Mubashir, M. S., Shao, L., & Seed, L. (2013). A survey on fall detection: Principles and approaches. *Neurocomputing, 100*, 144–152. doi:10.1016/j.neucom.2011.09.037

Muir, S. W., Berg, K., Chesworth, B., & Speechley, M. (2008). Use of the Berg Balance Scale for predicting multiple falls in community-dwelling elderly people: A prospective study. *Physical Therapy*, *88*(4), 449–459. doi:10.2522/ptj.20070251 PMID:18218822

Nimbalkar, S. P. (2016). Real-Time Data Pre-processing Technique in Web Usage Mining. *International Journal of Innovative Research in Computer*.

Otis, M. J. (2012). *Toward an augmented shoe for preventing falls related to physical conditions of the soil. In Systems, Man, and Cybernetics (SMC)* (pp. 3281–3285). IEEE.

Schwendimann, R. B., Bühler, H., De Geest, S., & Milisen, K. (2006). Falls and consequent injuries in hospitalized patients: Effects of an interdisciplinary falls prevention program. *BMC Health Services Research*, *6*(1), 69. doi:10.1186/1472-6963-6-69 PMID:16759386

Shumway-Cook, A. B. S. (2000). Predicting the probability for falls in community-dwelling older adults using the Timed Up & Go Test. *Physical Therapy*, 896–903. PMID:10960937

Staranowicz, A. B. (2013). Evaluating the accuracy of a mobile Kinect-based gait-monitoring system for fall prediction. In *International Conference on Pervasive Technologies Related to Assistive*. ACM.

ur Rehman, M. H. (2016). Big data reduction methods: a survey. *Data Science and Engineering*, 265-284. doi:10.1145/2504335.2504396

Vellas, B. J., Wayne, S. J., Romero, L., Baumgartner, R. N., Rubenstein, L. Z., & Garry, P. J. (1997). One-leg balance is an important predictor of injurious falls in older persons. *Journal of the American Geriatrics Society*, *45*(6), 735–738. doi:10.1111/j.1532-5415.1997.tb01479.x PMID:9180669

Weiss, A. S., Shimkin, I., Giladi, N., & Hausdorff, J. M. (2010). Automated detection of near falls: Algorithm development and preliminary results. *BMC Research Notes*, *3*(1), 62. doi:10.1186/1756-0500-3-62 PMID:20205708

Zakrzewska, D. M.-L. (2009). *Methods and Supporting Technologies for Data Analysis*. Springer.

KEY TERMS AND DEFINITIONS

Chronicle Component: A component to analyze the data event.
Data Reduction: Process of minimizing the amount of data.
Fall Prediction: A technique to predict a fall occurrence.
Health Care: The organized provision of medical care.
Real-Time: The actual time during a process or event occurs.

Chapter 5
Smart Senior Residences:
How to Improve Services Efficiency and Quality by Exploiting Big Data and Ambient Intelligence

Bruno Bouchard
Université du Québec à Chicoutimi (UQAC), Canada

Kevin Bouchard
Université du Québec à Chicoutimi (UQAC), Canada

Sebastien Gaboury
Université du Québec à Chicoutimi (UQAC), Canada

Abdenour Bouzouane
Université du Québec à Chicoutimi (UQAC), Canada

ABSTRACT

Population aging is the most significant social transformations of our century. In this context, affordable senior housing with supportive services is a key component to the world's long-term care continuum. One of the main issues is how to cost-efficiently provide adapted (and increasingly complex) care services in senior residences to an exponentially growing number of people considering staff shortage. The rise in operating costs (energy, food, etc.) forces companies to find new ways to stay competitive. In that context, this chapter tries to propose avenues of solutions by giving some answers to a simple question: how to optimize the work of the staff to meet the growing demand considering the context of staff shortage. More precisely, this chapter studies methods and strategies to exploit Ambient Intelligence and Big Data to increase the number of residents an employee can support by automating a part of his daily work.

DOI: 10.4018/978-1-5225-5222-2.ch005

Copyright © 2018, IGI Global. Copying or distributing in print or electronic forms without written permission of IGI Global is prohibited.

INTRODUCTION

The world is actually facing the worst demographic crisis of its history (He et al., 2016). Virtually every developed country is now experiencing population aging. It is poised to become one of the most significant social transformations of the twenty-first century, with implications for nearly all sectors of activities, including labor and financial markets, the demand for goods and services, such as housing, transportation and social protection, as well as family structures and intergenerational ties (United Nations, 2015). As an example, in Canada, the median age was 26.2 years old in 1974, according to *Statistics Canada* (2017), but the Canadian population reached the median age of 39.9 years in 2011. This situation can be explained by the decline of the average number of children per woman, the increase in life expectancy and the aging of the baby boomer generation. Ultimately, the number of Canadians aged 65 and over is projected to increase from 5 to 10.4 million between 2011 and 2036. By 2051, almost 25% of the Canadian population is expected to be 65 years of age, as shown in Figure 1 (Statistics Canada 2011). Another important element is seniors' people are living longer. According to a study by the Canadian Institute for Health Information (CIHI, 2011), they also live longer. Indeed, most people under the age of 85 feel that they have no limitations on their functional abilities. As of age 85, the situation is rapidly changing and almost 25% of people aged 85 and over report having average (15%), serious (5%) or total (5%) limitations. Note that functional abilities include both basic activities of everyday life (e.g. walking, washing, eating, etc.), as well as everyday instrumental activities such as shopping or preparing meals. The limitation most often mentioned by people was the inability to do housework without help (14%). For its part, the inability to prepare its meal was mentioned by nearly 5% of the elderly. In terms of cognitive impairment and dementia, in 2011, according to the Alzheimer Society of Canada, 747,000 people had Alzheimer's disease or related illness, or 14.9% of those aged 65 and more. Among those aged 85 and over, this rate is even 33%. By 2031, this figure could reach 1.4 million.

Figure 1. Population by age group in Canada, observed and projected (Statistics Canada 2011)

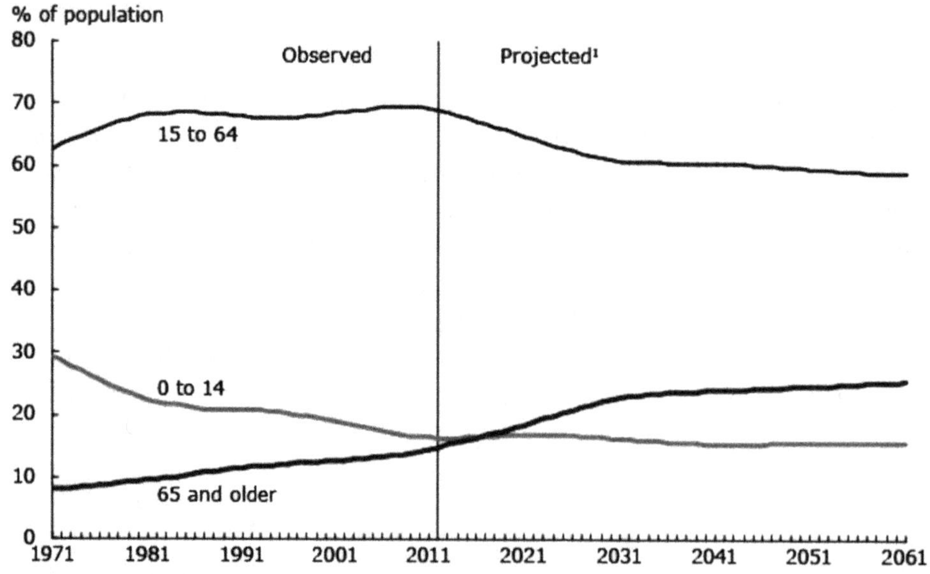

1. The M1 projection scenario combines medium fertility, life expectancy, immigration and internal migration observed from 1981 to 2008.

As a result, the Government of Canada, like others around the world, is deeply concerned since seniors' accommodation and care are a major part of the health budget. To meet this challenge, the number of adapted accommodation and services has increased considerably in the last few years, especially in the private sector, due to the budgetary constraints faced by the public sector. On the other hand, for-profit companies now offer more and more services to accommodate severe cases of impairments. For example, in 2013, according to the Canada Mortgage and Housing Corporation (CMHC) National Seniors' Housing Survey (CMHC, 2013), there were 2,579 private residences in Canada in 2013 with 205,112 residents, an increase of 1.5% compared to 2012. Note that the number of places in residences has also increased from 204,496 in 2012 to 208,301 in 2013, an increase of 1.9%. The majorities of places available in these residences (85.1%) are occupied by residents which pay rent and receives adapted services (help for taking medication, bathing, food service, etc.) each day.

The consequence of that aging problem is that affordable senior housing with supportive services will remain a key component to the world's long-term care continuum. However, many challenges arise for the public sector and the private service providers. One of the main problems is that they are both facing budget problems, leading to the fundamental question: how to cost-efficiently provides adapted (and increasingly complex) care services in senior homes to an exponentially growing number of persons considering the problem of staff shortage (Bouchard B. et al., 2017)? In addition, the rise in operating costs (energy, food, etc.) forces companies to find new ways to remain competitive in the face of competition (Ashrafi et al., 2014). Although, the recent technological advancements in the fields of Artificial Intelligence (AI), Ambient Intelligence (AmI), Sensors, and Big Data, might be considered as a very promising avenue for finding solutions to these issues. From that point of view, two major challenges arise:

1. How to optimize the work of the staff to meet the growing demand considering the context of staff shortage. More precisely, how can we exploit the technology of AmI, AI and Big Data so that an employee can support more residents and so that a part of his work can be done automatically?
2. How to use ubiquitous sensors and actuators to help the staff doing their job more efficiently by giving them key information and a support to their tasks (e.g. prevention of falls, detection of leaks and errors, identification of abnormal behavior, guidance in the completion of activities of everyday life, etc.)?

In the case of the first challenge, time optimization is a key element in managing the employee work plan for productivity improvement (Berry et al., 2004). In that regards, learning the behavior of the working staff is an essential component to be able to observe the most performing scheme and transmit the knowledge to the other employees. In addition, some services (e.g.: wake-up call, reminder and guidance for taking medication, frequency of needs, etc.) could be achieved, at least in part, automatically or semi-automatically to optimize the work schedule. Other issues are also raised. For instance, during an incident or an emergency, the staff must gather at a specific location, leaving several areas and some clients with limited or no supervision. The intervention time in case of another problem is then increased in these situations, in addition of creating an environment enhancing the chance of accidents. On all these points, intelligent services based on ubiquitous sensors could greatly help.

In the case of the second challenge, the main difficulty is mainly to improve the quality of service for the benefit of the users by giving better Business Intelligence (BI) tools, or decision support systems, to the staff and the managers (Groves et al. 2013). For example, falls are one of the main problems in senior residences (AC, 2014), along with fire and water damage. The detection (or even better, the prediction) of falls in real time is a major issue that has been studied extensively in the recent literature (Mubashir et al., 2013). In a service improvement framework, companies want not only to be informed in real time of this type of situations, but also to be able to prevent them (e.g.: to detect in advance the emergence of conditions leading to a fall). Thus, the challenge is to recognize, using sensors, a set of "abnormal" situations (Bouchard B. et al., 2007), such as falls, abnormal displacements, erratic behavior, unusual frequency of going to the bathroom, etc.). Thereafter, when the recognition is completed, the issue is to analyze the data with statistical tools and datamining algorithms (Berry et al., 2004) in order to identify the preconditions leading to this type of situation, with the aims of using these information for prevention. Finally, the challenge also includes the need to present the inferred information (discovered patterns, recognized situations, predictions, etc.) in a comprehensive way to the user (staff member or manager) (Homann et al., 2014).

As one can see, investigating these issues is a very complex task. However, we can summarize and formulate the problem with this question: how can we improve services efficiency and quality while exploiting Big Data and Ambient Intelligence by creating AI and BI tools for the benefit of the staff and the manager of smart residences? This question remains mostly uninvestigated in the literature since most works focus on how technology can directly help the patients, not the people working to care for them (Bouchard B. et al., 2017). In the remainder of this chapter, a walkthrough of each aspect of the problem is written for the savvy reader in order to be able to provide guidelines and cues on where to start, what to do, and how to do it.

WORK ORGANIZATION IN A SENIOR RESIDENCE

Before investigating how technology can help improve the efficiency in a senior residence, the structure of this kind of organization have to be analyzed (Carayon et al., 2006; Wickramasinghe 2009; Carayon 2012; Horwitz-Bennett 2014). In this section, a summary of the working organization of a standard senior residence is produced based on the literature and the authors' knowledge. The objective here is simply to give a functional understanding to the reader for him to be able better understanding the technological issues that are raised later in the chapter. It is very important because it directly influence the specific needs for new technological tools. The schema in Figure 2 summarizes the global organization of a senior residence.

Residents

As the reader can observe on Figure 2, the patients and the healthcare workers are at the center of the organization. They both share the same physical environment, in which they evolve, live and work. Residents perform their Activities of Daily Living (ADL), while being assisted by the caregivers. The persons living in a senior residence are usually semi-autonomous individuals needing different levels of supervision and/or specific care services. Some residences try to have only residents with minor needs, which are mostly able to take care of themselves. In those residences, the services provided are minimal: surveillance, medical emergency, laundry, meals, etc. However, most residences now open their doors to clients with higher needs. For instance, some housing facilities accept residents with cognitive impairment (Alzheimer's disease, head trauma, etc.). Other residences host persons with physical limitations (e.g.: mobility) or other mild to severe health problems. These kinds of clients require advanced care services

Figure 2. Organization of a senior residence (Carayon 2012)

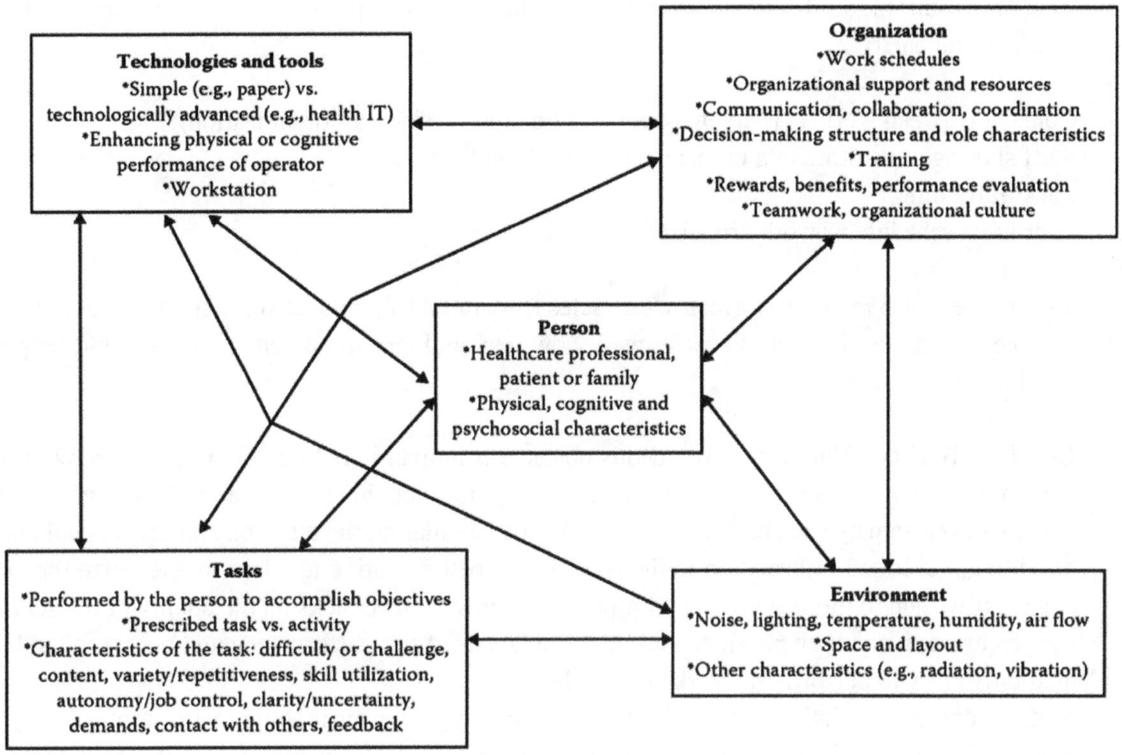

(assistance in taking medication, bathing service, increased surveillance, etc.). It should be noted that a large number of businesses have a very heterogeneous clients' base leading to complex organizational challenges to meet the various needs of all these different types of individuals.

Professionals

Professionals' employees have various tasks to complete in order to provide services to patients. These tasks have specific characteristics: difference in complexity, repetitiveness, skill utilization, autonomy/job control, clarity or uncertainty, feedback, etc. In addition, employees work inside an organizational structure, which gives them work schedules, supervises them, provides technological tools, ensures coordination and decision-making, clarifies their job specification, gives them adequate training, rewards, and performs evaluation. In this chapter, the focus is set on the need for technology of these two groups: the professionals and the managers. As we noted earlier, most of literature in the field of smart technology in healthcare focus on the patients' side of the problem (Bouchard B. et al., 2017), trying to answer the question: how to develop assistive technologies to help improving the patients quality of life inside the residence? However, many works have been done to improve the staff efficiency in other fields, such as management (Wickramasinghe 2009), architecture (Horwitz-Bennett 2014), human factors and ergonomic (Carayon 2012), etc. Therefore, the question here is: what must/can be improved, by the technology, in the course of the work of the staff and the management and, more specifically, how Big Data and Ambient Intelligence can be exploited to do that?

Research has been conducted to identify performance obstacles, specifically among staff in senior residence. The results highlights several works factors that can hinder performance and quality of service by the staff (Carayon 2012):

1. Conflict between workers (personal conflicts / methods of work / organization);
2. Staff shortage (resulting in a unmanageable workload);
3. Lack of training;
4. Poor work schedule or work organization.

These are the fourth major performance obstacles from the staff perspective. In light of these results, it is possible to foresee, for each obstacle cited, how new ambient intelligent services could help alleviating these barriers.

1. **Conflicts Between Workers:** Even if this obstacle is human in nature, it can be soften by development of new intelligent services for the staff. For instance, having a system, based on sensors, able to follow, step by step, each task of a worker by calculating the duration and delays could help providing fact-based information to the staff on the better routine to adopt to maximize the efficiency. If we add to the system a way for patient to provide feedbacks on the quality of the service they received, it can then provide a qualitative analysis of the performance and point out the best qualitative way to perform the work efficiently.
2. **Staff Shortage:** Assistive services can provide a way to perform some tasks automatically or semi-automatically (e.g.: reminding a patient to take his medication, monitoring that he completes some important daily activities, performing surveillance, etc.), using, for instance, sensors, screens, speakers and lights. Reducing the burden on the shoulder of the staff can lead on operating with a reduced staff.
3. **Lack of Training:** Having historical data about the work done by the staff, as mentioned, can be very useful to help creating technological guided training for staff. Having learned the pattern of work used by the best workers, the system could be able to create automatically or semi-automatically a step by step guided training for the new staff so they can learn how do the job like the best. It also allows providing very useful business intelligence tools to the managers about the forces and the weakness of the work of a specific employee in order to provide coaching and help, thus reducing the expensive training costs.
4. **Poor Work Schedule or Work Organization:** The work schedule is a sequence of tasks, including a series of atomic sub-tasks, which an employee must perform in the course of his work during the day. This schedule include many constraints: specific time for giving medications, ordering dependency (before giving a bath, you must unclothe the person), emergency and priorities, etc. With adequate data provided by sensors, it is possible to create a system that will analyze and automatically optimize work schedule. For example, based on its location information (trajectory) in the building, an employee could be suggested to inverse the order of two or more subtasks to reduce unnecessary walks.

RELATED WORK

Researchers from all disciplines have been working over the last few decades over making the shift in healthcare toward the technological era. One aspect of this transition is to build smarter residences in order to reduce hospital admissions and the need for constant healthcare professional supervision. While there has been a plethora of research investigations addressing various, but very specific health issues (e.g.: monitoring of asthma (Adams et al. 2003) or falls detection (Majumder et al. 2013)), the real-world implementation of smart residences has yet to gain traction. Moreover, the current literature on decision support systems and data analytics exploiting these new threads of knowledge, is very scarce. Indeed, most research teams, including our, tend to focus solely on user-centered design, and, therefore, put less emphasis on the management and staff perspective. Unfortunately, it was not possible to find research works leveraging decision support systems using smart environments for the management of senior residence. Therefore, the literature review presented in this chapter revolved around two closely related topics: tools for decision support in healthcare applications and smart homes.

Tools for Decision Support

Using decision support systems for healthcare is not a new idea. They are actually one of the key applications of earlier expert systems in AI. For example, a large body of the literature on this topic concerns computer assisted diagnosis. These systems, including the well-known MYCIN expert system (Shortliffe et al. 1975), were based on knowledge written in formal logic by human experts and a series of simple, yet expressive, IF-THEN rules for reasoning. Although, they usually do so for very specific diagnosis investigations, expert systems are still thriving in some applications, often even improving over the specialists' performances (Boguševičius et al. 2002). Their success has been refrained, however, by the complexity inherent to the construction of their knowledge base and the black box coupling of the inference rules. To name a few of their very wide applications range, they have been used to reduce inappropriate prescribing in primary care (Tamblyn et al. 2003) or to improve the search of missing elderly with dementia (Lin et al. 2006). However, systems in the likes of what this chapter is discussing are still in embryo stage.

On the other hand, the team of Groves (2013) published a report on the emergence and the importance of Big Data as a game changer for the future of healthcare, which strongly support the hypotheses formulated in this chapter. In addition to the classic user centered design of system, they propose new value pathway for Big Data in health care. They say that this revolution can enable: 1) Better choosing strategy for care provider (through analytics) and 2) Better value with payors and providers continuously enhancing services while preserving or maintaining quality. They claim that the main priority to secure the success of such endeavors in the future is to ensure consistent and comprehensive data capture, and reinforcing the culture of information sharing (Bouchard et al. 2016). The team of Chae (2003) is one example of strong leverage of Big Data information in healthcare. They have conducted a study on the quality of healthcare services from large datasets of hospital patients. They exploited a decision tree to classify over inpatient mortality using several characteristics (age, sex, disease classes, etc.). Their team then developed a decision support system to monitor the trends of quality indicator in order to potentially improve quality of care and savings on cost. Another decision support system from Eveborn et al. (2006), which is called Laps Care, is based on optimization techniques and is used to automate the planning of visit schedule. This type of system can help the management of hospitals or other healthcare facilities and is, therefore, a step in the right direction.

Perhaps the closest system to the idea shared by the authors of this paper, is the one from Moatamed et al. (2016). In their paper, they propose a small transportable kit made of a smart watch and few Bluetooth Low Energy (BLE) beacons. With this small set of sensors, they enable patients in a rehab facility to equip their room in the fashion of an *ad hoc* smart home. Statistics on their whereabouts and their postures in the rehabilitation center are then presented to doctors and nurses to help manage their condition. Their results are, however, very preliminary and nothing has been said regarding the use of such system for the management team. A similar system has been proposed by Zhang et al. (2015). It consists of a phone app designed around the patient to help him monitor his health status. It also provides a report the associated physician with necessary data facilitate remote services. However, it has not been designed to support the management staff through comprehensive dashboard and data analytics. Finally, while we have not been able to identify a decision support platform copping with the management of a senior residence, the research of Anderson et al. (2003) support the importance of good management to enhance the care quality in nursing homes. The study suggests nursing home administrators need to be willing to go counter culture for effective self-organization.

Smart Homes

The researches on smart homes cover more ground with respect to supporting elders. The systems are generally focusing on *monitoring* rather than decision support, but their purpose is closer to the topic of this chapter. Monitoring in the field is the act of using sensors, whatever the type, in order to provide some methods to evaluate the state of the residents. Monitoring may involve decision support, and in some way always help professionals who are using such systems. The Table 1 summarizes few of the characteristics of some of the most renowned smart home teams.

The first characteristic describe the *(I) Type of infrastructures* the teams possess. A living lab is a smart home where humans, who are not a lab member, spend long time living into. In comparison, the prototyping infrastructures are one where the goal is to test and develop new techniques and new systems. In addition to their prototyping infrastructure, the LIARA (Bouchard K. et al. 2017) and Gator Tech (Helal et al. 2005) teams also have developed simulators in order to increase the prototyping speed. GOODIES (Augusto et al. 2017) and CASAS (Cook et al. 2013) have transportable version of their smart homes. The second characteristic, *(II) Activity recognition*, describes the type of focus each team has regarding the difficulties related to the recognition of the ongoing activities in the smart home. Teams are usually either focusing on knowledge driven methods or data driven methods with the exception of the LIARA which tackle the problem from both sides. CASAS is a pioneer in using machine learning techniques for this task and they were the first to work on using the models for prediction in addition to recognition. The *(III) Sensors* used by the smart homes teams is extremely important in determining what type of services can be provided and the granularity of activity recognition. It ranges from very simple technologies such as passive infrared motion sensors and electromagnetic contact to much more complex sensors such as smart power analyzer or ultrasonic sensors. This chapter discuss their significance in broad details in the next section entitled "Selecting adapted and useful sensors". Note that both AHRI (Kientz et al. 2008) and IATSL (Mihailidis et al. 2011) lab focus on vision based sensors in their infrastructures.

The themes surrounding research on smart home are diverse. We only surveyed the teams working on smart homes for assistance, but smart homes are also deployed as architectural enhancement and

Table 1. Summary of the properties of each of the most renowned smart homes research teams. [1] (Lapointe et al. 2013) [2] (Jones et al. 2015)

Research teams	(I) Type of insfrastructure	(II) Activity recognition	(III) Sensors	(IV) Main focus	(V) Decision Support Systems	(VI) Quality of services
CASAS	Transportable - Prototyping - Living	Temporal - Prediction - Coarse grained	Small number, mostly PIR and contacts	Aging in place - Data mining		Clinical evaluations of technology
DOMUS	Prototyping - Living	Logical - Ontology	Large number, binary to very complex (heterogeneous)	Cognitive orthosis - Health telematics		Clinical evaluations of technology
LIARA	Prototyping - Simulation	Spatiotemporal - Fine-grained	Large number, binary to very complex (heterogeneous)	Activity recognition - Cognitive assistance		On prompting [1]
GatorTech	Living lab - Simulation	Varied - Coarse grained	Large number, binary to very complex (heterogeneous)	Middleware - Context awareness		
AHRI	Prototyping - Living	Not a primary focus	RFID - Vision based technology	Aging in place - Better home living		
SERG	Prototyping	Knowledge driven	Small number, mostly PIR and contacts	Mobile-based self-managing tools	Self-managing chronic disease - Emerging work	
GOODIES	Transportable - Prototyping	Not a primary focus	Project specific	HCI - Context awareness		On ethic [2]
IATSL	Prototyping	Not a primary focus	Camera and other vision based technology	Aging in place - Dementia	Telerehab - Few related works	Clinical evaluations of technology

better energy management. The *(IV) Main focus* of the IATSL, CASAS and AHRI is on aging in place, while DOMUS (Giroux and Pigot 2013) and LIARA focus on cognitive support. The other teams have a more heterogeneous range of projects. All the teams are involved in *(V) Decision support systems* to some extent, however, this topic is generally not in the priority of the researchers. SERG (Rafferty et al. 2017) and IATSL seem to have done some specific projects regarding that topic. The lack of research projects regarding that topic among the smart home research teams could be explained by the fact that most of the them are mainly composed of engineers/computer scientists which usually prefer focusing on algorithms and more challenging issues or of clinicians who focus on the end users. Still, as we argue in this chapter, decision support systems could be the entry door of assistive technology to be economically viable and to provide useful services. Finally, the last characteristic is the *(VI) Quality of services*. Obviously, most researchers are concerned with the quality of the services their prototypes are providing, but we only put in this category the teams who specifically emphasized on this aspect in some of their projects. For instance, GOODIES have conducted research on the ethics of ambient intelligence for assistance (Jones et al. 2015) and LIARA has evaluated the efficiency of prompts according to the resident cognitive profile (Lapointe et al. 2013). DOMUS, IATSL and CASAS have conducted extensive clinical studies to evaluate the quality of the technology.

The advised reader should keep in mind that the literature review presented in this chapter only offer a glimpse of the vast extend of projects related to healthcare improvement through the use of technology. It aimed to show, however, from what type of research could be inspired a decision support system taking benefits from Big Data and ambient intelligence to improve services efficiency/quality in senior residence.

SELECTING ADAPTED AND USEFUL SENSORS

A key element to enable the use of ambient intelligence to build decision support system to improve services delivery in smart senior residences is to adequately select the sensors to install in the smart environment. The argument of the type of services that can be delivered is, for one, very convincing to make. However, the truth of the impact of the sensors goes beyond these considerations. It might seem very compelling to equip the residence with as many sensors as possible, but this strategy would result in high cost overhead. Therefore, we argue that sensors should be instead minimized in the residence, hence making the case for meticulous choice. Still, it must be kept in mind that the cost used to evaluate the sensors should not be simply the direct cost (i.e.: cost of one sensor), but the overall cost of using the technology versus the gain in knowledge from it. It follows that, for instance, an expensive depth camera could be in fact cheaper than equipping every resident with cheap passive RFID for the task of gesture recognition. There are two other main characteristics that should be taken into account in addition to the overall cost of the technology. The first one, the quality of data, is the direct consequence of the reasoning we just made. The goal is to install sensors that will, *reliably*, provides us with rich data to perform as many tasks as possible. The last criterion, a bit more controversial and even more subjective, is the acceptability toward the employees and the residents. Despite the importance of this issue, there are very few studies regarding the acceptability of the sensors (Demeris et al. 2008). The empirical evidence seems to suggest the sensors might be perceived as invasive if they are visible, especially if they look like camera (Mäkela et al. 2007). The LIARA team is working on a project to provide further cues on sensors acceptability in the future, but we invite other researchers to further investigate this topic. The authors of this chapter are less inclined to use vision-based technology for these concerns, but the team think there is no single technology that stand out. Consequently, it results that no consensus exist among the scientists. Therefore, we advise the readers to carefully consider the advantages and the inconvenients of each type of sensors and make their own informed decision.

Sensors Options: As we discussed before, there has been a large range of sensors exploited in smart homes in the literature. While the point of this chapter is not to provide a thorough description of each of them, it seems necessary to introduce the main types before proceeding with the remainder of this section. The most commonly used sensors are the Passive InfraRed motion sensors (PIR) and electromagnetic contact. PIR work simply by detecting heat in the form infrared radiation. The heat is focused on a sensor using Fresnel lens that enables to cover a wide range (or a specific shape) with the PIR. It simply says if there is a motion detected in the area covered or not. Electromagnetic contact is a binary sensor made of two pieces. One of the piece is a magnet that closes the sensor circuit when it is near the second piece (the door, window or cabinet is closed). Other well-known sensors are temperature, light and humidity sensors, all of which, a pretty much self-explanatory. Tactile mat or tactile floor are also sometime used. The later less frequently because the installation require major house renovation and the cost is prohibitive. Nevertheless, these sensors provide a binary information (something on it or not) with varying granularity (depending on the size and number of tiles). Similarly to PIR, they can often be triggered by pets. Next, there is the wide range of radio technology that can act as sensors and which include, but not exhaustively, Bluetooth beacons, NFC/RFID and WiFi. While they possess different properties, they all are based on emitted radio waves which propagate through space, using a well-defined channel, in order to carry an information. Their specifications enable more or less information to be carried, at different power levels (thus consuming different amount of energy) within a certain distance. NFC and RFID can work in passive mode, the chip not possessing any internal power and harvesting the latent energy of the radio wave. WiFi and Bluetooth have the advantage of being widely used by resident (through their internet capabilities or their smart phone). Finally, wearable sensors are also related and wide-spread in smart home research. The Inertial Measurement Unit (IMU), which include an accelerometer, a gyroscope and sometime a magnetometer, is the most commonly exploited. To abstract the details, the IMU is simply made of sensors able to calculate a force over a body, such as the acceleration for example. The Table 2 summarizes the strengths, the weaknesses and the usage of many of these sensors.

Useful Services

The sensors can be used for a multitude of services. The first one, that we name ambient information, can enable to have a quick idea of the state of the residence and ensure its comfort and minimal security (Ricquebourg et al. 2006). Sensors such as temperature and light sensors, can provide information on the general state, but are less important than flow sensors which can help detect and prevent water damage. Similarly, equipping the residence with smart smoke detector can provide prompt information on a dashboard for any person monitoring the residence. The second service is context awareness (Alam et al. 2012). Context awareness is a general service that enable systems to adapt their behavior depending on the current state of the smart environment. In consequence, it usually relies on time and space to work. Many sensors can contribute to context awareness, but BLE beacons are specifically designed for that propose. The third service is the tracking. Research on tracking are very extensive and we could not even hope to begin summarizing them properly in this small section. Tracking generally means *online* localization of

Table 2. Summary of sensors strengths and use.

Sensing Tech.	Strengths	Weaknesses	Used for
RFID	• High granularity information • Cheap and small passive tags • Tags are robust	• Expensive system • Complex to use	• Resident tracking • Small and big objects tracking • Gestures, gait analysis
BLE beacons	• High longevity of the battery • Long range • Very easy to use	• Inaccurate • Require a wearable (watch, phone, etc.) • Performance depends on installation quality	• Resident tracking • Context aware services • Gait analysis
PIR	• Cheap and well-established • Their effect area is well-defined	• Animals can trigger them • Timing of the triggering is important	• Resident tracking • Gait analysis
WiFi	Most residence/building are already equipped with the tech.	• Require learning for every new configuration • Require a wearable (watch, phone, etc.) • High battery consumption	Resident tracking
Depth camera	• Rich information • Wide range of prices	• Installation is complex • More adapted to specific solution than general one	• Resident tracking • Objects tracking • Gestures
IMU	• Embedded in most wearable (watches, phone, etc.) • Tons on literature on their use	• Limited applications • Require a wearable	• Resident Tracking • Gesture • Gait analysis

the resident (Au et al. 2013). WiFi, BLE beacons, RFID, PIR are all technologies used for that purpose. The current most popular technique is to learn a radio map with current WiFi infrastructure and to use that same map to pinpoint the precise location of the user. In that case, a wearable is used and often an IMU can help improve the tracking. Tracking can also mean online *objects* localization (Fortin-Simard et al. 2015). In that case, the tracking follow one to several daily life objects that can be used for several activities of daily living or for telehealth. Only passive RFID and camera can be used for that purpose. For camera, the precision is higher, but the range is generally limited and the configuration carefully fixed. For RFID, the precision and accuracy is lower, although adjustable, but the tracking can be done for several objects in a larger area. However, objects tracking in a large residence can potentially require a large number of antennas and readers, hence being a costly enterprise. The fourth service is a direct consequence of tracking. In smart homes, especially for telehealth of human computer interaction, it can be useful to perform gesture recognition. It is generally done with vision based technology (Patsadu et al. 2012), but can also work with passive RFID. Finally, the last service, but nonetheless, is gait analysis. Gait analysis is a method to assess the way a person walks and to highlight bio mechanicals abnormalities (Seel et al. 2014). IMU is often used for that task, but to compute the walking speed active infrared, Ultrasonic sensors, RFID and even BLE beacons can be exploited.

EFFICIENT MONITORING IN THE SENIOR RESIDENCE

Being able to monitor the activities of the staff and the residents is key step toward improving service efficiency and quality while exploiting Big Data (Bouchard B. et al. 2017). Evidently, intelligent algorithms and services can do nothing to help the staff if they do not have any data as input to process. However, there is so much things that can be monitored (bathroom utilization, medication taking, staff movements, etc.) and so many ways to do it (e.g.: we can monitor bathroom utilization by compiling the number of time a person use it per day, or we can monitor how much time he/she spends each time, of which path she/he uses to go there). Therefore, the question is: what should we monitor in priority to improve the efficiency and how should we do it?

The Staff

The first persons who should be monitored in a smart residence is the staff. Why? Because they do most of the work and it is precisely that work that need to be optimized (Carayon et al., 2006). More specifically, the task is to monitor the caregivers' work with the residents, because it is where the work can be optimized (for instance, a care can take more or less time) and it is where the quality of service can be improved. In a standard senior residence, each caregiver has a work schedule for the day, which take approximatively the form of the one shown in Table 3. The schedule gives information about the time required to achieve each task, about the resident, a description of the task itself, and the resources needed to be prepared before the task. In addition, after completing a task, the employee has to mark it in the form of yes/no or to check a box. She/he also has to sign the sheet to acknowledge the completion of the work.

The work schedule (or work plan) is the key component that one should want to monitor. To do that, we need to be able to:

Table 3. A simplified example of work schedule

Friday 12, Work Schedule						
Time	**Resident**	**Room**	**Task**	**Ressources**	**Completed**	**Comment**
08:00	John Smith	A3001	Give a bath	Soap, towels, ...	Y	
08:20	Jenna Marbles	B2024	Giving medication (see med profile)	Med profile, medication	Y	
09:00	Erik Jones	A2030	Laundry service	Laundry carrier	N	No laundry
09:15	Marty McFly	A3030	Give a bath	Soap, towels, ...		
...						

1. Keep track of the caregiver position and movements
2. Know when a task begin and end (therefore knowing how much time it took to give the care)
3. Receive a computable feedback from residents on the quality of the work

Time is the key to optimize work. Time is money. Taking more time to give a care result in a more expensive business and to a reduced capacity to serve an increased number of residents. However, taking less time (saving money) but giving poor cares is unacceptable. Therefore, we need to collect data about the time and the quality of service, and process the data to give avenues of optimization. For instance, if ten caregivers give services to residents, monitoring them can result in finding that two of them are quicker at giving a certain care more efficiently. One can then ask them for the method they are using to do it, and after that teach the other ones. It can also be useful for training new employees to the best practices. Finally, monitoring the position of the caregiver can be very insightful. Time is often wasted by using suboptimal paths for displacements. For instance, one caregiver might go to a room, realize that he need a resource like a soap, which is really far away from that room, resulting in a lot of inefficient displacements.

Now, how can we monitor these key elements? First, we need to keep track of the task beginning and end to monitor the performance of the staff. To do that, a simple tablet (e.g. Ipad or Androïd) can be used to show the work schedule instead of a paper. The electronic version of work schedule should be linked to an employee account, so we can keep track of the performance over the time for each one. When the employee finished a task, he could simply check a box on the tablet screen with his finger. In the same way, the resident should have access to the account on some kind of web intranet. This way, he could be able to fill his profile (for instance food restrictions, activities preferences, etc.) and to provide feedbacks on the care he received. The feedbacks' form could include a text commentary section, but it must has a quantitative type of notation (e.g. 1 to 5 stars). This way, these data would be computable so the system would be able to provide charts, graph and other form of visual tools to monitor the performance of the staff in terms of execution quality and speed. Finally, the position of the staff should be monitored. The more precise is the tracking, more useful is the data. We can simply monitor the room where the employee is at each moment or we can precisely track is movements. The best way could be to provide a tablet to each employee to carry the work schedule and others new BI tools and to attach some form of tracking device on the tablet (e.g. RFID or BLE beacons). We can also track the tablet position using its WiFi connection.

Residents

Concerning the residents, the key element is monitoring their positions and their biometric signs: blood pressure, heart rate, skin temperature, etc. In addition, having them wearing an accelerometer is very useful for the specific use of detecting and preventing falls. Ideally, having each resident wearing a smart wrist can do the trick. A well-chosen wrist could monitor the biometric signs we need and to send the data to an ambient intelligent system that will link them to the patient's profile. The position can be monitored by using that wrist by using WiFi positioning or by adding a small sensor (e.g.: BLE beacons) to the wrist. Having the position of each resident would be very useful because it would allow the system to automatically take care of monitoring the restricted areas and to avoid patient leaving the site without proper authorizations. The data concerning the biometric signs could be use by the system to monitor decline in the health of patients, to prevent incident by anticipating problems (e.g. observing unusual changes in the signs). Visual tools should be developed so the caregiver could get on his tablet a resume of the patient's health monitoring using these data.

PRAGMATIC DATA PROCESSING AND VISUALIZATION

Knowing what to observe and how to deploy adequate sensors in the work environment to monitor it is not sufficient. In order to have a useful system able to help improving the work efficiency, one needs to process the gathered data with algorithmic tools provided by the field of artificial intelligence (Russell & Norvig 2009), and to present it properly to the staff and people in charge. There are four main processing services needed. We will now describe them and suggest an appropriate algorithmic approach that could be used to develop such services. The reader can also consult Table 4 for a visual summary.

- **Real-Time Monitoring of the Ongoing Tasks (Staff), Health (Resident), Activities and Abnormalities**: Real-time monitoring (Al-Shaqi et al. 2016) is essential if one want to have a system that will be useful on a day-to-day basis. For instance, monitoring the ongoing tasks while the staff perform them could be very useful. A manager could, as an example, knows in real-time the progression of the job, be immediately aware of any delay or problem, and act accordingly

Table 4. Types of needed services vs suggested algorithmic approaches

Type of service	Targeted user	Examples of application	Algorithmic model
Real-time monitoring	Staff	Monitoring biometric signs (resident), monitoring task achievement (staff), detecting abnormal situation, etc.	Symbolic (logical) approach, markov model
Machine learning	Managers, Staff	Statistics (tasks everage time), best paths, employee profile, behavior change, patterns, performance evaluation and comparison	Time series analysis, Datamining models, Behavior Change Detection (BCD)
Optimization	Managers, Staff	Optimizing work schedules, automated task repartition, etc.	Metaheuristics (ex. genetic algorithms)
Decision support	Managers	Dash boards, performance metrics, etc.	Efficient visual representation

(e.g. adding a caregiver in the afternoon to compensate). The real-time monitoring challenge corresponds to the so-called plans/activities recognition problem that has been well studied in the field of artificial intelligence (Carberry 2001). This problem can be summarized as the process of interpreting low-level actions (which are detected by sensors placed in environment) and to match it with the corresponding high-level task (included in some kind of tasks library). More precisely, it need four processing steps (Roy et al. 2013): (1) gathering sensor inputs, (2) interpreting and merging sensor data to get useful information, (3) identifying basic actions performed, and (4) interpreting high-level behavior. In the literature, there are mainly two type of algorithmic approaches used to solve this problem (Bouchard B. et al. 2007). The first type is logical approaches consisting of using, for instance, first-order logic (Smullyan 1995), in order to formalize the recognition of activities by an inference process. In order to take into account uncertainty in activity recognition, the second type make use of approaches based on probabilistic models, such as Markov model (Rabiner 1990). For a fine-grained overview of that challenge and a complete literature review, the reader should consult (Roy et al 2013).

- **Learning the Best Practice, Best Routes, Profiles, Performance, Patterns, etc:** Deploying a network of sensors in the working environment will necessarily results in having a large quantity of historical data. This unstructured pile of data is not so much useful without proper processing. It is why it requires applying machine-learning techniques (Witten et al. 2011) on it to learn and extract useful and often subtle information, which is often hidden to the naked eyes. As an example, suppose that you have the historical data concerning the performance (e.g. the time spent for each task on the work schedule) of each employee for three month. It is a huge amount of data and it is very difficult to look at it clearly. Of course, one could synthetize the data by creating graph representing, for instance, fluctuation in the performance of the staff. However, it is not enough to identify unobvious patterns that can help optimizing the work. For instance, applying a datamining algorithm on the data pile could lead to identify a certain pattern; such each time an employee do the task A after the task B, then the task B take longer than usual to perform. Knowing that information allows investigating the cause of that delay, which can simply be that the task A require moving a long distance from the required resource needed for task B, which cause the extra time. With that knowledge, manager can better organize work schedules to optimize the order of the tasks to avoid that, or to change the working practice (e.g. asking workers to bring the needed material for task B before doing task A). In the literature (Cook, Feuz et al. 2013), most of the works exploit datamining techniques by making use of the concept of time series analysis (Aminikhanghahi et al. 2017). Time series analysis can be used for clustering, classification, query by content, anomaly detection as well as forecasting. Recently, Dr. Diane Cook of Washington State University (WSU) proposed to use a model called Behavior Change Detection (BCD) (Sprint et al. 2016) in order to track changes in routine behavior. Her team quantitatively compare two or more time periods, or windows, of activity labeled data. If the two time windows contain significantly different activity information then this may indicate a significant behavior change. That kind of inferred information could be very useful in the context of work optimization.
- **Optimization of the Work:** Once we learned the patterns and identified problematic situations, we want to optimize the work schedule and the working practice accordingly. For optimizing the practice, no algorithmic approach can really help. One must relies on the staff and the management by using standard techniques of continuous improvements, such as the practices of Kaizen in Lean Management (Byrne & Womack 2012). However, concerning the optimization of, for

instance, the work schedule, one can certainty take profit of an algorithmic approach based on Metaheuristics (Yang 2010). There are several variables to take into account while creating a work schedule: the distance between rooms and resources (you want to minimize the walking distance to save time), employees' performance (certain employee are better and faster at performing specific task), employees qualifications (some employees could be accredited to performs certain tasks, such as giving medication), etc. There variables should be taken into account in creating the work schedules in order to optimize them. The algorithm could provide the manager with several optimized propositions of work schedules. Thereafter, the manager could simply use one of the proposition directly or edit one of them to adjust it to his needs. To develop such a tools, one could use an approach based on a Genetic Algorithm (GA), which is commonly used to generate high-quality solutions to optimization and search problems by relying on bio-inspired operators such as mutation, crossover and selection (Mitchell 1996).

- **Decision Support Tools for Business Intelligence (BI):** Decision support tools is the final essential ingredient needed to help the managers and the staff using all the processed data. One of the best BI tool is the dashboard (Few 2006). A dashboard consists in a single screen that give the user a synthetic view of the information that matters most. It can transform raw data into critical information that jumps out to your users, who can better understand and act on it in a fraction of the time it would otherwise take them. Dashboard design can mean the difference in taking important decisions. It allows presenting the learned data in a simple yet efficient way.

CONCLUSION

Nowadays, it is well known that senior housing with supportive services is a key component to the world's long-term care continuum (CIHI, 2011). As we discussed throughout this chapter, one of the main challenge is how to cost-efficiently provides such adapted care services in senior residences to an exponentially growing number of individuals. With the rise in operating costs and staff shortage, companies have to find new innovative solutions to meet the growing demands and to stay competitive (Ashrafi et al., 2014). Cleary, exploiting new technologies could be viewed as a potential solution.

In this chapter, we presented such avenues of solution based on technology, which take advantage on the new development on the field of the ambient intelligence and Big Data. The main idea of the chapter is to argue that we need much more research focused on developing decision support tools (in the fashion of Business Intelligence) to help the staff and the management in senior residences. These tools need to make a better uses of the multiple and useful data that can be provided by well-chosen ubiquitous sensors. In the literature (Demeris et al. 2008;Mihailidis et al. 2011; Oderandi 2012; Suresh et al. 2015; Bouchard B. et al. 2017), most of the work is concentrated on developing systems aiming to help the patient live a better life. The objective is very noble, but it does not solve the challenge that the companies are facing.

As a contribution, this chapter aimed to provide a set of guidelines for interdisciplinary researchers and practitioners of the field. First, it presented a synthetic view of the operation of a residence while highlighting the main elements representing an opportunity for technological optimization. Secondly, a comprehensive review of the literature of the field was presented. As the reader was able to assess, very few works are actually addressing the important issues raised in this chapter. Thereafter, the kinds of tasks which should be optimized using the ambient intelligence and ubiquitous sensors were described. That description took the form of a set of guidelines that aim to provide a clear path for futures researches. The chapter also provided a complete description of what kind of sensors could/should be used, which algorithmic approaches can be exploited, and what kind of visual tools could be developed. As a whole, this chapter constitutes a base of reference putting together all the foundations needed to address the problem: how can we improve service efficiency and quality while exploiting Big Data and ambient intelligence by creating AI and decision support tools for the benefit of the staff and the manager of smart residences?

REFERENCES

Adams, W. G., Fuhlbrigge, A. L., Miller, C. W., Panek, C. G., Gi, Y., & Loane, K. C. et al.. & Friedman, R. H. (2003). TLC-Asthma: an integrated information system for patient-centered monitoring, case management, and point-of-care decision support. In *AMIA Annual Symposium Proceedings* (Vol. 2003, p. 1). American Medical Informatics Association.

Al-Shaqi, R., Mourshed, M., & Rezgui, Y. (2016, May). Progress in ambient assisted systems for independent living by the elderly. *SpringerPlus*, *5*(1), 624. doi:10.1186/s40064-016-2272-8 PMID:27330890

Alam, M. R., Reaz, M. B. I., & Ali, M. A. M. (2012). A review of smart homes—Past, present, and future. *IEEE Transactions on Systems, Man and Cybernetics. Part C, Applications and Reviews*, *42*(6), 1190–1203. doi:10.1109/TSMCC.2012.2189204

Aminikhanghahi, S., & Cook, D. (2017). A survey of methods for time series change point detection. *Knowledge and Information Systems*, *51*(2), 339–367. doi:10.1007/s10115-016-0987-z PMID:28603327

Anderson, R. A., Issel, L. M., & McDaniel, R. R. Jr. (2003). Nursing homes as complex adaptive systems: Relationship between management practice and resident outcomes. *Nursing Research*, *52*(1), 12–21. doi:10.1097/00006199-200301000-00003 PMID:12552171

Ashrafi, N., Kelleher, L., & Kuilboer, J.-P. (2014). The impact of business intelligence on healthcare delivery in the USA. *Interdisciplinary Journal of Information, Knowledge, and Management*, *9*, 117–130.

Au, A. W. S., Feng, C., Valaee, S., Reyes, S., Sorour, S., Markowitz, S. N., & Eizenman, M. et al. (2013). Indoor tracking and navigation using received signal strength and compressive sensing on a mobile device. *IEEE Transactions on Mobile Computing*, *12*(10), 2050–2062. doi:10.1109/TMC.2012.175

Augusto, J., Kramer, D., Alegre, U., Covaci, A., & Santokhee, A. (2017). The user-centred intelligent environments development process as a guide to co-create smart technology for people with special needs. *Universal Access in the Information Society*, 1–16.

Berry, J. A., & Linoff, G. (2004). *Data Mining Techniques: For Marketing, Sales, and Customer Relationship Management*. Wiley.

Boguševičius, A., Maleckas, A., Pundzius, J., & Skaudickas, D. (2002). Prospective randomised trial of computer-aided diagnosis and contrast radiography in acute small bowel obstruction. *European Journal of Surgery*, *168*(2), 78–83. doi:10.1080/11024150252884287 PMID:12113275

Bouchard, B. (2017). *Smart Technologies in Healthcare*. CRC Press, Taylor & Francis. doi:10.1201/9781315145686

Bouchard, B., Bouzouane, A., & Giroux, S. (2007, July). A Keyhole Plan Recognition Model for Alzheimers Patients. *Journal of Applied Artificial Intelligence, Taylor & Francis*, *22*(7), 623–658. doi:10.1080/08839510701492579

Bouchard, K., Bouchard, B., & Bouzouane, A. (2017). *Practical Guidelines to Build Smart Homes: Lessons Learned, Opportunistic Networking: Vehicular, D2D and Cognitive Radio Networks*. CRC Press, Taylor & Francis.

Bouchard, K., Gaboury, S., Bouchard, B., Bouzouane, A., & Giroux, S. (2016). Smart Homes in the Era of Big Data. In *Trends in Ambient Intelligent Systems* (pp. 117–137). Springer. doi:10.1007/978-3-319-30184-6_5

Byrne, A., & Womack, J. P. (2012). *The Lean Turnaround: How Business Leaders Use Lean Principles to Create Value and Transform Their Company*. McGraw-Hill.

Canadian Institute for Health Information (CIHI). (2011). *Les soins de santé au Canada 2011: Regard sur les personnes âgées et le vieillissement*. Author.

Canadian Mortage and Housing Coporation (CMHC). (2013). *Report, National Seniors' Housing Survey*. Author.

Carayon, P. (Ed.). (2012). *Handbook of Human Factors and Ergonomics in Health Care and Patient Safety*. CRC Press, Taylor & Francis.

Carayon, P., Schoofs, A. H., Karsh, B.-T., Gurses, A. P., Alvarado, C. J., & Smith, M. (2006). Flatley, Work system design for patient safety: The SEIPS model. *Quality & Safety in Health Care*, *15*(suppl_1), 50–58. doi:10.1136/qshc.2005.015842

Carberry, S. (2001). *Techniques for Plan Recognition, User Modeling and User Adapted-Interaction*. Academic Press.

Chae, Y. M., Kim, H. S., Tark, K. C., Park, H. J., & Ho, S. H. (2003). Analysis of healthcare quality indicator using data mining and decision support system. *Expert Systems with Applications*, *24*(2), 167–172. doi:10.1016/S0957-4174(02)00139-2

Cook, D., Crandall, A. S., Thomas, B. L., & Krishnan, N. C. (2013). CASAS: A smart home in a box. *Computer*, *46*(7), 62–69. doi:10.1109/MC.2012.328 PMID:24415794

Cook, D., Feuz, F., & Krishnan, N. (2013). Transfer learning for activity recognition: A survey. *Knowledge and Information Systems*, *36*(3), 537–556. doi:10.1007/s10115-013-0665-3 PMID:24039326

Demiris, G., Hensel, B. K., Skubic, M., & Rantz, M. (2008). Senior residents perceived need of and preferences for smart home sensor technologies. *International Journal of Technology Assessment in Health Care*, *24*(1), 120–124. doi:10.1017/S0266462307080154 PMID:18218177

Eveborn, P., Flisberg, P., & Rönnqvist, M. (2006). Laps Care—an operational system for staff planning of home care. *European Journal of Operational Research*, *171*(3), 962–976. doi:10.1016/j.ejor.2005.01.011

Few, S. (2006). *Information Dashboard Design: The Effective Visual Communication of Data*. O'Reilly.

Fortin-Simard, D., Bilodeau, J. S., Bouchard, K., Gaboury, S., Bouchard, B., & Bouzouane, A. (2015). Exploiting passive RFID technology for activity recognition in smart homes. *IEEE Intelligent Systems*, *30*(4), 7–15. doi:10.1109/MIS.2015.18

Giroux, S., & Pigot, H. (2013). Smart homes for people suffering from cognitive disorders. *Computer Science and Ambient Intelligence*, 225-262.

Groves, P., Kayyali, B., Knott, D., & Van Kuiken, S. (2013). The 'big data' revolution in healthcare. *The McKinsey Quarterly*, *2*, 3.

He, W., Goodkind, D., & Kowal, P. (2016). *An Aging World: International Population Report*. National Institute on Aging (NIA).

Helal, S., Mann, W., El-Zabadani, H., King, J., Kaddoura, Y., & Jansen, E. (2005). The gator tech smart house: A programmable pervasive space. *Computer*, *38*(3), 50–60. doi:10.1109/MC.2005.107

Homann, M., Banova, V., Oelbermann, P., Wittges, H., & Krcmar, H. (2014). Towards User Interface Components for Dashboard Applications on Smartphones. In G. Memmi & U. Blanke (Eds.), *Mobile Computing, Applications, and Services. MobiCASE 2013. Lecture Notes of the Institute for Computer Sciences, Social Informatics and Telecommunications Engineering* (Vol. 130, pp. 19–32). Springer. doi:10.1007/978-3-319-05452-0_2

Horwitz-Bennett, B. (2014). *Staff Support: Designing Optimal Healthcare Work Environments*. Healthcare Design Magazine.

Jones, S., Hara, S., & Augusto, J. C. (2015). eFRIEND: An ethical framework for intelligent environments development. *Ethics and Information Technology*, *17*(1), 11–25. doi:10.1007/s10676-014-9358-1

Kientz, J. A., Patel, S. N., Jones, B., Price, E. D., Mynatt, E. D., & Abowd, G. D. (2008). The georgia tech aware home. In *CHI'08 extended abstracts on Human factors in computing systems* (pp. 3675–3680). ACM.

Lapointe, J., Verreault, A., Bouchard, B., Bouchard, J., Potvin, A., & Bouzouane, A. (2013). How to maximize the effectiveness of prompts in assistive technologies according to the particular cognitive profile of people with alzheimer. *International Journal of Smart Home*, *7*(5), 19–38. doi:10.14257/ijsh.2013.7.5.03

Lin, C. C., Chiu, M. J., Hsiao, C. C., Lee, R. G., & Tsai, Y. S. (2006). Wireless health care service system for elderly with dementia. *IEEE Transactions on Information Technology in Biomedicine*, *10*(4), 696–704. doi:10.1109/TITB.2006.874196 PMID:17044403

Majumder, A. J. A., Rahman, F., Zerin, I., Ebel, W. Jr, & Ahamed, S. I. (2013, March). iPrevention: Towards a novel real-time smartphone-based fall prevention system. In *Proceedings of the 28th Annual ACM Symposium on Applied Computing* (pp. 513-518). ACM. doi:10.1145/2480362.2480462

Mäkelä, K., Belt, S., Greenblatt, D., & Häkkilä, J. (2007). Mobile interaction with visual and RFID tags: a field study on user perceptions. In *Proceedings of the SIGCHI conference on Human factors in computing systems* (pp. 991-994). ACM. doi:10.1145/1240624.1240774

Mihailidis, A., Boger, J., & Kautz, H. (2011). *Technology and Aging, Assistive Technology Research Series* (Vol. 21). IOS Press.

Mitchell, M. (1996). *An Introduction to Genetic Algorithms*. Cambridge, MA: MIT Press.

Moatamed, B., Shahmohammadi, F., Ramezani, R., Naeim, A., & Sarrafzadeh, M. (2016). Low-cost indoor health monitoring system. In *Wearable and Implantable Body Sensor Networks (BSN), 2016 IEEE 13th International Conference on* (pp. 159-164). IEEE.

Mubashir, M., Shao, L., & Seed, L. (2013, January). A survey on fall detection: Principles and approaches. *Elsevier Neurocomputing*, *100*(16), 144–152. doi:10.1016/j.neucom.2011.09.037

Oderanti, F. O. (2012). *Commercialisation of Assisted Living Technologies and Services: A Framework for Sustainable Business Models*. Cardiff, UK: BAM.

Patsadu, O., Nukoolkit, C., & Watanapa, B. (2012). Human gesture recognition using Kinect camera. *International Joint Conference on Computer Science and Software Engineering (JCSSE)* (pp. 28-32). IEEE.

Rabiner, L. (1990). A Tutorial on Hidden Markov Models and Selected Applications in Speech Recognition. *Proceeding of the IEEE, 77*(2).

Rafferty, J., Nugent, C. D., Liu, J., & Chen, L. (2017). From activity recognition to intention recognition for assisted living within smart homes. *IEEE Transactions on Human-Machine Systems*, *47*(3), 368–379. doi:10.1109/THMS.2016.2641388

Ramos, C. (2008). Ambient Intelligence: The Next Step for AI. *IEEE Intelligent Systems*, *23*(2), 15–18. doi:10.1109/MIS.2008.19

Ricquebourg, V., Menga, D., Durand, D., Marhic, B., Delahoche, L., & Loge, C. (2006). The smart home concept: our immediate future. In *1st IEEE International Conference on E-Learning in Industrial Electronics* (pp. 23-28). IEEE. doi:10.1109/ICELIE.2006.347206

Roy, P., Bouchard, B., Bouzouane, A., & Giroux, S. (2013). *Ambient Activity Recognition in Smart Environments for Cognitive Assistance. International Journal of Robotics Applications and Technologies.*

Russell, S., & Norvig, P. (2009). Artificial Intelligence: A modern approach (3rd ed.). Academic Press.

Seel, T., Raisch, J., & Schauer, T. (2014). IMU-based joint angle measurement for gait analysis. *Sensors (Basel, Switzerland)*, *14*(4), 6891–6909. doi:10.3390/s140406891 PMID:24743160

Shortliffe, E. H., Davis, R., Axline, S. G., Buchanan, B. G., Green, C. C., & Cohen, S. N. (1975). Computer-based consultations in clinical therapeutics: Explanation and rule acquisition capabilities of the MYCIN system. *Computers and Biomedical Research, an International Journal*, *8*(4), 303–320. doi:10.1016/0010-4809(75)90009-9 PMID:1157471

Smullyan, R. M. (1995). *First-Order Logic*. Dover Publications.

Spring, G., Cook, D., Fritz, R., & Schmitter-Edgecombe, M. (2016). Detecting Health and Behavior Change by Analyzing Smart Home Sensor Data. *IEEE International Conference on Smart Computing*.

Statistics Canada. (n.d.). *2016 Census*. Statistics Canada Catalogue no. 98-316-X2016001. Author.

Statistics Canada. (2011). Canada Year Book 2011 Catalogue no. 11-402-X. Author.

Suresh, S., & Sruthi, P. V. (2015). A review on smart home technology. *IEEE International Conference on Green Engineering and Technologies (IC-GET)*, 1-8.

Tamblyn, R., Huang, A., Perreault, R., Jacques, A., Roy, D., & Hanley, J. et al. Laprise, R. (2003). The medical office of the 21st century (MOXXI): Effectiveness of computerized decision-making support in reducing inappropriate prescribing in primary care. *Canadian Medical Association Journal*, *169*(6), 549-556. PMID:12975221

United Nations. (2015). *World Population Ageing. Dep. of Economic and Social Affairs*. Population Division.

Wickramasinghe, N., Bali, R. K., Gibbons, M. C., Choi, J. H., & Schaffer, J. L. (2009). A systematic approach: Optimization of healthcare operations with knowledge management. *Journal of Healthcare Information Management*, *23*(3), 44–50. PMID:19663164

Witten, H., Frank, E., & Hall, M. (2011). *Data Mining: Practical Machine Learning Tools and Techniques* (3rd ed.). Morgan Kaufmann.

Yang, X. (2010). *Engineering Optimization: An Introduction with Metaheuristic Applications*. Wiley. doi:10.1002/9780470640425

Zhang, Y., Liu, H., Su, X., Jiang, P., & Wei, D. (2015). Remote mobile health monitoring system based on smart phone and browser/server structure. *Journal of Healthcare Engineering, 6*(4), 717-738.

Chapter 6
Security Issues and Challenges Related to Big Data

Jaimin N. Undavia
CHARUSAT University, India

Atul Patel
CHARUSAT University, India

Sheenal Patel
CHARUSAT University, India

ABSTRACT

Availability of huge amount of data has opened up a new area and challenge to analyze these data. Analysis of these data become essential for each organization and these analyses may yield some useful information for their future prospectus. To store, manage and analyze such huge amount of data traditional database systems are not adequate and not capable also, so new data term is introduced – "Big Data". This term refers to huge amount of data which are used for analytical purpose and future prediction or forecasting. Big Data may consist of combination of structured, semi structured or unstructured data and managing such data is a big challenge in current time. Such heterogeneous data is required to maintained in very secured and specific way. In this chapter, we have tried to identify such challenges and issues and also tried to resolve it with specific tools.

INTRODUCTION

The term "Security" refers to the mechanism to avoid risk of unauthorized access and use. A specific resource or process is always called for the purpose to resolve risk. When security is in concern with big data then the size of the big data is always considered a challenging task to provide security.

As Big Data is too big, fast and versatile, traditional systems cannot compile them with the same approach that was used with database system. It was easy to analyze the tradition database as it contains only structured data and thus such method cannot be used to analyze unstructured data. So, it becomes the most prominent challenge to offer security to such unstructured and massive amount of data – Big Data.

DOI: 10.4018/978-1-5225-5222-2.ch006

Copyright © 2018, IGI Global. Copying or distributing in print or electronic forms without written permission of IGI Global is prohibited.

All the characteristics of the Big Data are the challenges in self. In the early era data is structured having a same pattern, uniform speed, and clean; so traditional technologies behave well. But these days' traditional tools and technologies are not sufficient to analysis Big Data.

SECURITY ISSUES IN BIG DATA

As the name suggests, Big Data is the term which describes massive amount of data which may be in structured and unstructured form. These data are used in business on day-to-day basis. Here, the amount of data is not only important but how organization uses this data is important. Such data can be analyzed and used for decision making process for strategic business moves and forecasting in various perspectives.

The "Big Data" term is relatively new and describes the act of gathering and storing massive amount of data for the purpose of analytics. The concept gained momentum in the early 2000s when industry analysts articulated the now-mainstream definition of big data as the three Vs:

Big Data – the term which reveals the fact that it has enormous amount of data availability. Such large volume of data is always combination of both structured and unstructured natured data. In recent days, these data overwhelm business at a very high extent.

Introduction to Security in Big Data

Recent trends of most of the corporates prove that the data is the most important asset of them. Each and every section or department within the company have faith in data which are generated within the company (Moura & Serrao, n.d.). Amount and versatility increased in the data yield some more difficulties in the maintenance of the same. Such huge amount of data can be analyzed using traditional analysis so a new paradigm is introduced known as Big Data.

Big Data is a collection of huge amount of data and they are characterized by four different basic V's. These V's are Volume, velocity, variety and variability. Some authors have added some more characteristics depending upon their understanding and research outcome such as value and complexity. The term refers the data which is collected by the companies and government. This data is about us or about surrounding of us (Schmitt et al., 2013). Such huge amount of data is not only required to maintain and manage because this data is being manipulated and updated every day with another huge amount of fresh data. This phenomenon characterizes the following founding properties of Big Data.

Table 1. Characteristics of Big Data

Characteristic of Big Data	Meaning	Related Challenge
Volume	Size of data which is converting from terabytes to petabytes and so on.	Such increasing data needs to secure
Velocity	Speed at which the data has arrived	Increasing in data at rapid speed became difficult
Variability	Different speed of data from various sources	It is challenging to accommodate data from different sources & speed
Veracity	Produces data of different pattern	Accommodate data from different sources

Once you are in the field of Big Data then you have to consider some serious issues related to it like security and privacy. Such issues are required to be considered because of different data sources and formats, streaming nature of data acquisition, cloud based infrastructure and inter-cloud migration as well. The attack surface of entire system is increased because of the use of large scale cloud infrastructure, different software platforms, large computer networks, etc.

In the field of Big Data, it is not only important to acquire large volume of data but what you do with these data is really matters (Shirudkar & Motwani, 2015). Correct methodology must be adopted by the company or organization to collect data from various sources of different formats and nature to improve volume, value and versatility of data. Corrective approach is required to adopt to offer security and privacy to that data.

As described before, each of the characteristic of Big Data come with some inherent challenges with them. Volume is the characteristic which represents the volume of data and in case of Big Data this volume is very huge. Data are converted from terabytes to petabytes at a very rapid speed. Velocity presents the frequency at which data is being arrived, changed or updated. Big Data is repository of huge amount of complex data so there may be number of sources to produce the data and each source has its own speed to evolve the data and send it to the data repository. Each connected data source is not bound to produce data of similar type or at a similar speed. Such versatile sources produce data with lot of noise, which reflects the characteristic Veracity. Each characteristics of big data is a challenge itself.

In early days, when data were of same pattern, adequate and uniform speed, noiseless, that time traditional analytical technique and tools were sufficient to work upon. But when such complex data is required to manage and maintain against various aspects, then related challenges have been evolved for such a huge amount of data.

Main challenges related to big data are listed below (Ghosh & Nath, 2015):

1. Initially organization has to choose and select the relevant and important data in context of their application and requirements.
2. After getting adequate data source, organization has to establish secure connections with data points. Big Data must be connected with several transaction points and to maintain secured connection with them is a big hurdle for the concerned organizations.

Figure 1. Big Data Security Challenges

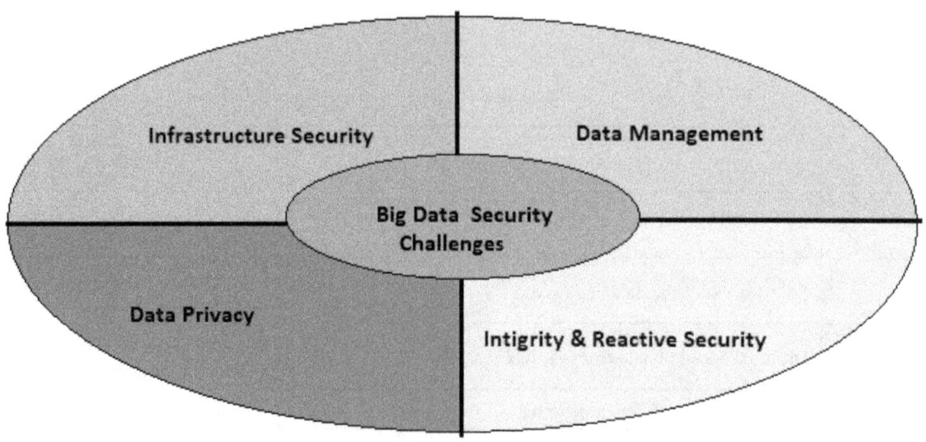

3. Then organization has to maintain the data volume by creating power grid operations.
4. Another significant challenge for the organization is to leverage Big Data. For that, one has to work across different departments like finance, IT and engineering. So, data within these departments has to be cooperative across.
5. Another and most important angle related to Big Data is the security concern of such huge, valued and sensitive data. This is the biggest challenge for the companies who are tend to take advantages from Big Data.

Main Security Concern in Big Data

Many business organizations and academic institutes are using these Big Data for the various purposes like future planning, marketing, research to know consumer behavior, consumer usage pattern, marketing plan and strategy, etc. Sensitivity and role of the data within the business is very high. So, to establish a reciprocal approach for this data of high sensitivity is essential. If proper security approach is not being adopted by the concern organization, then it would result in some serious legal repercussions and reputational damage as well (Subaira, 2016).

In recent times, many businesses are tending to use this Big Data but they are not considering this data as asset to them so they are violating some serious considerations like security. Such security breaks may yield in some serious legal issues and reputation of the business may fall down like anything.

This is the new era in term of research and technology. Now-a-days, companies are storing and using petabytes of data for the various purposes. They are storing this data about their customers, business plans, market surveys and many other aspects are being stored and used for analysis. When such a huge amount of data is stored then it becomes more important to establish a secure way to filter out or classify the data as and when needed against the different and versatile demand of the application and situation as well. To make such sensitive data secured, organizations are using different techniques such as encryption, logging, honeypot detection, etc. To detect and protect your data in advance, you must have to stick to Big Data style analytics. Such techniques are useful to detect threats in early stages with the help of some sophisticated pattern analysis and by analyzing multiple data sources.

When issues are related to Big Data, then not only security is main concern, to provide data privacy is also a major challenge to most of the organizations and industries. As the use of Big Data increased in the industry, many organizations have started to face the issues related to data privacy. Privacy is not the necessity but its liability, so companies have to adopt privacy defense approach. Security does not offer any additional advantage to the organization while privacy become asset to the organization. And this will be help-full to all the stack holders of the organization. At this point, companies are responsible to maintain balance between data privacy and data security.

TOP 10 CHALLENGES IN BIG DATA SECURITY

We have entered into an era which produces bulk of data either by IoT devices, human interactions on internet or data repositories of organizations. Big data cannot be compared to traditional database system as big data is actually a large collection of heterogeneous data, much faster and a way too bigger in size. When such a bulk of data is to be analyzed it becomes challenging to satisfy its security aspects. Here we will see few Security challenges of Big Data. According to CSA Big Data Security WG, online publication "Top Ten Big Data Security and Privacy Challenges", Security challenges can be categorized as below (Alliance Cloud Security, 2013):

Infrastructure Security

Secure Computations in Distributed Programming Frameworks

When massive amount of data is available for computing then distributed programming frameworks are used for parallel computing. MapReduce framework is the most common example of such framework. It divides an input file into small chunks of input. Then a mapper comes into picture and reads the data within each chunk. It also computes the data and generates the output in the form of key-value pair. Then reducer collects each result corresponding to each unique chunk and combines the result which belongs to unique key. Then it outputs the result.

Securing the mappers and securing the data from malicious mapper is the main concern over here as incorrect result from mappers is difficult to judge and then after this incorrect result yields in incorrect

Figure 2. MapReduce Framework

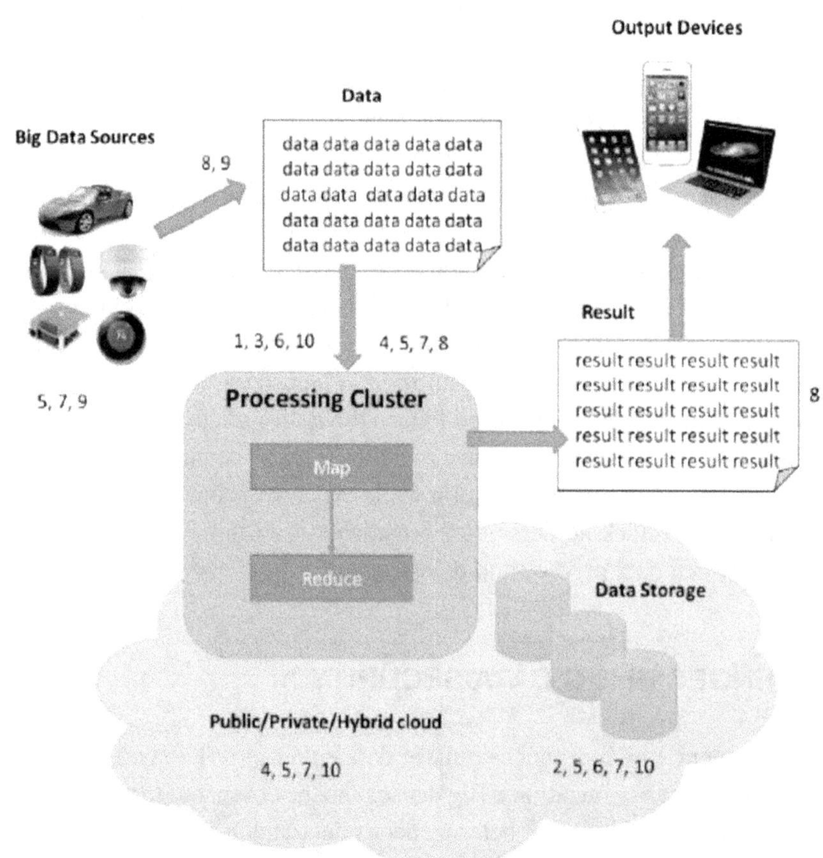

aggregate result. Working with large data sets, it is very difficult to detect malicious mapper and eventually they damage essential data also. Private records within these massive data needs to be reciprocated from such malicious mappers. MapReduce computations are responsible to look after such malicious activities by reintroducing altered copies (Alliance Cloud Security, 2013).

Security Best Practices for Non-Relational Data Stores

Many challenges related to Big Data have been handled by non-relational database like NoSQL without concerning much over the security issues. Such databases do not have any explicit security enforcement but they are embedded with such security code in middleware. Transactional integrity and complex integrity constrains can be trained in NoSQL as it hampers with its target to provide better performance and scalability. NoSQL databases have weak authentication techniques and weak password storage mechanisms. They use HTTP Basic- or Digest- based authentication and are subjected to man-in-the-middle attack. REST (Representational State Transfer) based on HTTP is prone to cross-site scripting, cross-site request forgery and injection attacks like: JSON injection, array injection, view injection, REST injection, GQL (Generalized Query Language) injection, schema injection and others. NoSQL is unsupportive of blocking with the help of third party as well. Authorization techniques in NoSQL provide authorization at higher layers only. Due to lenient security mechanism, database like NoSQL does provide only database level security checks. It does not provide security check from the data sources. Such databases have risk from internal threats as well. They do have poor logging and log analysis methods so such threats may go unnoticed (Alliance Cloud Security, 2013).

Secure Data Storage and Transactions Logs

Multi-tiered storage media is being used to keep data and transaction logs. With the increase in data, scalability and accessibility issues become more important to consider and they are subject to auto-tiering for Big Data storage. In such mechanism, IT managers are completely unaware with the fact that where and how data is being stored and what kind of security measures have been taken. Some storage service providers can have mechanism to search potential usage pattern and activity of users. But they are not able to break into the data overcoming the encipherment. Authentication mechanism must be safe enough to determine which user has right to use which part of data. But sometimes, user may access each other's data by exchanging the keys and entire security mechanism may fall down. The service provider must have adequate rollback mechanism specially in multi-user environment. Data loss or damage in data may result in conflicts within the organization (Demchenko, Ngo, & Membry, 2013).

Auto-tiering for Big Data storage is introduced to solve the issue of scalability and accessibility. It does not keep track and record of the data where they are stored as like in multi-tiered storage media where the data manager knew which data resided where and when. Some clues may be found by the untrustworthy database service provider where they can predict user's activity and database transactions.

End-Point Input Validation/Filtering

Many different sources can give numerous data from their devices. Especially when an organization is following Bring Your Own Device (BYOD) model, the chances of malicious inputs become higher in such cases. In an organization network many systems would collect data from billions of software applications and hardware devices. While collecting the data the main challenge comes in picture is the validation of these data. Trusting the data becomes the main question whether the data collected is genuine or not. Second question may arise is validating the source of input data, such end-point devices are difficult to identify. Third question may arise is how to filter these malicious inputs from such a huge collection. Thus validating inputs and filtering the data becomes the formidable challenge modelled by untrusted sources.

Access Control and Policy

Granular Access Control and Data Centric Access Policies

Data for big data analytics, machine learnings and cloud computing are always focusing on handling different schemas of data at various levels of security. The security that actually matters from the standpoint of access control is confidentiality. Secrecy is preventing the data from the people who do not have the authority to view it. Sometimes the data that are not to be shared with others are swept away to more restrictive area where it can gain guaranteed confidentiality. Data handling requires corporate and privacy policies as well as agreements. Managing these restrictions have always incurred cost increase for such application development. Moreover, very few people will help in analysis of such applications. Thus granular access control should be adapted for such analytical systems to maintain high level of security environment.

Cryptographically Enforced Access Control and Secure Communication

In any organization data security is obligatory part that each data source has to accomplish. To ensure that only authorized person is accessing the most sensitive data, the data should be encrypted. Cryptography is the cryptanalysis theory of encrypting the data before storing it. Only authorized users can decrypt the data else others cannot read such encrypted data. A lot of research has been done in this area and multiple algorithms have been developed to encrypt the data and provide security to the data. Still to ensure authentication of data these algorithms have to be made effective, scalable and more efficient. Usually cloud stores data without encrypting. The main problem of encrypting such a large set of data arises here. Sometimes this policy restricts the user to perform the basic operations on data like searching records or sharing. One technique i.e. Attribute-based encryption (ABE) can lessen this problem by applying public key cryptosystem. This system works on keys to unlock the data of attributes. On the other side we also have data that is unencrypted and less sensitive. These data should be shared using some cryptographically secured communication framework, sharing of such data can be useful for analytics.

DATA MANAGEMENT

Real-Time Security/Compliance Monitoring

To maintain real time security is always a challenging task. Real time security monitoring system can give number of alerts generated by the security device which can either be related or can be just a false positive which are usually ignored by humans. As big data consists of data increase in volume, however we might have an opportunity to expand big data technology that may provide faster analytics of varied data.

By doing this most organizations and government would be benefitted in various ways. They may have solutions to various question like- Do we have any threats to our data? Second question may arise like who is accessing- which data from which resource and at what time? They may also have question like - Do we need to start plan B because of occurrence of Action A?

Health industry can also be largely benefitted from big data technology, by reducing the frauds related to claims and becoming more precise with the expenditures of claims.

Granular Audits

The main aim of real time security monitoring system is to get notification of attack at the moment it takes place. But sometimes due to any reason we might not be able to receive the notifications because of missed true positives. To get the details of missed attacks one should go through auditing. Auditing the information is thoroughly examining the details to understand what was wrong and what had actually happened. Auditing is not new concept in this term but the scope of auditing and the granularities may differ. Big Data contains a huge collection of data thus auditing these data can really be a challenging task for the one who is performing it. Moreover, different firms require different types of auditing, like marketing organizations would require social media content of people to enhance their online advertisements and sales.

Data Provenance

Provenance of data is the information about the ownership of data or in other words it gives origin and creation of data which would be useful for the accuracy and authentication of data.

Big Data applications that includes provenance supported programming environment may generate provenance graphs in large quantity and these graphs may generate complexity in provenance metadata. It becomes complicated to understand metadata dependencies for security purpose from these provenance graphs. Thus, we need to have very good computational algorithms to understand the such provenance graphs. Many applications have history of such provenance data in form of digital records, these can be the details about its creation.

e.g. Determining the accuracy of data sources for researchers is important. The process of assessment is time sensitive and should be performed faster. Thus it requires faster algorithms to process provenance metadata.

Privacy and Confidentiality

Scalable and Composable Privacy-Preserving Data Mining and Analytics

Data that is collected by many organizations or any government agencies is constantly under supervision of some mining agencies and analysts to obtain knowledgeable information. A malevolent insider can harm these datasets and obtain private information of customers. In the same way, intelligence agencies also require large number of datasets from various data sources which can be blogs, chat history, routers, websites, etc. We need to have a robust, efficient and scalable privacy mining algorithms to rise the chance of accumulating only appropriate data of users. Big data is popularly known for its invasive privacy policies and trending marketing. The major challenge comes in picture is to preserve privacy of user because anonymizing data for analytics is not sufficient to preserve user privacy. In recent example of AOL who have released anonymized search log which was mainly used for academic purpose, but it had easily identified users by their searches. Thus it becomes essential to create new policies, techniques or guidelines for preventing unintended disclosures of user.

ADDRESSING SECURITY ISSUES IN BIG DATA

In the preceding sections, we have seen what Big Data is, what are top 10 challenges for the Big Data and now we will emphasize on how to deal with such challenges to make sure security concerns of the Big Data.

We have observed that, this Big Data technology compelling the existing traditional technologies to change in order to suit to new requirements and technology. If we adopt the change in the way we were using the technology, then we must design new security approach for emerging security challenges. This section of the chapter will highlight some approaches to deal with newer version of the security issues related to Big Data.

We have discussed in preceding sections that characteristics of the Big Data such as veracity, volume, variety and dynamicity have a huge impact on Big Data Security. Before we proceed with the possible solutions of the security and privacy issues related to Big Data, let's list out the main concerns of it (Tarekegn, 2016).

1. Security and privacy are big concern in Big Data because Big Data is the data which are subject to change and upgrade every second as it is connected with the continuous source of the data.
2. Another main concern to provide security to Big Data is that now Big Data is widely accessible. Data are shared by various organizations or individuals like students, doctors, scientists, business officials, researchers, government agencies and other interested people. So, sharing of such sensitive data on large scale for variety of purposes requires high level of security (Schmitt et al., 2013).
3. Lacking of basic knowledge in how to provide security to such a huge mass is the major concern of Big Data security and privacy (Schmitt et al., 2013).
4. Full proof policies are not designed to confirm data security and privacy (Schmitt et al., 2013).
5. Current security and privacy technologies have limited capabilities. They are more suitable to provide security to static data while in case of Big Data, data grows at rapid speed (Schmitt et al., 2013).
6. Companies approach towards the security of Big Data is very lethargic and so as misuse of such data becomes very common practice by the unauthorized agencies or personals.

Addressing Big Data Privacy and Security Issues

As stated earlier, most of the security threats in Big Data are because of its characteristics of volume, variety and velocity. The difference in nature of data sources, format of data, different speed of data flow combined with the streaming nature of data acquisition and high volume of data create unique security risks (Gaddam, n.d.).

As far security in Big Data is concerned, there are following 5 major concerns.

1. Data Management
2. Identity & Access Management
3. Data Protection & Privacy
4. Network Security
5. Infrastructure Security

Reliable Proposed Framework for Big Data Security and Privacy Issue

Data Management

This component is further divided into 3 sub components: Data Classification, Data Discovery & Data Tagging (Gaddam, n.d.).

Data Classification

Effective data classification is the most significant way to achieve security in Big Data Environment. When organization works with huge volume of data, they must be in position to classify the data in terms of which data is the most important, which requirescryptographical protection, which fields required

Figure 3. Big Data Security Framework

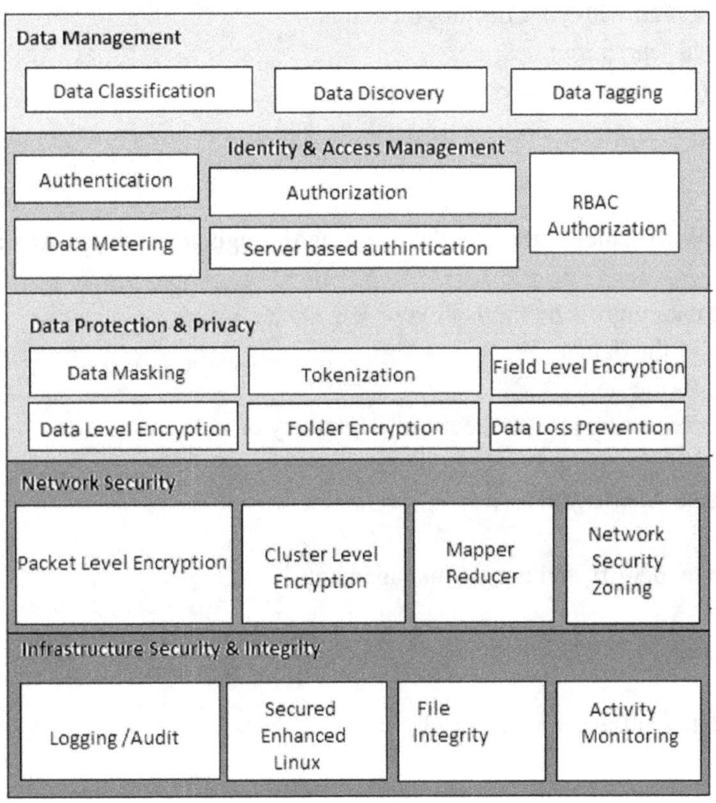

more priority for the sake of security, etc. Successful security initiatives are then considered after this précised and defined classification.

Following are the core items which can lead to successful classification matrix of your environment.

1. Encourage your reader to go beyond the symbolic policy level exercise by identifying level of security required to your data resources of different types.
2. Deploy efforts on security control assessments. Determine location of data, number of users and their access rights, measures of security, etc.
3. Determine value of the data to the attacker.
4. Determine Agreement and Expenses Impact
5. Determine impact to the stockholders

Data Discovery

Lack in situational awareness for the sensitive data may lead the organization to significant risks. Data marking, Data Redaction, Tokenization or encryption key are the major concern to leave data at secure level.

Structure and unstructured kind of data must be reciprocated and protected from the malicious activities. Some crucial exercise listed here for effective data discovery exercise.

1. Emphasize on data protection at later stage by defining and validating proper data structure.
2. Collect Metrics.
3. Convey proposed data structures to the concerned security team to design adequate security model.
4. Decide the work plan with your development team.
5. Build conditional search routines.
6. Identify protected data and means of its work.

Data Tagging

Follow following steps to achieve effective data tagging through ingress or egress methods.

1. Identify all the data ingress methods in your Big Data cluster.
2. Know the flow of the data.
3. Identify all egress method.
4. Decide whether reporting jobs are required separately or not.

Identify and Access Management

Follow Hadoop step to identify and access management.

User Entitlement and Data Metering

1. Tie policy to data not the access methods.

2. Leverage attributes
3. Perform data Metering

RBAC Authorization

Define uniform policy for Role based Access Control.

1. Manage data access by role but not by the user
2. Manage user groups through their common role

Data Protection and Privacy

Following are security measures to protect the data.

1. Application level cryptography
2. Transparent Encryption
3. Data Making

Network Security

Security measures must be taken when data is on transmission. This is part of network level security. Following are the controls that when implemented in a Big Data cluster can ensure properties of data confidentiality.

1. Packet level encryption using TLS from the client to Hadoop cluster
2. Packet level encryption using TLS within the cluster itself. This includes using https between NameMode to Job Tracker to DataNode.
3. Packet level encryption using TLS in the cluster (e.g. mapper-reducer)
4. Use LDAP over SSL (LDAPS) rather than LDAP when communicating with the corporate enterprise directories to prevent sniffing attacks.
5. Allow your admins to configure and enable encrypted shuffle and TLS/https for HDFS, MapReduce, YARN, HBase UIs etc.

Infrastructure Security and Integrity

This layer has following sub-components:

Logging/Audit

All system/ecosystem changes unique to Hadoop clusters need to be audited with the audit logs being protected.

Secured Enhanced Linux

SELinux was created by the United States National Security Agency (NSA) as a set of patches to the Linux Kernel using Linux Security Modules (LSM).

Conclusion on Security and Privacy Issues

Some key recommendations are listed out to work with security risks associated with Big Data.

1. Always try to select reputed and experienced vendor and products that have provided its security services to similar or larger organizations for at least more one year.
2. To obtain a reliable security is tough but still there are many key pillars that can help us to achieve honest security are accountability, access-control centric, balanced network centric and data centric security.
3. Usually security for data is incorporated after the storage process, but we can use Data centric security like cell-level security or labelled security which is the latest flair of securing the data. With such data centric techniques, we add security constrictions into the data itself or into the application codes.
4. Facilities of securing the data should be externalizedwhenever possible or required. Use other techniques like data masking and redaction that obscures the data for security purpose, tokenization technique that surrogates sensitive data with less delicate ones, services with granular control can also be used to access Hadoop. These techniques can be assimilated at the time of ingestion of data to their specified storage location.
5. Data provenance can be achieved by harnessing the logs and audit clusters. This can be done thru data management tools like Zettaset Orchestrator, OSS Apache Falcon, Cloudera Navigator and many other that can assist with the origins of data which might be useful to ensure the level of authentication.

Big Data Other Issues

Privacy and Security

This concept of big data is sensitive and technical. Information shared on large external data-set can be personal data of a person which he/she might not want to share with the data owners.

Various organization collects information about users for expanding their business and the users are not aware about this.

Certain people suffer from adverse moment without knowing that they are being discriminated nor they could even fight back due to law implementation of Big Data. Increase in Social stratification where an educated person could enjoy big data predictive analysis whereas on contrary less educated people are easily recognized and treated badly (Katal, 2013).

Data Access and Sharing of Information

For better efficiency, decision making and business intelligence it is necessary that data should be available in specified format and within stipulated time duration. Accurate decisions are taken only if the data is complete, accurate and available in time. Importance to make data available in standardized manner increases the complexity of data managers. To expand the business, data sharing among the business organizations might not be possible. Sharing their client data among business organizations threatens the culture of competitiveness.

Storage and Processing Issues

Storage of massive data which is produced by various sources like sensors, social media, and various websites is not sufficient as day by day these data keeps on increasing in size. As demands of these data are high one option can be thought of storing these data on cloud so that network and servers can access it easily. But the problem of uploading these data can be a question, as to store these data on cloud one need to upload such a massive data on network. Only uploading these data cannot solve the problem, further these data should also be analyzed thoroughly to obtain useful information. Such terabytes of data may take more time to get uploaded in cloud and moreover these data keeps changing quickly.

Cloud stores its data in distributed grading which makes it firm to analyze data. Moving the data for processing is also another major question. We can solve this problem by processing the data in storage place and transferring the results to some other locations or the other is to transfer the important data for analyzing to some other location and then process it. But both techniques require provenance of data. Finding an element from such a huge amount of data would be difficult to scan so the solution can be to give indexes to the data while storing it saves large time.

Analytical Challenges

Analytical challenges are the most prominent challenges for the people who deals with the Big Data. As far as analytical challenges are concerned, the challenges are as under (Katal, 2013).

1. How can we get maximum benefit out of available data?
2. What is the need to store all data? Is it required to store all the data?
3. How to find an effective method to deal with such a huge data?
4. How to identify task relevant data?
5. How to identify important data points?

Analysis is considered to be one of the trickiest tasks in the field of Information Technology. It requires vast experience and commonsense to judge the situation. When dealing with such a huge mass, Big Data is having some implicit analytical challenges. Analytics in Big Data becomes more challenging as it is combination of structured, unstructured and semi structured data. Thus analytics requires large number of advanced skill. Selection of suitable analytical techniques is also an important consideration to make. For such decision making incorporate massive data volumes in analysis or determine upfront which Big Data is relevant with (Katal, 2013).

Skill Requirement

Big Data is relatively recent concept and needs to be handled with emerging tools and technology. It does not require only technical skill set but it is also important to handle these Big Data with some expertise in analytical skill. The skill set is also extended to research capability, interpretive capability and must have ability to have clear vision of the expected outcome or result. To develop such capabilities, organizations have to conduct various training program for that. On the other hand, universities need to introduce this recent term Big Data in their curriculum so that industry may get skilled candidate to work with.

Technical Challenges

Technical challenges are further divided into following 3 sub challenges.

Fault Tolerance

Rework is very costly in the recent fields like Big Data. Such technology must be implemented with the aids of effective fault tolerance so that any damage or bug must not compel the organization to rollback to initial phase of the implementation. Fault tolerance is extremely difficult job and it is near to impossible to have 100% reliable software product or framework. So, the prime focus on not to have most reliable infrastructure but to have most reliable with minimum chance of failure.

Researchers have found two methods to deal with fault tolerance in the field of Big Data.

1. Divided the whole computation into small chunks, let them do computing individually and then integrate their results. If any particular node is not working as per the expectations, then this particular task needs to be restarted.
2. Sometimes it is not possible to divide the task into small chunks because some processes are recursive in nature or some computations are dependent on the intermediate result of another part of process. In such case restarting the whole process becomes very tedious job. In such case, we can improvise the process by adding suitable checkpoints at particular places. Here, system performance is being checked at regular intervals and if something unexpected happens then only we have to restart the work up to the last check point only.

Quality of Data

Costing is the most significant factor when we are storing such a huge amount of data. This huge amount of data incurred huge cost for storage. On the other hand, it is also important to have more amount of data because good amount of data results in better decision making process in business. Business Leaders will always want more and more data storage whereas the IT Leaders will take all technical aspects in mind before storing all the data (Katal, 2013).

Big Data actually target quality of data than the irrelevant data to be stored for betterment in decision making process. In such case certain questions become extremely important to answer like,

- How to determine relevant data?
- How much data would be enough?
- How to validate the accuracy of the result which is drawn from the available amount of data?

Heterogeneous Nature of Data

Unstructured data is unstructured in terms of their sources. Such data may come from any of the sources like social media sites, streaming file, flat file, database file, PDF file etc. Structured data on the other hand is always organized into highly mechanized and manageable way. So, it becomes cumbersome to handle unstructured data as they are available in variety of format. It is challenging task for IT managers to integrate such data at minimum cost possible.

Scalability

Recent processor technology has really boost up the processing speed and headache of parallel processing is removed because of it. Now the major concern is parallelism within the single node. In past the techniques which were used to do parallel data processing across data nodes aren't capable of handling intra-node parallelism. This is because of the fact that many more hardware resources such as cache and processor memory channels are shared across a core in a single node. The scalability issue of Big data has led towards cloud computing, which now aggregates multiple disparate workloads with varying performance goals into very large clusters. This requires a high level of sharing of resources which is expensive and also brings with it various challenges like how to run and execute various jobs so that we can meet the goal of each workload cost effectively. It also requires dealing with the system failures in an efficient manner which occurs more frequently if operating on large clusters. These factors combined put the concern on how to express the programs, even complex machine learning tasks. There has been a huge shift in the technologies being used. Hard Disk Drives (HDD) are being replaced by the solid state Drives and Phase Change technology which are not having the same performance between sequential and random data transfer. Thus what kind of storage devices are to be used is again a big question for data storage.

REFERENCES

Alliance Cloud Security. (2013). *Top Ten Big Data Security and Privacy Challenges*. Alliance.

Demchenko, Ngo, & Membrey. (2013). *Big Security for Big Data: Addressing Security Challenges for the Big Data Infrastructure*. Academic Press.

Ghosh & Nath. (2015). Big Data Security Issues and Challenges. *International Journal of Innovative Research in Advanced Engineering, 2*, 15-20.

Moura & Serrao. (n.d.). *Security and Privacy Issues of Big Data*. Academic Press.

Munaye. (2016). Big data: Security issues, challenges and future scope. *International Journal of Computer Engineering & Technology, 4*(7), 12-24.

Schmitt, C., Shoffner, M., Owen, P., Wang, X., Lamm, B., & Barker, M. J. (2013). Security and Privacy in the era of Big Data. *RENCI, 1*.

Shirudkar & Motwani. (2015). Big-Data Security. *International Journal of Advanced Research in Computer Science and Software Engineering*, 1100-1109.

Subaira, A.S., Gayathri, R., & Sindhujaa, N. (n.d.). Security Issues and Challenges in Big Data Analysis. *International Journal of Advanced Research in Computer Science and Software Engineering, 6*, 530-536.

Wazid & Goudar. (2013). *Big Data: Issues, Challenges, Tools and Good Practices*. Institute of Electrical and Electronics Engineers.

Chapter 7
Big Data Analysis for Cardiovascular Diseases:
Detection, Prevention, and Management

Miguel A. Sánchez-Acevedo
Universidad de la Cañada, Mexico & Universidad Popular Autónoma del Estado de Puebla, Mexico

Zaydi A. Acosta-Chí
Universidad de la Cañada, Mexico

Beatriz A. Sabino-Moxo
Universidad de la Cañada, Mexico

José A. Márquez-Domínguez
Universidad de la Cañada, Mexico

Rosa M. Canton-Croda
Universidad Popular Autónoma del Estado de Puebla, Mexico

ABSTRACT

In the healthcare field, plenty of clinical data is generated every day from patient records, surveys, research papers, medical devices, among others sources. These data can be exploited to discover new insights about health issues. For helping decision makers and healthcare data managers, a survey of research works and tools covering the process of handling big data in the healthcare field is included. A methodology for CVD prevention, detection and management through the use of tools for big data analysis is proposed. Also, it is important to maintain privacy of patients when handling healthcare data; therefore, a list of recommendations for maintaining privacy when handling healthcare data is presented. Specific clinical analysis are recommended on those regions where the incidence rate of CVD is high, but a weak relation with the common risk factors is observed according to historical data. Finally, challenges which need to be addressed are presented.

DOI: 10.4018/978-1-5225-5222-2.ch007

Copyright © 2018, IGI Global. Copying or distributing in print or electronic forms without written permission of IGI Global is prohibited.

INTRODUCTION

Big Data term could be relative to the context, but quantities starting from petabytes are always considered as Big Data. Every second, a lot of data is generated from several sources: traditional databases, text files, remote data, mobile devices, sensors, etc. The way in which data is presented can be classified as structured, semi-structured, and unstructured data. In order to analyze the collected data, it is required to prepare it; starting with an exploration, followed by description, and then visualizing the data with graphs. Good results in the analysis phase can be guaranteed with quality of data. Quality of data is achieved by removing data with missing values, merging duplicate records, generating best estimates for invalid values, and removing outliers. After data preparation, a set of analysis techniques can be applied to discover relevant information; most used techniques are: classification, clustering, regression, graph analytics, and association analysis. All the stages involved in big data processing allow the generation of new insights that could be used to take actions for solving the problem under study.

According to the World Health Organization (WHO, 2016), cardiovascular disease (CVD) is the main cause of death in the world; the organization estimates that more than 17.5 million people died of CVD in 2012, and this number has increased in last years. Coronary heart disease, cerebrovascular disease, peripheral arterial disease, rheumatic heart disease, congenital heart disease, deep vein thrombosis, pulmonary embolism, heart attacks, and strokes are the most common CVDs, while coronary heart disease is the leading cause of premature death. The probability of suffering a coronary heart disease is increased by risk factors like unhealthy diet, physical inactivity, tobacco use, and harmful use of alcohol; also, those risk factors alter normal blood conditions of pressure, glucose, and lipids, and generate overweight and obesity. Solutions to this problematic seems easy: not smoking, eat healthily, and exercise; however, people is not motivated to perform those activities and it is necessary to identify the reasons of this behavior in order to establish public politics that contribute to reduce CVD. There are regions in the world where CVD has increased, but a lack of resources in healthcare institutions reduce the possibility of identifying the roots of the problem; nevertheless, some risk factors are easily observable (poverty, stress, age, gender, overweight, obesity, tobacco use, etc.) and can guide to a more deeper analysis in regions where insufficient information is available; on the other hand, health issues with known risk factors can be addressed with proposed solutions in regions with similar characteristics.

Nowadays, it is possible to access data related to CVD in several databases around the world, National Cardiovascular Disease Database, Coronary Artery Disease Gene Database, Ensanut, Centers for Disease Control and Prevention, and ONEdata, to name a few. With those data available, tools for big data analysis can be employed for discovering new correlations among data that could not be observed before. For those countries where a lack of resources limits the number of clinical analysis that can be performed in the population, big data analysis can contribute to identify common characteristics with people in other regions of the world and select more pertinent analysis to be performed. This chapter proposes a methodology for using healthcare databases to detect CVD risk factors, determine the high profitable actions for preventing CVD based on risks detected, and identify what are the best clinical analysis and drugs for treatment of CVD according to historical success cases. Although great advances have been achieved in big data field, there are issues that have not been addressed yet. A CVD can be originated by several factors and not always presenting the same symptoms, making its detection more difficult; therefore, challenges to be addressed are presented.

BACKGROUND

Data generated in the healthcare field is processed with the objective to identify, diagnose, detect and prevent possible diseases. However, integrating data (text, images, video) into structured data sets requires legal, business, and technical challenges. Although a lot of health data around the world is available, most are stored in individual repositories. Information from clinics and hospitals is kept within the healthcare provider's limits. In addition, the data stored inside a hospital is almost never integrated into multiple IT systems. A great challenge when working with health data is to integrate data obtained from electronic medical records, vital signs, laboratory, medication information, doctor's notes, medical publications, among others sources (Big Data Value Association, 2016). To achieve this, big data technologies provide a good approach.

Big data in health refers to data collected from individuals which is related with their health and is generated in high volumes (Auffray et al., 2016). Big data technologies have already made some impact in fields like medical diagnosis from imaging data in medicine and quantifying lifestyle data in the fitness industry. In biology and cardiovascular medicine, significant changes have been made in the way of accessing, extracting, organizing, integrating, modeling information, and how they affect basic scientific research and clinical care. Heart disease is a major health problem; this is the leading cause of death worldwide. Early detection of heart diseases is a subject that has much relevance in medical research. In recent decades, advances have been made in therapies for the treatment and prevention of cardiovascular diseases. The need to measure and study the results of health care has increased, as well as the administration of cardiovascular treatment. Unfortunately, these researches have shown that there is poor quality of care, high variation in patient outcomes, and care costs (Lampropulos et al., 2013; Krumholz, 2008; Fisher et al., 2003). Alexander and Wang (2017) mention that it is necessary to evaluate large datasets for extracting information that can be used in the prediction, prevention and management of chronic diseases. Health management for very large scale population, cardiovascular disease risk prediction, precision medicine using genomic information, and clinical decision support are areas that can be improved with big data technology (Antman et al., 2015; Rumsfeld, et al., 2016).

Motwani et al. (2016) demonstrated that analysis through machine learning using a large data registry improved cardiovascular outcome prediction in patients with suspected coronary artery disease compared with the conventional risk scoring method. Similarly, Loghmanpour et al. (2016) examined the Bayesian network algorithm model, showing superior prediction of right ventricular failure following left ventricular assist device therapy over the currently available risk prediction model. Vaishali and Kalaivani (2016) proposed to develop a centralized patient monitoring system using big data. The proposed system receives medical records as input; then extracts the required information by using the mapreduce technique; next, features like RR, QRS, and QT intervals are analyzed; finally, the system indicates whether the patient status is normal or abnormal.

In the United States, federal resources have been assigned to support the use of big data for advancing biomedicine. Several NIH Centers of Excellence have been established for transforming the culture of research. Data science promise to improve cardiovascular investigations (Scruggs et al, 2015). The research community is interested in predicting heart attacks since this prediction can help to save a vast amount of lives; but also, opens the possibility to develop personalized medicine (Alexander and Wang, 2017). Changes on disease detection, prevention and management will be introduced by the use of big data technologies.

TOOLS AND FRAMEWORKS FOR HEALTHCARE DATA MANAGEMENT

Effective manipulation of big data in the healthcare field requires specialized tools for identifying all possible correlations which could guide to the discovery of the leading diseases causes. Actions addressed to decrease the known factors of CVD remains poor, and the obtained results are not relevant as expected; moreover, the reasons that justify failures are not always clear. In order to help with big data manipulation, several tools have been designed. Those tools reduce the time for analyzing big data and generate insights about undetected relationships.

IBM Watson is a cloud platform with tools that can be used in health, including genomics, drug discovery, health patient engagement, oncology, and care manager. Researchers have used those tools for heart failure detection (Guidi, Miniati, Mazzola, and Iadanza, 2016) and exploration of patterns of cancer incidence (Tsoi et al., 2017). Gathered structured data can be integrated and uploaded to this platform for performing analysis and identify correlations that could be difficult to observe in the raw data. Although there exist institutions which are in charge of recollecting and maintaining structured data in the healthcare field, about 80% of data remains unstructured (Stonová, 2014). Several frameworks have been proposed for processing unstructured data like GATE, Apache UIMA, DKPro, Open NLP, NeOn Toolkit, and cTakes (Ostankov, Röhrbein, and Waltinger, 2014). Wiki-Health is a web platform developed to discover information of health and fitness (Li, Wu, Guo, Lee, and Guo, 2014). The platform allows users to store data obtained from sensors like Fitbit, Zephyr, Nike+ Fuelband, Withings, electroencephalogram devices, etc. and provides tools to obtain information from the stored data through a web interface. Predefined graphs show relevant discovered information, and an editor to execute R commands can be used to obtain further information from the data. Another platform for integrating data of patients, plans, locations, products, providers and employees, which are collected from several devices is Informatica (Informatica, 2012). This platform is composed by several tools to perform analysis over integrated data. The Centers for Disease Control and Prevention have published an interactive atlas of heart disease and stroke (2017) where information about coronary heart disease, acute myocardial infarction, cardiac dysrhythmia, heart failure, hypertension, and all stroke is visualized over a US map. A platform widely used for developing applications is Apache Hadoop. Researchers at the Chungbuk National University developed a health care system for disease detection and prediction based on Hadoop (Li, Park, Batbaatar, Piao, and Ryu, 2016). The system analyzes information collected from a mobile health sensor network, captured by user, or imported from other databases. For analyzing the data and generating a prediction, a Multivariate Adaptive Regression Splines (MARS) model is used.

Every day, tools with better capabilities in managing big data appears. Therefore, it is necessary to establish a methodology, which guides to decision makers and policy makers about what data has to be analyzed in order to prevent, detect, and manage CVD. The World Health Organization (2016) has designed a set of recommendations and protocols for detecting, preventing, and managing CVD: to prevent CVD it is necessary to maintain control over tobacco use, hypertension, high blood cholesterol and diabetes; detection can be performed through clinical measurements, simple laboratory testing, CVD risk assessment charts, and blood pressure measurement; management of CVD requires access to core set of affordable medicines and basic technology, total cardiovascular risk assessment, decentralized community based and patient-centered care, patient data collection and programed evaluation in order to offer quality of life to people with chronic diseases.

METHODOLOGY FOR DETECTION, PREVENTION AND MANAGEMENT OF CARDIOVASCULAR DISEASES

The World Health Organization has identified a set of risk factors that influence directly in CVD. The first step in order to establish politics for detection, prevention, and management of CVD is to identify which of those factors are present in the population under study. Factors can be detected by non-invasive methods, associated factors or clinical analysis (Figure 1). Among factors that can be detected through non-invasive methods, there are no modifiable (age, gender, family history, and social history), and modifiable (diet, physical activity, tobacco exposure, alcohol intake, waist circumference, body mass index, and blood pressure). Because of CVD could be the result of other diseases, there exists factors that have to be monitored like high blood pressure, overweight, obesity, diabetes mellitus, chronic kidney disease, familial hypercholesterolemia, and atrial fibrillation. Finally, some factors can be detected only through clinical analysis like blood lipids, inflammatory markers, glomerular filtration rate, albuminuria, and medical conditions or treatments. In following sections, a methodology for identifying those factors through big data sets is proposed.

Detection

Detecting CVD risk is a process which requires to analyze several factors on patients or healthy persons. The risks assessment can be performed through the identification of risk factors, imaging methods or methods like fibrinogen, homocysteine, and lipoprotein-associated phospholipase 2.

Figure 1. Risk factors and their detection

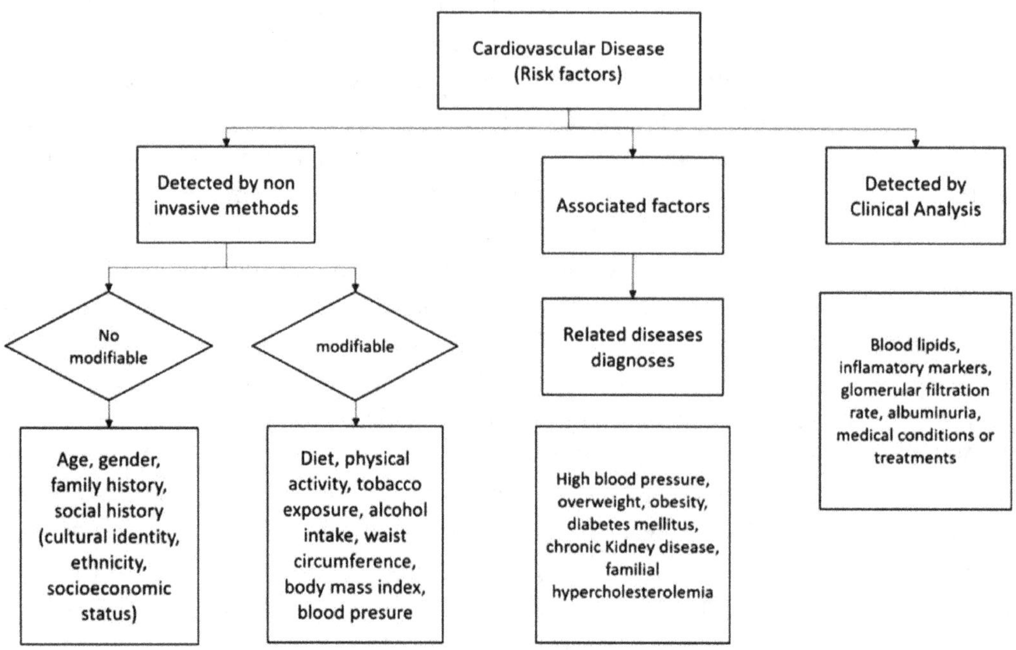

According to the European guidelines on cardiovascular disease prevention in clinical practice (2012), for patients 20 to 79 years of age who are free from clinical atherosclerotic cardiovascular disease (AS-CVD), the first step is to assess ASCVD risk factors: Age, gender, race/ethnicity, current smoker (yes/no), any family history of heart attack in first degree relative (parent/sibling/child) (yes/no). Diabetes, total and HDL cholesterol, use of lipid lowering medication (yes/no), systolic blood pressure (mmHg), and use of antihypertensive medication. For patients outside this age range, providers should refer to applicable clinical practice guidelines and adult primary prevention guidelines.

The assessment of cardiovascular risk is not necessary for specific subgroups of asymptomatic individuals at unusually high risk, such as those with genetically determined extreme values of traditional risk factors, hypercholesterolemia, hypertension and others diseases like diabetes, chronic kidney disease, obstructive sleep apnoea, and erectile dysfunction. The parameters are presented below:

1. Diabetes and age >60 years
2. Diabetes with microalbuminuria (>20 mcg/min or urinary albumin: creatinine ratio [UACR] >2.5 mg/mmol for males, >3.5 mg/mmol for females)
3. Moderate or severe chronic kidney disease (CKD) (persistent proteinuria or estimated glomerular filtration rate [eGFR] <45 mL/min/1.73 m^2)
4. A previous diagnosis of familial hypercholesterolemia
5. Systolic blood pressure (SBP) ≥180 mmHg or diastolic blood pressure (DBP) ≥110 mmHg
6. Serum total cholesterol (TC) >7.5 mmol/L

There are others methods for diagnosis that are used as a complement to the risk assessment.

1. Imaging studies: Measurement of carotid intima-media thickness and/or screening for atherosclerotic plaques by carotid artery scanning, measurement of ankle–brachial index, computed tomography for coronary calcium, and exercise electrocardiography.
2. Measurement of inflammatory and thrombotic biomarkers: high-sensitivity C-reactive protein (CRP) and homocysteine, fibrinogen, homocysteine and lipoprotein-associated phospholipase 2 (LpPLA2)
3. Genetic testing (Deoxyribonucleic acid (DNA)-based tests for common genetic polymorphisms)
4. Assessment of psychosocial risk factors such as low socioeconomic status, lack of social support, stress at work and in family life, depression, anxiety, hostility, and the type D personality.

The application of some of those methods will depend on the level of risk:

- **Moderate Risk:** High-sensitivity-C-reactive protein (CPR), homocysteine, measurement of ankle–brachial index, computed tomography for coronary calcium, and exercise electrocardiography.
- **High Risk of a Recurrent Acute Atherothrombotic Event:** lipoprotein-associated phospholipase 2 (LpPLA2).

The genetic testing is not recommended, because the testing do not add significantly to diagnosis, risk prediction, or patient management but the psychosocial risk factors can be assessed through data mining to improve treatment adherence.

There exist several databases where those information is stored and can be used to perform an automated analysis in order to identify accurately CVD risk levels. For example, the Dartnet Institute provides a dataset containing records of blood pressure, LDL, Total Cholesterol, HDL, among others, obtained from patients of several institutions in the United States. In the United Kingdom the same data can be obtained from the Consumer Data Research Centre (CDRC). In Europe data is collected by the European Genome-phenome Archive and the European Society of Cardiology. Others datasets can be obtained from diverse institutions around the world, which can be used for identifying CVD risks levels by regions following the next methodology (Figure 2).

1. **Datasets Merging:** Collect all data available which include most factors as possible of those described above. A more accurate assessment is obtained when multiple risk factors are analyzed. More data available increases accuracy.
2. **Identify People with Established CVD and Exclude:** When data is collected from several sources, data about persons which are currently under CVD treatment could be included. So, exclude them and continue working with the remaining registries.
3. **Age Classification:** Separate men and women older than 45 in two independent groups. Although they are at the same risk level, the risk could be increased by independent factors like menopause, diabetes, and birth control pills in women; on the other hand, more than 50% of men who suffered cvd not presented symptoms, so their risk is high and constant monitoring over every factor has to be performed. Include those registries in the high level risk and continue working with the remaining registries.
4. **Risk Assessment and Risk Stratification:** For classifying the remaining registries consider the next groups:
    a. people with very high levels of individual risk factors:
        i. Without established CVD who have a total cholesterol ≥ 8 mmol/l (320 mg/dl) or low-density lipoprotein (LDL) cholesterol ≥ 6 mmol/l (240 mg/dl) or TC/HDL-C (total cholesterol/high density lipoprotein cholesterol) ratio >8
        ii. Without established CVD who have persistent raised blood pressure (>160–170/100–105 mmHg)
        iii. With type 1 or 2 diabetes, with overt nephropathy or other significant renal disease
        iv. With renal failure or renal impairment

The risk estimation using Framingham Risk Equation (Anderson, 1991), it is a set of steps described below.

1. Compute an interim number a that is based on risk factor measurements.

$$a = 11.1122 - 0.9119 x log\left(SBP\right) - 0.2767 x\, smoking - 0.7181 x log\left(cholesterol\,/\,HDL\right) 0.5865 x\, ECG - LVH$$

HDL, high density lipoprotein; SBP, diastolic blood pressure, CHD, coronary heart disease; ECG-LVH, left ventricular hypertrophy by electrocardiography.

2. Computing a second interim value m, is different for men and women (Table 1).

Table 1. Computing of second interim value for men and women.

Men:	$m = a - 1.4792 x \, log\left(age\right) - 0.1759 x \, diabetes$
Woman:	$m = a - 5.8549 + 1.8515 x \left[log\left(age \,/\, 74\right)\right] 2 - 0.3758 x \, diabetes$

3. Compute μ and σ for both sexes

$$\mu = 4.4181 + m$$

$$\sigma = exp\left(-0.3155 - 0.2784 x \, m\right)$$

4. Choose the number of years for which you wish to predict (from 4 to 12) and call it t

$$u = \frac{log\left(t\right) - \mu}{\sigma}$$

5. The predicted probability for t is

$$p = 1 - exp\left(-e^{u}\right)$$

Compute for systolic blood pressure (SBP) and diastolic blood pressure (DBP) with the equations and calculate the average. The Table 2 presents categories to describe calculated absolute cardiovascular risk and the regular review at intervals according to the initial assessed risk level:

Prevention

The European guidelines on cardiovascular disease prevention in clinical practice (Perk, J. et al, 2012), recommend:

1. Adoption of a healthy lifestyle: smoking cessation, healthy diet, increased physical activity, management of psychosocial factors, weight reduction.

Table 2. Absolute cardiovascular risk

Categories	Score	Regular Review
Low Risk	<10% probability of CVD	every 2 years
Moderate risk	10% to 15% probability of CVD	every 6 to 12 months
High risk	>15% probability of CVD	according to clinical context

Figure 2. CVD Detection from big data

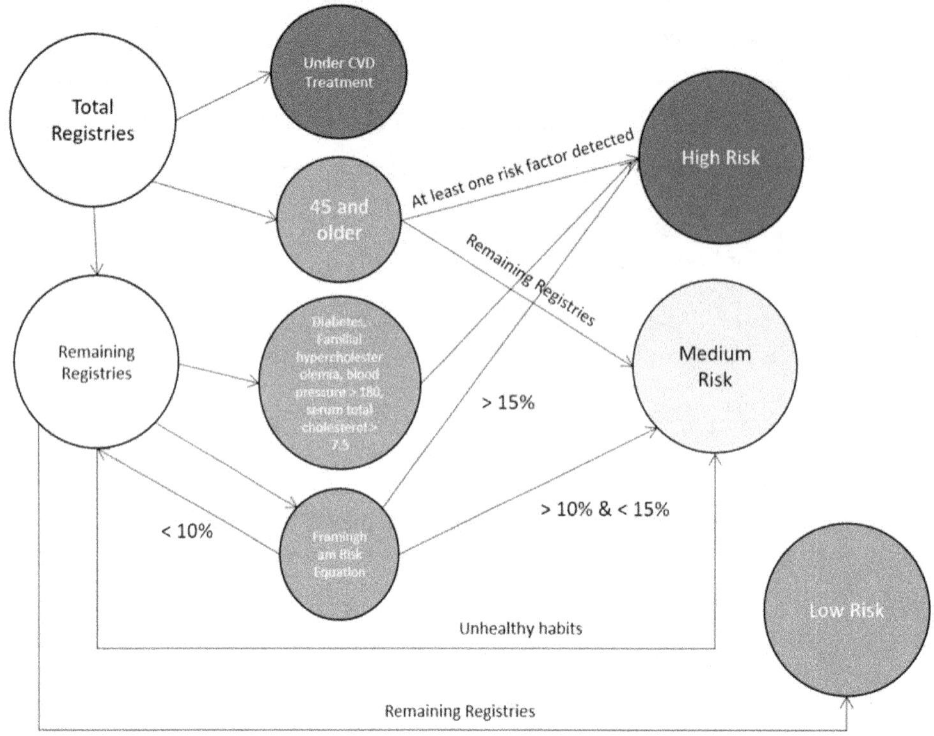

2. Management of hypertension, type 2 diabetes and hyperlipidemia (Table 3).
3. Antithrombotic therapy: dual antiplatelet therapy with a P2Y12 inhibitor added to aspirin, clopidogrel, dipyridamole plus aspirin, aspirin alone.
4. Interventions to ensure medication adherence and cardiovascular disease prevention programmes (nurse, physician, cardiologist and others).

Aspirin or other antiplatelet therapy is not routinely recommended for primary prevention of CVD, however the American College of Chest Physicians, proposes for antithrombotic therapy and prevention of thrombosis:

Table 3. Management of hypertension

Hypertension	Type 2 Diabetes	Hyperlipidemia
Lifestyle measures, antihypertensive drug treatment (diuretics, angiotensin-converting enzyme [ACE] inhibitors, calcium antagonists, angiotensin receptor antagonists, and beta-blockers), risk stratification using SCORE, antiplatelet therapy.	Targeted glycated haemoglobin (HbA1c), Statins, Avoiding hypoglycaemia and excessive weight gain, metformin as first-line therapy, establishing targets for blood pressure and low-density lipoprotein (LDL)-cholesterol levels	Establishing target levels of total plasma cholesterol and LDL-cholesterol, intervention strategies based on total cardiovascular risk and LDL-cholesterol level, statins, lifestyle interventions.

Primary Prevention

1. **Aspirin Therapy:** 75-100 mg/aspirin for persons aged 50 years or older without symptomatic cardiovascular disease. Individuals who value preventing an MI substantially higher than avoiding a gastrointestinal (GI) bleed will be, if they are in the moderate or high cardiovascular risk group, more likely to choose aspirin.

Secondary Prevention

1. **Choice of Long-Term Antithrombotic Therapy in Patients With Established Coronary Artery Disease (CAD):** Recommends long-term single antiplatelet therapy with aspirin 75 to 100 mg daily or clopidogrel 75 mg daily over no antiplatelet therapy and suggests single over dual antiplatelet therapy with aspirin plus clopidogrel.
2. **Choice of Antithrombotic Therapy Following ACS:**
    a. For patients in the first year after an ACS who have not undergone percutaneous coronary intervention (PCI):
    b. For patients in the first year after an ACS who have undergone PCI with stent placement:
    c. For patients with ACS who undergo PCI with stent placement, the expert panel refers to "Antithrombotic Therapy Following Elective PCI," below for recommendations concerning minimum and prolonged duration of treatment.
    d. For patients with anterior MI and left ventricular (LV) thrombus, or at high risk for LV thrombus (ejection fraction <40%, anteroapical wall motion abnormality), who do not undergo stenting:
    e. For patients with anterior MI and LV thrombus, or at high risk for LV thrombus (ejection fraction <40%, anteroapical wall motion abnormality), who undergo bare-metal stent (BMS) placement:
    f. For patients with anterior MI and LV thrombus, or at high risk for LV thrombus (ejection fraction <40%, anteroapical wall motion abnormality) who undergo drug-eluting stent (DES) placement:

Management

Lifestyle to Reduce Cardiovascular Risk

1. Dietary Pattern
    a. Intake of vegetables, fruits, and whole grains, low-fat dairy products, poultry, fish, legumes, nontropical vegetable oils, and nuts;
    b. Limits intake of sweets, sugar-sweetened beverages, and red meats.
2. Adapt this dietary pattern to appropriate calorie requirements, personal and cultural food preferences, and nutrition therapy for other medical conditions (including diabetes).
3. Achieve this pattern by following plans such as the Dietary Approaches to Stop Hypertension (DASH) dietary pattern, the U.S. Department of Agriculture (USDA) Food Pattern, or the AHA Diet.

4. Aim for a dietary pattern that achieves 5% to 6% of calories from saturated fat.
5. Reduce percent of calories from saturated fat.
6. Reduce percent of calories from *trans*-fat.

Blood Pressure (BP)

1. Dietary pattern
2. Lower sodium intake.
3. a. Consume no more than 2,400 mg of sodium/d; b. Further reduction of sodium intake to 1,500 mg/d can result in even greater reduction in BP; and c. Even without achieving these goals, reducing sodium intake by at least 1,000 mg/d lowers BP.
4. Combine the DASH dietary pattern with lower sodium intake.
5. Drug monotherapy with any one of the following agents: Angiotensin-converting enzyme (ACE) inhibitor, angiotensin receptor blocker, calcium channel blocker, low dose thiazide or thiazide-like diuretic. If monotherapy does not sufficiently reduce blood pressure add a second agent from a different pharmacological class (NGC, 2013).
6. Blood pressure-lowering therapy in people with diabetes should preferentially include an ACE inhibitor or angiotensin receptor blocker and if it does not sufficiently reduce blood pressure add one of the following: calcium channel blocker or low-dose thiazide or thiazide-like diuretic. In people with CKD should begin with an ACE inhibitor or angiotensin receptor blocker (NGC, 2013).

Physical Activity

Aerobic physical activity: 3–4 sessions per week, lasting on average 40 minutes per session, and involving moderate- to vigorous-intensity physical activity: to reduce LDL-C and non-high-density lipoprotein cholesterol (non–HDL-C) and to lower blood pressure.

Dyslipidemia

1. Mediterranean dietary model and to eat fish as a source of omega-3 acids and unsaturated fats as part of the Mediterranean diet.
2. Daily consumption of fruit and vegetables
3. Alcohol consumption must not exceed 2 units* daily of alcohol in men and 1 unit daily in women: 1 unit of alcohol is equal to 1 small glass of wine, 1 beer, half a glass of brandy or one coffee with brandy. 2 units of alcohol are equal to 1 glass of wine, a glass of brandy, or one rum and Coke highball or similar.
4. Aerobic-intensive exercise such as walking, running, moderately strenuous swimming for at least 30 minutes, five days per week; or strenuous activity for at least 20 minutes, three days per week.
5. If there are overweight or obesity, the recommendation is to reduce calorie intake and to increase physical activity.
6. Dieting and physical activity is recommended for prior 6 months to beginning the drug therapy.

7. Drug therapy: Statins should be used as first-line therapy.
   a. **Primary Prevention:** Therapy should begin with low to mild dose statin in patients with isolated levels of total cholesterol higher than 320 mg/dl and/or LDL-c levels of 240 mg/dl. If the individual has intolerance to statins is to insist on non-drug therapy and to lower the dose or change to another statin (Ezetimibe, bile acid binding resin and Nicotinic acid).
   b. Secondary prevention depends of the cardiovascular disease: treatment with mild statin doses in patients with ischaemic heart disease, individuals discharged from hospital after acute coronary syndromes, in patients with ischaemic ictus of atherothrombotic origin and no ischaemic heart disease and patients with peripheral arterial disease and related comorbidity.
   c. If low-density lipoprotein cholesterol (LDL-C) levels are not sufficiently reduced on maximally tolerated dose of statin, one or more of the following may be added: ezetimibe, bile acid binding resin, nicotinic acid.

If triglyceride levels remain elevated, treatment with one of the following may be considered:

- Fenofibrate (especially if high-density lipoprotein [HDL] is below target), nicotinic acid, fish oil.

A set of recommendations for every risk level is presented in Table 4.

Table 4. Recommendations for CVD absolute risk

	<10%	10% to <20%	20% to <30%	≥ 30%
Classification	Low risk	Moderate risk	High risk	Very high risk
Smoking			Nicotine replacement therapy and/or nortriptyline or amfebutamone (bupropion)	
Antihypertensive drugs	Persistent blood pressure ≥140/90			Persistent blood pressure ≥130/80
	Should continue lifestyle strategies to lower blood pressure and have their blood pressure.		Are unable to lower blood pressure through lifestyle strategies.	Should reduce blood pressure and risk of cardiovascular disease through drugs.
Antiplatelet drugs	For individuals in this risk category, the harm caused by aspirin treatment outweighs the benefits. Aspirin should not be given to individuals in this low-risk category.	For individuals in this risk category, the benefits of aspirin treatment are balanced by the harm caused. Aspirin should not be given to individuals in this risk category.	For individuals in this risk category, the balance of benefits and harm from aspirin treatment is not clear. Aspirin should probably not be given to individuals in this risk category.	Individuals in this risk category should be given low-dose aspirin.
	Should be advised to follow a lipid-lowering die.	Should be advised to follow a lipid-lowering diet.	Adults >40 years with persistently high serum cholesterol (>5.0 mmol/l) and/or LDL cholesterol >3.0 mmol/l, despite a lipid-lowering diet, should be given a statin. (1+, A).	Individuals in this risk category should be advised to follow a lipid-lowering diet and given a statin. (1++, A) Serum cholesterol should be reduced to less than 5.0 mmol/l (LDL cholesterol to below 3.0 mmol/l) or by 25% (30% for LDL cholesterol), whichever is greater.

PRIVACY AND SECURITY IN HEALTHCARE DATA MANAGEMENT

Based on results presented by the Ponemon Institute (2016), the data breaches in healthcare have been increased in last years, and they estimate a more than $2.2 million cost to healthcare industry. Their report shows that the common causes of data breaches are criminal attacks, employee negligence, third-party snafus, stolen computing devices, mobile device insecurity, and use of public cloud services. All those threats are scaled when working with big data tools, since all information is collected and made available through a unique platform for further analysis. For ensuring privacy and security on governmental data, The United State Congress enacted the Health Insurance Portability and Accountability Act in 1996 (HIPAA, 1996). This document establishes that physical or mental health condition of an individual in past, present and future has to be protected. The rules established in the act, gives to health care providers the responsibility of ensuring the good management of information for maintaining privacy and security of data.

The Office of the National Coordinator for Health Information Technology (2015) established a set of features that information tools, used in the healthcare field, have to provide: encryption, auditing functions, backup and recovery routines, unique user ID's and strong passwords, role or user-based access controls, auto time-out, emergency access, amendments and accounting of disclosures. Moreover, in order to reduce risks at data manipulation, the data used for analysis has to be unrelated from patients. Garfinkel (2015) defines de-identification as the process to move data linked to a specific individual to a set of data that cannot be related to individuals; between these two sets, other 3 sets are established: data that can be unambiguously linked to a specific individual, data that can be ambiguously linked several individuals, and data that cannot be linked to any individual. With this classification of data, de-identification reduces the privacy risk by moving data linked to a specific individual to one of the other sets. For performing this movement, Emam and Malin (2015) proposed a process of eleven steps: 1) determine direct identifiers in the dataset, 2) mask (transform) direct identifiers, 3) perform threat modeling, 4) determine minimal acceptable data utility, 5) determine the re-identification risk threshold, 6) import (sample) data from the source database, 7) evaluate the actual re-identification risk, 8) compare the actual risk with the threshold, 9) set parameters and apply data transformations, 10) perform diagnostics on the solution, and 11) export transformed data to external data set.

The methodology proposed above offers good results when working with structured data, but every day a lot of unstructured data is also generated from the healthcare field, which needs to be analyzed too. Researchers of MIT (Douglas, Clifford, Reisner, Long, Moody, and Mark, 2005) proposed an algorithm for removing names, geographic subdivisions, dates, ages, phone numbers, social security numbers, and medical record numbers from free-text nursing notes. Also Dehghan, Kovacevic, Karystianis, Keane, and Nenadic (2015) proposed a machine learning algorithm to identify names, profession, locations, contacts, ids, ages, and dates from clinical narratives. However, many of the data generated in the healthcare field, come from radiology, ultrasonography, tomography, magnetic resonance imaging, among other areas where the resultant data are images. Medical images are stored and shared with DICOM standard. This standard, allows to maintain together the identity data and the image. For working with images while the risk of identification is reduced, a de-identification process has to be performed over DICOM images. Aryanto, van Kernebeek, Berendsen, Oudkerk, and van Ooijen (2016) proposed to eliminate or pseudonymise header information, and remove pixels that could contain sensitive data. This process has to be performed before transmitting images over network to prevent privacy breaches.

CHALLENGES IN HEALTHCARE DATA USE

Great advances in storing, retrieving, and analyzing big data in the healthcare field have been achieved in last years; however, those approaches, as this work too, have focused on a specific group or area into the healthcare field. For gaining accuracy and confidence in data analysis, it is required to include data from every available source and provide tools to manage and analyze such data. Most platforms are designed to manipulate structured data or unstructured data in text format. It is required to develop applications that mix audio, web, video, pictures, databases, data obtained from mobile apps, and data obtained from sensors. Collecting data from several sources is challenging, more when every developer follows their own formats to store them. It is required to establish standards for generating, storing and retrieving data related to healthcare in order to increase the availability of data, and reduce the complexity of integrating all generated data for later analysis. When data is obtained from mobile devices, wearable sensors, and clinical records, the user's' privacy has to be maintained; also, secure protocols for collecting that information are required to avoid the identification of persons through use patterns or data location. Some categories where improvements can be proposed are described below.

- **Data Format:** Collected data is stored in structured, semi-structured, and unstructured format. Complexity arises when information has to be discovered through diverse data sources due to every source represents data in different ways according to the needs of the institution where it is generated. Standards about data format and tools for transforming them among formats have to be proposed in order to reduce the handling complexity.
- **Frameworks:** A lot of data is generated every second in the healthcare field; however, a pre-processing stage, semi-automated in some cases, is performed before sharing data for further analysis. If decision makers want to use updated data, it is necessary to be tracking every source, transform, clean, and upload data to some platform or application for performing the analysis. This behavior establishes the necessity of developing frameworks which could gather, preprocess, clean, and standardize all generated data, in such a way that the user can make use of the data through a simple interface.
- **Privacy and Security:** Since data comes from many sources and has to be distributed over the Internet, it is required to remove data fields that can be used for identifying individuals. De-identification techniques need to be standardized in order to determine what values have to be removed for maintaining privacy. When data is transmitted over networks, it is susceptible to be intercepted by intruders. Mechanisms are required, which allow to determine in what point over the network data was extracted; also, to know what data was stolen is important for identifying the risk to which users could be exposed. That information can be used by authorities to identify intruders and avoid a redistribution of stolen data.
- **Data Sharing:** Healthcare data is generated from sources who are located in many places around the world. Vast majority of institutions have access to Internet; however, there are regions where Internet connection is not available; in such cases, government could propose policies for transmitting health data through satellite in order to maintain the collection of updated data. Store all data in only one place is risky and unfeasible; this situation requires data sharing mechanisms which allow to gather information from every source when required in order to generate better

analysis. While bigger the sets of data transmitted are, more bandwidth is required to maintain the data transmission velocity. Network protocols could be established to share healthcare data; those protocols could select better routes for transmission according to the location where the data is required. All those approaches will improve real time big data applications in the healthcare field.

CONCLUSION

Production of large amounts of data in the healthcare field, opens the possibility to have a change in the way of diagnosing diseases. The diagnosis can be supported with information about accurate family history and group of patients with same symptoms in other regions of the world; also, treatments with good historical results can be applied over patients with similar characteristics. Including Big Data in the healthcare field contributes to the reduction of costs and the increasing of the effectiveness of treatments since a lot of information for supporting the decision-taking process is available. This chapter presented some advances in managing big data in the healthcare field, and a set of sources where data related to healthcare field can be obtained. A methodology was proposed, for including big data in the detection, prevention and management of the CVD. A list of challenges to be performed in order to take more advantage of the available data was presented, and some recommendations to maintain privacy and security of patients were included.

REFERENCES

Anderson, K. M., Wilson, P. W. F., Odell, P. M., & Kannel, W. B. (1991). An updated coronary risk profile: A statement for health professionals. *Circulation*, *83*, 357–363. doi:10.1161/01.CIR.83.1.356

Perk, J. et al.. (2012). European guidelines on cardiovascular disease prevention in clinical practice. *European Heart Journal*, *33*(13), 1635–1701. doi:10.1093/eurheartj/ehs092

Alexander, C. A., & Wang, L. (2017). Big data analytics in heart attack prediction. *The Journal of Nursing Care*, *6*(393). doi:10.4172/2167-1168.1000393

Antman, E. M., Benjamin, E. J., Harrington, R. A., Houser, S. R., Peterson, E. D., Bauman, M. A., & Wayte, P. et al. (2015). Acquisition, analysis, and sharing of data in 2015 and beyond: A survey of the landscape. *Journal of the American Heart Association*, *4*(11), e002810. doi:10.1161/JAHA.115.002810 PMID:26541391

Aryanto, K. Y. E., van Kernebeek, G., Berendsen, B., Oudkerk, M., & van Ooijen, P. M. A. (2016). Image de-identification methods for clinical research in the XDS environment. *Journal of Medical Systems*, *40*(4), 1–8. doi:10.1007/s10916-016-0431-7 PMID:26811074

Auffray, C. (2016). Making sense of big data in health research: Towards an EU action plan. *Genome Medicine*, *8*(71), 1–13. doi:10.1186/s13073-016-0323-y PMID:26750923

Big Data Value Association. (2016). *Big Data Technologies in Healthcare, Needs, opportunities and challenges*. TF/Healthcare subgroup.

Centers for Disease Control and Prevention. (2017). *Interactive atlas of heart disease and stroke*. Retrieved from the Centers for Disease Control and Prevention website: https://nccd.cdc.gov/dhdspatlas/

Dehghan, A., Kovacevic, A., Karystianis, G., Keane, J. A., & Nenadic, G. (2015). Combining knowledge and data-driven methods for de-identification of clinical narratives. *Journal of Biomedical Informatics*, *58*(1), S53–S59. doi:10.1016/j.jbi.2015.06.029 PMID:26210359

Douglas, M. M., Clifford, G. D., Reisner, A., Long, W. J., Moody, G. B., & Mark, R. G. (2005). De-identification algorithm for free-text nursing notes. *Proceedings of Computers in Cardiology*, *05*, 331–334.

Emam, K. E., & Malin, B. (2015). Appendix B: concepts and methods for de-identifying clinical trial data. In *Sharing Clinical Trial Data: Maximizing Benefits, Minimizing Risk* (pp. 203–256). Institute of Medicine of the National Academies.

Fisher, E. S., Wennberg, D. E., Stukel, T. A., Gottlieb, D. J., Lucas, F. L., & Pinder, E. L. (2003). The implications of regional variations in Medicare spending. Part 1: The content, quality, and accessibility of care. *Annals of Internal Medicine*, *138*(4), 273–287. doi:10.7326/0003-4819-138-4-200302180-00006 PMID:12585825

Garfinkel, S. L. (2015). *De-identification of personal information. National Institute of Standards and Technology Internal Report 8053*. Department of Commerce. doi:10.6028/NIST.IR.8053

Guidi, G., Miniati, R., Mazzola, M., & Iadanza, E. (2016). Case study: IBM Watson Analytics cloud platform as analytics-as-a-service system for heart failure early detection. *Future Internet*, *8*(32), 1–16. doi:10.3390/fi8030032

HIPAA. (1996). *Health Insurance Portability and Accountability Act of 1996. 104th United State Congress*.

Informatica. (2012). *Healthcare data management: expanding insight, increasing efficiency, improving care*. Informatica Corporation.

Krumholz, H. M. (2008). Outcomes research: Generating evidence for best practice and policies. *Circulation*, *118*(3), 309–318. doi:10.1161/CIRCULATIONAHA.107.690917 PMID:18625906

Lampropulos, J. F., Gupta, A., Kulkarni, V. T., Mody, P., Chen, R., Bikdeli, B., & Dharmarajan, K. (2013). Most important outcomes research papers on variation in cardiovascular disease. *Circulation: Cardiovascular Quality and Outcomes*, *6*(2), e9–e16. doi:10.1161/CIRCOUTCOMES.113.000185 PMID:23481532

Li, D., Park, H. W., Batbaatar, E., Piao, Y., & Ryu, K. H. (2016). Design of health care system for disease detection and prediction on Hadoop using DM techniques. In *Proceedings of the 2nd International Conference on Health Informatics and Medical Systems* (pp. 124-129). Las Vegas, NV: WORLDCOMP.

Li, Y., Wu, C., Guo, L., Lee, C. H., & Guo, Y. (2014). Wiki-Health: a big data platform for health sensor data management. In A. Moumtzoglou & A. Kastania (Eds.), *Cloud Computing Applications for Quality Health Care Delivery* (pp. 59–77). Hershey, PA: IGI Global. doi:10.4018/978-1-4666-6118-9.ch004

Loghmanpour, N. A., Kormos, R. L., Kanwar, M. K., Teuteberg, J. J., Murali, S., & Antaki, J. F. (2016). A Bayesian model to predict right ventricular failure following left ventricular assist device therapy. *JACC: Heart Failure*, *4*(9), 722–725. doi:10.1016/j.jchf.2016.04.004 PMID:27289403

Motwani, M. (2017). Machine learning for prediction of all-cause mortality in patients with suspected coronary artery disease: A 5-year multicentre prospective registry analysis. *European Heart Journal*, *38*, 500–507. doi:10.1093/eurheartj/ehw188 PMID:27252451

National Guideline Clearinghouse. (2013). *Guideline summary: 2013 AHA/ACC guideline on lifestyle management to reduce cardiovascular risk: a report of the American College of Cardiology/American Heart Association Task Force on Practice Guidelines*. Rockville, MD: Agency for Healthcare Research and Quality (AHRQ). Available: https://www.guideline.gov

Niño, M., & Illarramendi, A. (2015). Understanding big data: Antecedents, origin and later development. *DYNA New Technologies*, *2*, 1–8. doi:10.6036/NT7835

Ostankov, A., Röhrbein, F., & Waltinger, U. (2014). LinkedHealthAnswers: towards linked data-driven question answering for the healthcare domain. In *Proceedings of the Ninth International Conference on Language Resources and Evaluation* (pp. 2613-2620). Reykjavik, Iceland: ELRA.

Ponemon Institute. (2016). *Sixth annual benchmark study on privacy & security of healthcare data*. Ponemon Institute LLC.

Rumsfeld, J. S., Joynt, K. E., & Maddox, T. M. (2016). Big data analytics to improve cardiovascular care: Promise and challenges. *Nature Reviews. Cardiology*, *13*(6), 250–359. doi:10.1038/nrcardio.2016.42 PMID:27009423

Scruggs, S. B., Watson, K., Su, A. I., Hermjakob, H., Yates, J. R. III, Lindsey, M. L., & Ping, P. (2015). Harnessing the heart of big data. *Circulation Research*, *116*(7), 1115–1119. doi:10.1161/CIRCRESAHA.115.306013 PMID:25814682

Stonová, M. (2014). Unstructured data in healthcare. *International Journal on Biomedicine and Healthcare*, *2*(1), 34–36.

The Office of the National Coordinator for Health Information Technology. (2015). *Guide to privacy and security of electronic health information*. HHS.

Tsoi, K. K. F., Chan, F. C. H., Hirai, H. W., Leung, G. K. S., Kuo, Y. H., Tai, S., & Meng, H. (2017). Data visualization on global trends on cancer incidence an application of IBM Watson Analytics. In *Proceedings of the 50th Hawaii International Conference on System Sciences* (pp. 3283-3288). Waikoloa, HI: UH Mānoa Shidler College of Business. doi:10.24251/HICSS.2017.397

Vaishali, G., & Kalaivani, V. (2016). Big data analysis for heart disease detection system using map reduce technique. In *Proceedings of the 2016 International Conference on Computing Technologies and Intelligent Data Engineering* (pp. 1-6). Kovilpatti, India: IEEE. doi:10.1109/ICCTIDE.2016.7725360

World Health Organization. (2016). *HEARTS: Technical package for cardiovascular disease management in primary health care*. Geneva, Switzerland: World Health Organization.

ADDITIONAL READING

Copper, T., & Collman, J. (2005). Managing information security and privacy in healthcare data mining: state of the art. In H. Chen, S. S. Fuller, C. Friedman, & W. Hersh (Eds.), *Medical Informatics, 8* (pp. 95–137). Springer. doi:10.1007/0-387-25739-X_4

NVPDA. (2012). *Guidelines for the management of absolute cardiovascular disease risk.* National Stroke Foundation.

KEY TERMS AND DEFINITIONS

Big Data: A term used to reference a large data sizes, usually in the range of petabytes and up.

Cardiovascular Disease: Class of diseases related to heart conditions, blood vessels state, and circulation.

Data Mining: Set of techniques employed to extract data from several sources.

Data Science: Discipline that uses data mining and statistic to discover information hidden on raw data.

De-Identification: Process of removing identifiers from data which allow to identify unambiguously to an individual.

Structured Data: Set of data stored in an organized way like a database or in XML format.

Unstructured Data: Set of data extracted directly from texts, pictures or videos, where there is not a predefined structure.

Chapter 8
Improvement of Railway Transportation System Using IoT Applications and Services

Sudesh Kumar
Indira Gandhi National Tribal University, India

Ram Shringar Raw
Indira Gandhi National Tribal University, India

ABSTRACT

In this chapter, the authors have introduced the use of Internet of Things (IoT) applications and services in Indian Railway Transportation System (IRTS). Railway transportation infrastructure is one of the most important factors for the development of any country. India is a developing country and we have a vision to transform India into a developed nation by 2020 using different technologies and tools. Therefore, we need to adopt smart and secure technology for advancement in each area especially in railway transportation for growth and betterment of the country. Further, authors has introduced Vehicular Ad-Hoc Network (VANET) concept for automatic railway gate controlling system to reduce number of accidents over railway premises and enhance the system components for the Indian railway transportation system to provide the comfort, security, safety and infotainment services to the passengers.

1. INTRODUCTION

By railway statics 2014 Synopsis, railway transported 8.397 billion passengers and over 106 million tonnes of freight annually. Most probably, passenger rail traffic globally is expected to double by 2020, posing a challenge for train operators and commuters' alike. As tens of thousands of sensors have been already deployed along with rail roadsides, rail tracks, and on trains in many countries, but in India it's not implemented up to the mark. Everyone has a story about how a broken down train ruined their day. But with recent advancements in maintenance, improving the reliability because of IoT applications, trains themselves has become smart device with sensor nodes on critical parts such as brakes, wheels and engines. Tracks are also benefitted from IoT where some train networks have thousands of sensor

DOI: 10.4018/978-1-5225-5222-2.ch008

Copyright © 2018, IGI Global. Copying or distributing in print or electronic forms without written permission of IGI Global is prohibited.

nodes deployed across their systems, measuring track stress and condition, air and track temperatures, and other variables that have predictive value to maintenance teams.

In recent year the Internet of Things (IoT) is receiving much research attention and effort from industry and academia worldwide. It is provided the back born to the modern society. The IoT is the inter networking of physical devices, vehicles or nodes (also referred to as "connected devices" and "smart devices"), buildings, and other items embedded with electronics, software, sensors, actuators, and network connectivity that enable these objects to collect and exchange data.

The Internet of Things term is introduced by Kevin Ashton executive director of the Auto-ID Centre Massachusetts Institute of Technology (MIT). The IoT is a computing concept that describes the idea of everyday physical objects being connected to the internet and being able to identify themselves to other devices and share the information and date. The term is closely identified with RFID (Radio-frequency identification uses electromagnetic fields to automatically identify and track tags attached to objects) as the method of communication, although it also may include other advanced sensor technologies, wireless technologies or QR (Quick Response) codes (Ashton, K. 2009). In the five-year span between 2015 and 2020, IoT will grow faster than any other category of connected devices, according to a new Cisco report, (Figure 1) the number of machine-to-machine (M2M) connections should grow nearly 2.5-fold, from 4.9 billion in 2015 to 12.2 billion in 2020 (Cisco, VNI. 2017).

In short, the IoT refers to the rapidly growing network of connected objects that are able to collect and exchange data using embedded sensors. In IoT environment, an entity uses a remote like smart phone, Tablet, smart watch or device etc. to send a command, or a request for information over a network to an IoT device. Then the device performs the command and sends information back over the network to be

Figure 1. Global M2M Connections / IoT growth by vertical
Source: Cisco VNI Global IP Traffic Forecast, 2015–2020

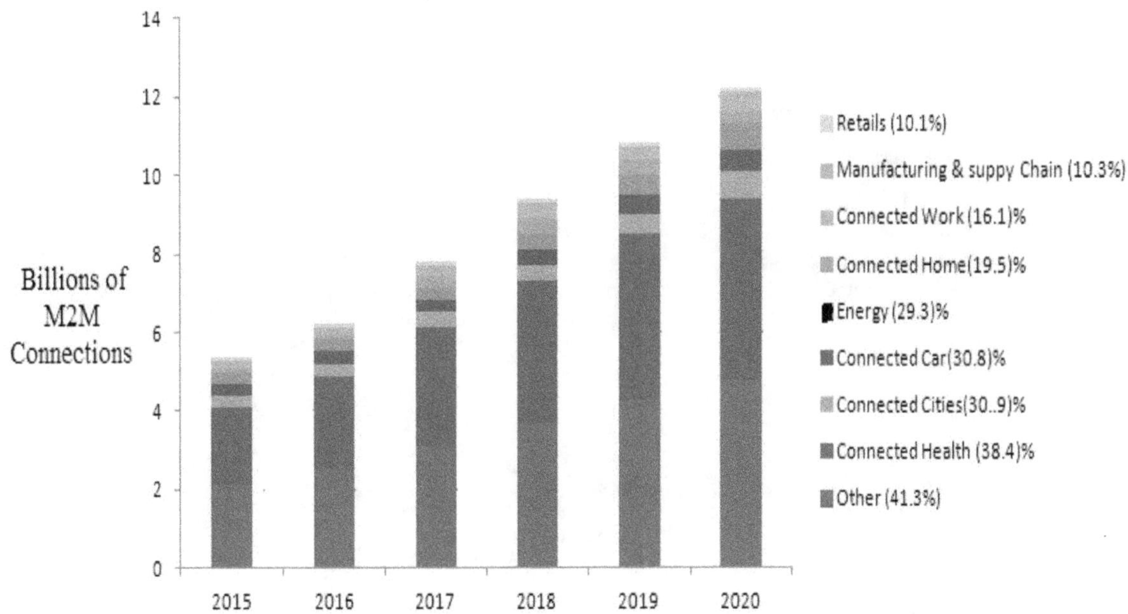

**For a more accurate representation see the electronic version.*

analysed and displayed on the remote. There are multiple locations in which the data generated by the IoT device can be analyse and stored, including the cloud, a local data base, on the remote, or locally, on the IoT device itself (Figure 2).

IoT devices is going beyond laptops and smart phones; it is going towards connected smart home, cars, connected wearable, smart industries, agriculture, smart cities, transportation and connected health care. According to the Gartner report, by 2020 connected devices across all technologies will reach to 20.6 billion. These devices will bridge the gap between physical and digital world to improve the quality, value and effective productivity of life and society. Because of actively growing field, below authors will discuss some popular applications of IoTs which show how it will transform our lives.

Now a day's Smart home is the most popular application of IoT infrastructure. Which are allowing homeowners to monitor and control a wide range of useful applications such as improved energy efficiency, access control, security & privacy, fire detection and home monitoring, etc. Consider a real scenario before reaching home you could switch on air conditioning and switch off lights even after you have left home, also unlock the doors to family members or friends for temporary access even when you are not at home. Amazon Echo is popular example, which works through its voice assistant, in which users can talk to in order to perform a variety of functions. Users can tell to playing music, provide a weather report, and get sports scores, order a cab and many more.

With the continuously growth of population, demand for food supply is extremely raised. The Governments of India are helping farmers to use advanced techniques and technology to increase quality food production. IoT is one of the fastest growing technologies which can help to Smart farming. New advance IoT applications, increasing the quality, quantity, sustainability and cost effectiveness of agricultural production. Sensing for soil moisture with nutrients and controlling water usage of plant are some simplest uses of IoT. It is also includes smart GPS based remote controlled robot to perform tasks like weeding, spraying, moisture sensing, keeping vigilance, etc. into the field of agriculture to overcome farmer work.

Figure 2. Basic Working environment of IoT devices

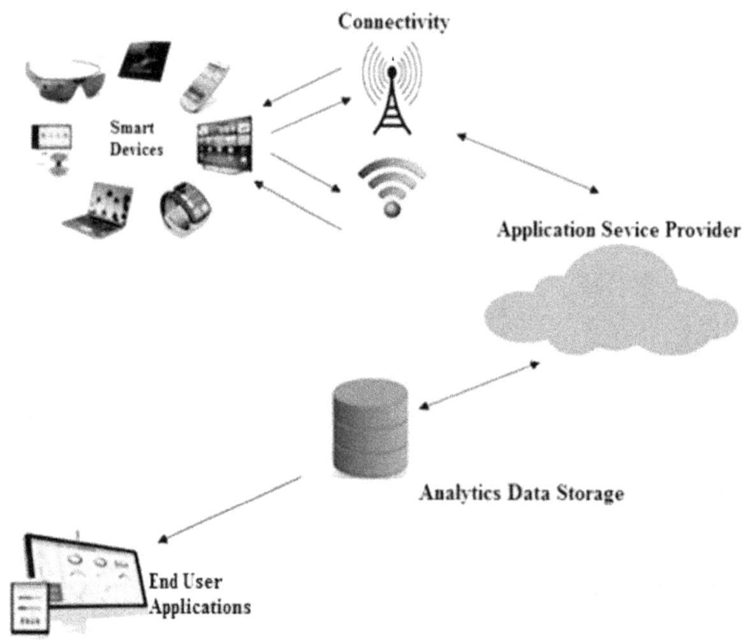

IoT application for wearable remains a hot topic too. These devices have explosive demand in markets all over the world. Companies like Google, Samsung have invested heavily in building such smart devices, because of the huge demand of these high energy efficient or ultra-low power and small sized. FuGeX is a deloitte award-winning wearable IoT application development company in India and USA. Basically wearable devices are installed with sensors and software which collect data and information about the users. This data is later reprocessed to extract important and essential insights about the user. These attractive devices broadly cover fitness, health and entertainment requirements fields. The apple watch and other smart watches on the market have turned our wrists into smart phone holsters by enabling text messaging, phone calls, and many more.

A smart city is an urban development vision to integrate multiple Information Communication Technology (ICT) and IoT solutions in a secure fashion to manage a city's assets like traffic, transportation, library, schools, hospitals, water supply management, waste management, smart surveillance and environmental monitoring all are examples of internet of things applications for smart cities. IoT will solve major problems faced by the people living in cities. The Spanish city Barcelona is one of the foremost smart cities in the world after it implemented several IoT initiatives that have helped enhance smart parking and the environment.

Researcher shows IoT in health care will be massive in coming years. The main objective to uses of IoT devices is empowering peoples healthy life by wearing connected devices. IoT in health care is a heterogeneous computing, wireless communicating system of applications and devices that connects patient and wellness providers to diagnose, monitor, track and store vital statics and medical data. Large figure of advantages of IoT devices in the field of healthcare likes.

Figure 3. Popular applications of Internet of Things

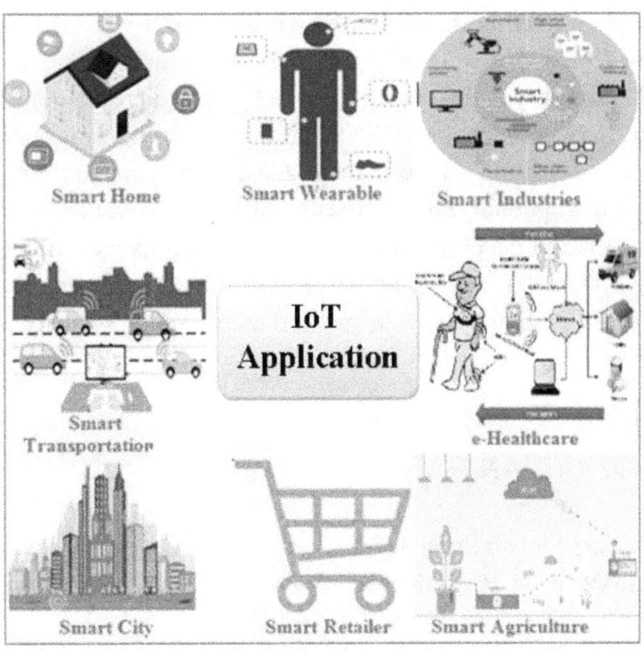

- It is reduced health care costs by allowing medical staff to remotely work together and instantly access patient data.
- Headset that measure brainwaves.
- BP and Glucose monitors
- Monitor the consumption of medicines on time.
- This application now lets patients schedule their appointments without the need to visit a doctor's office and wait for a receptionist.
- Wireless sensor embedded in medical equipment, dispensing systems, surgical robots and device implants.
- Transform the patient data generated in an ambulance during the transit to the hospitals and doctors in real time, therefore making the emergency care more efficient.

  In India, IOT can also aid in monitoring the supervision of the rural and tribal health care units, can prepare the skilled doctors available remotely and make the health care more affordable.

It offers an opportunity for retailers to link with the customers to enhance the in-store experience. The smart phone is solution for retailers to remain united with their consumers even out of the store. They can also track consumers' path through a memory board and improve store layout and place premium products in high traffic regions.

With billions of things already connected to the internet, It sustains a great potential to transform industries, businesses, decision making, digitalisation, network centric, automated, improving quality, automation, validation, security etc. in the area of growing smart industries.

The IoT initiatives to commute hassles, secure, safe and simplify transportation for millions around the world with the help of IoT platform. By utilising this platform building an intelligent transportation system is very easy which provides real-time vehicle tracking and optimization of logistics and public transit systems, Asset management and tracking, Web based queries and reports.

The future of IoT is more riveting than this where billions of things will be blabbing to each other and human interface will get lost. Not only IoT applications are enhancing our comfort, but they likewise present us more control to simplify daily routine work and personal project. The main aim of this chapter is to first identify the primary component of IRTS and then offers the solutions for improvement these components with the help of IoT and sensor network technology. Furthermore, proposed a concept by applying VANET technology, popular applications of MANET (Mobile Ad-hoc Network) which is a promising field for research and development of wireless networks and IoT technology for automatic railway gate controlling system to reduce the number of accidents and enhance the system components of the Indian railway transportation system to provide the comfort, security, safety and infotainment services to the passengers.

2. COMPONENTS OF INDIAN RAILWAY

On 26th February 2015, Shri Suresh Prabhu, Minister for Railways presented the Rail Budget in Lok Sabha, which was acclaimed by the Prime Minister for the technology-driven measures announced. The

Rail Budget 2015 proposed all-embracing use of Information Technology and e-Governance initiatives in Railway functioning. Corporate India termed the budget, as 'Technology-Enabled Traveller-Centric' (Rajnish Kumar, 2015).

Indian Railway was released official figures in 2012-13 on an average, on any given day, 12617 trains were running on Indian Railway tracks. The total number of passengers carried in 2012-13 was 8.421 billion and 23.07 million passengers were on the move on any given day. About 1.9% of India's total population was on trains, on any given day. Now present scenario, it gets a huge amount of data. Thus the huge of improvements are required to straighten to Indian railway. As tens of thousands of sensors have been already deployed along with rail roadsides, rail tracks, and on trains in many countries, but in India it's not implemented up to the mark. India is a developing country and we have a vision to transform India into a developed nation by 2020 using different technologies as tools.

Firstly authors describe main components of IRTS (M H Eiza et al., 2015) and then provide some solution of these components with the help of IoT technology and tools for improvement in this system.

2.1 Basic Components of IRTS

- **Trains:** Each train is composed by many coaches with powerful Engine, where different types of technologies are installed such as heat capacity/seats sensors, Security Camera, beacons, Wi-Fi, etc.
- **Stations:** Place where passengers can get on and off trains and/or goods may be loaded or unloaded, also different objects and systems can be found in a rail station including the rail information system, ticketing system, Wi-Fi, Waiting room, Toilets, Cameras, Check in/out system etc.
- **Tracks:** Tracks only interact with trains and the different zone of rail control system. Different sensor technologies are installed along the tracks to crack/fatigue detection, Out of round wheel detect, RFIDs etc.
- **Passengers:** This part is required the most improvement part of railway system. In India around 50 present uneducated passengers have travelled by train in everyday, so the providing to them smart knowledge of IoT is important task.
- **Railway Crossing Gate:** A railway crossing occurs where a railway line is crossed by a road or path on one level. Now each crossing required men power to open and shut the gate. Then, it is increasing the number of man's power for controlling it and some time human error can make the accidental situation.

Beloved given architecture will help to improve in various stages of Indian railway transportation system. Cloud computing creates a single platform to handle and integrate data from multiple sources and then through the WAN all are monitored by the central monitoring system. All components interact to each other and every component enabled with new smart technology like IoT, sensor, Wi-fi, Camera etc. so all components are become smart component like smart train, smart station, smart passenger, smart track, smart railway crossing gate etc.

Unaccepted circumstances can sometimes disrupt transportation such as like breakdowns, track disconnected, or inclement weather. IoT platform will enable to more easily notify to passengers and help them make alternate arrangements. We will discuss how to improve all these system components.

Figure 4. System Component Architecture Using IoT Devices

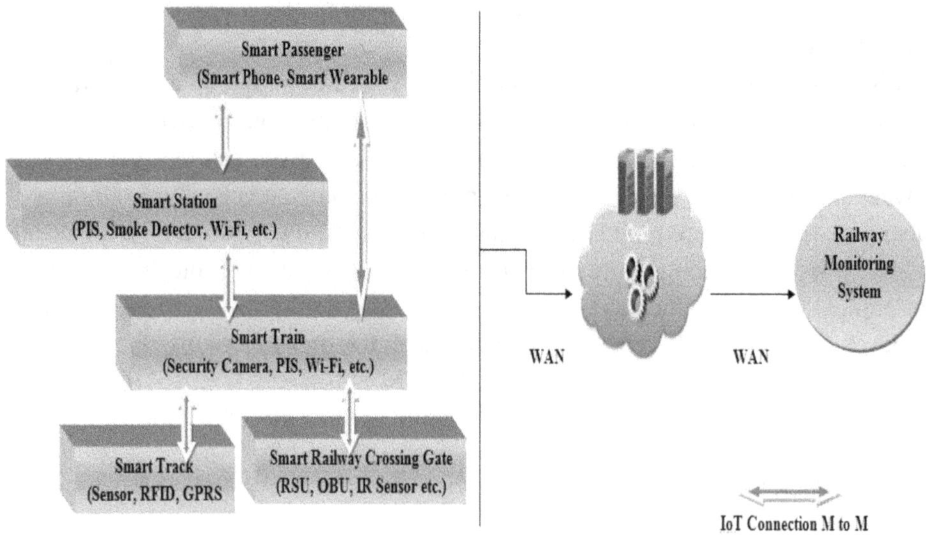

3. IMPROVEMENT FIELD

3.1 Smart Train

Indian Railway Minister Suresh Prabhu said "These new SMART (Specially Modified Aesthetic Refreshing Travel) coaches would cater to the emerging needs of our clients and also ensure lower unit cost of operations due to higher carrying capacity,". The benefit of creating IoT connected trains is various but it is facing a lot of challenges.

But once it is implemented the changes will improve the transportation worlds. Following are some points will improve the train to transform into smart train.

- Smart coaches are configured with passenger information systems (PIS) including audio announcements similar to metro train or planes.
- GPS-based wake up alert system will inform passengers when the train is about to reach their station.
- Every coach provides fully Wi-Fi facility.
- Speed of train needs to be improved.
- Every train with one special pantry car which have on-board self paid vending machines for water, coffee and Snacks for refreshment and it should be prepared to stick to the highest measure and should work through regular quality checks.
- Each coach also equipped smart bio-toilets with sensor-based taps, flushing systems and hand driers.
- For safety and security purpose each coach configured with automatic fire and smoke detection system and also with smart CCTV surveillance system.
- Interactive voice-based assistance from the train operators or conductors to be available.

- To reduce the risk of train collision, on-board train location and detection systems should be there to enable trains to be aware of the location of other trains.
- Some smart device to be available for speed monitoring and control as safety is major concern for passengers. This application have been developed that can display train velocity for drivers and report speeds back to central control systems.
- Enhance the availability of real time data so that Food and drinks can be easily refilled at the next upcoming station based on the items sold.
- Smart device to be used for controlling Temperature to avoid issues with for preserving the food quality over time.
- Real time data use for on board seat availability.
- Awareness should be created among the public and passengers about keeping trains and platforms clean and bigger dustbins in every compartment and they being emptied at every major station.
- Anti-collision devices and sensors should be made mandatory in all trains.
- Railways should acquire modern safety, monitoring and communication equipment with using this smart technology to prevent accidents.

The Global Positioning System is mainly funded and controlled by the U.S. Department of Defence (DOD). The system was initially designed for the operation of U. S. military. But today, there are too many civil users of GPS across the solid globe. GPS mainly devised to locate the place on earth, it helps to determine the location and another way, it is provides accurate and timely information to the controller. The inbuilt GPS module identifies the train location (latitude and longitude values) with a highest accuracy and transmits the information to the central Railway system via high speed internet connectivity like 4G or WiMAX. The availability of this information allows the train controller to take

Figure 5. Smart train embedded with IoT devices

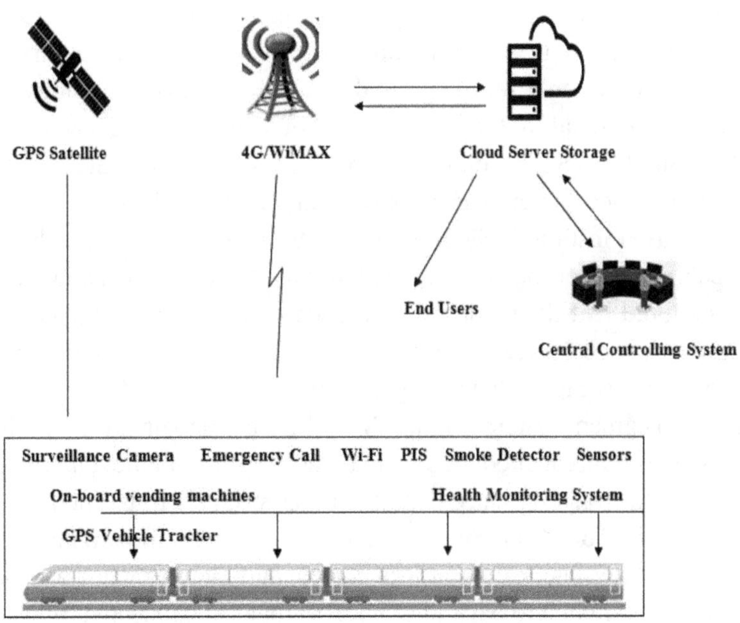

accurate decisions as for the train location. Positioning data can be further processed to provide visual positioning using maps to facilitate accurate scheduling with regards to train arrival and exit on each station (Seokju Lee, Girma Tewolde & JaerockKwon 2014).

Now discuss some IoT devices which are equipped with train for improvement in safety and comfort.

3.1.1 Surveillances Camera

An Internet protocol camera, or IP camera, is a smart IoT device and type of digital video camera which is commonly used for surveillances and can send and receive data via a computer network and the Internet. This IP based systems are becoming an absolute necessity for transportation. Effective video surveillance protects passenger safety and makes transportation services more effective. IP camera provides numerous features.

- Easy installation for different locations on board trains.
- Crystal-clean image quality in a wide dynamic range of dark and light environments.
- Creates a safer environment for passengers.
- High performance video streams for smooth video surveillance.
- Vibration, humidity, and dust resistant devices for harsh on-board environments.
- Secure data transmission through encryption and authentication methods.
- Remote accessibility which allows live video from selected cameras to be viewed on a computer system, smart phone and any other devices (with sufficient access privileges).
- Weatherproof (IP65) with temperature range of -30°C to +60°C (-22°F to +140°F)
- PoE (Power over Ethernet) to supply power through the Ethernet cable and operate without a dedicated power supply.
- Remote monitoring via using 3G/4G/GPRS/Wireless data communications.

A smart camera networks capable of carrying out advanced surveillance tasks with little or no human supervision (Faisal Qureshi & Demetri Terzopoulos. 2008). European countries adopted this smart technology in public transportation a very large scale (figure 6). This technology for the Indian transportation system is more beneficial for the improvement of safety purpose, each train is to be equipped with this IoT device having high configuration like Wi-Fi, visualizing, pixel ratio, Alarm Facility etc.

Although video surveillance camera has already been widely deployed in many public places like airports, hospitals, education institutes, shopping malls, train and bus stations, but Video surveillance systems on moving public transport however, are still offline (i.e., recorded and then analyzed at a later time). A centrally monitored real-time video surveillance system in running vehicles is a very typical task because of technological challenges mainly due to the limited throughput provided by the existing communication technologies at high vehicular speeds (Iftekhar Ahmad & Daryoush Habibi, 2011).

Integrated smart video camera system (Figure 7), real-time video data from multiple video cameras which is configured to smart train can produce an immediate live view of the status both inside and outside their train by the remotely railway vigilance department as well as a train operator. The train operator, whether working on-board or from a control room, can use the information to make loading and unloading passengers more efficiently, check the status of routes, and identify when a passenger train is full.

Real-time video data transmitted to base stations (BS) that are connected to a high speed wide area network (WAN). BSs then forward the video data to a central monitoring or control room where the

Figure 6. Video surveillance in public transportation by A. Soehnchen on March 7, 2016

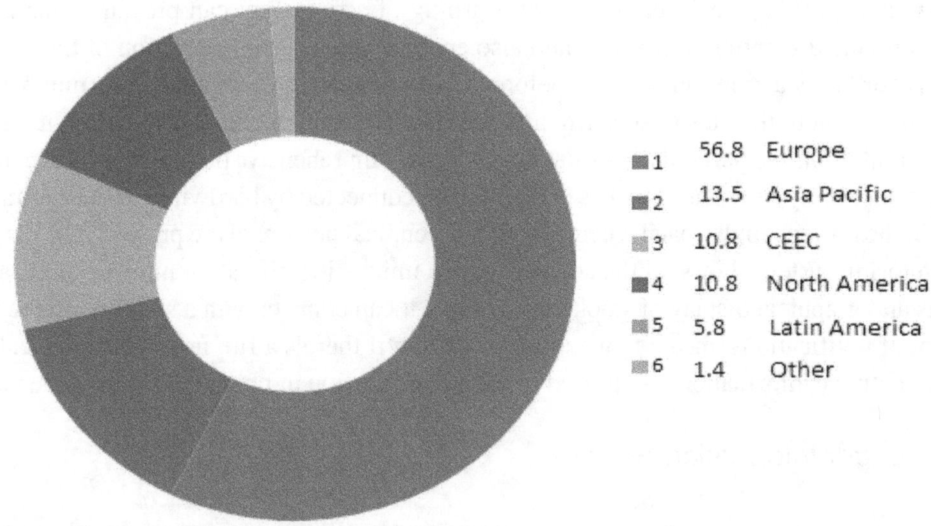

**For a more accurate representation see the electronic version.*

Figure 7. Framework for surveillance camera connected with vigilance department

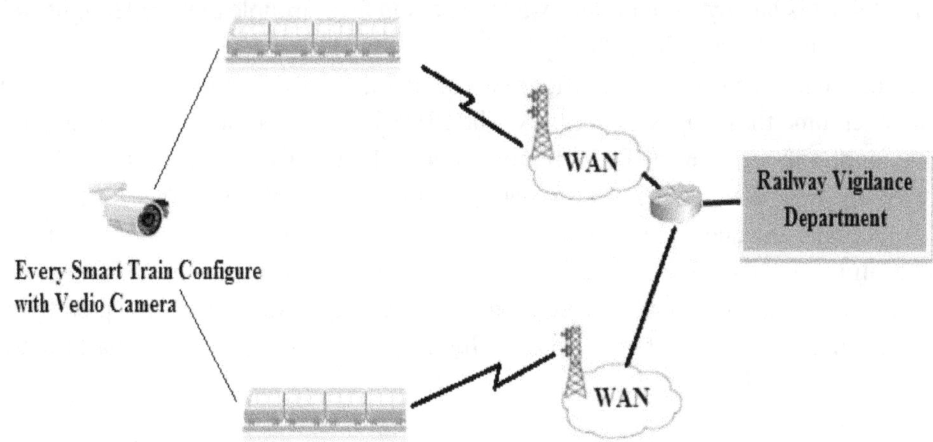

security experts monitor all these things. The IEEE 802.16 (Chuck, D. & Chang, J.M. 2010) also known as WiMAX, is designed to support high capacity, rapid deployment and high speed data rate, through this connectivity, all the real-time video data can be accessed by railway zone vigilance department. Vigilance department has video evidence in the unfortunate case that someone robs your Luggage or commits any other crime.

3.1.2 Smoke Detector System

A smoke detector is a device that senses smoke, typically use as an indicator of fire. In the railway transportation system, fire accidents are occurred due to electrical short circuits, wood materials, flammable materials, derailments, collision, etc. If every rail train is to be fitted with a smart smoke detector system, then it offers the earliest possible warning of a potential fire event by detecting smoke particles at the incipient stage of a fire. Therefore, early warning of a fire event can prevent panic and loss of life and minimizing disruption of services and also enables proactive investigation of the source of the smoke and accordingly action can be taken before the fire escalates. There are a large number of smoke detectors which is more than a smoke alarm and CO detector; they monitor dust, humidity, air quality, temperature, pollution, and particulate, so that we can get a comprehensive picture of the air in the domain.

The fire detection system in all coaches of rail is to be connected by hardwired to the central monitoring system in the power supply coach where electrical/technical personnel are present. The display of the central monitoring system shows all the coaches with a unique identification number on its screen, the alarm status and graphical display of smoke level. Also, it can connect with a smart phone to transmit a wide variety of notifications, meaning it can let you know if there's a fire in some coach, call the train operator and then the information also passed to the nearest station in-charge or fire brigade via internet.

3.1.3 Passenger Information System

Consider a real scenario in which supposes a person is travelling in train with family members and luggage. His destination point arrives at midnight 2:00 PM and they do not have any smart phone or any other smart equipment to know the exact status of the train. According to the arrival time, he puts himself alert half an hour before time. He later on finds out that the train is running late by 2 hours and another source tells it is late by 3 hours. This way the person faces trouble the whole night waiting when his station would arrive along with his family.

So, if each on-board train coach is configured with Passenger Information Display System (PIDS) then they can overcome these types of troubles. The PIDS is a method or technological gadget to give information to public about status of Train running / rescheduling / Cancellation etc. to the passenger in Person or remotely. It is provided Status of Reservation either on Public Telephone lines or on Internet. Also closely integrates the audio and visual functions for conveying the desired information to passengers and the central control unit controls these functions. Although the activities of the group date back to 1961 and it has been a long journey since then. This technique was already adapted by most of the countries but it is not yet properly implemented in Indian Railway system. Each smart train enabled by

Figure 8. Smart smoke detector connected by Ethernet to monitoring system

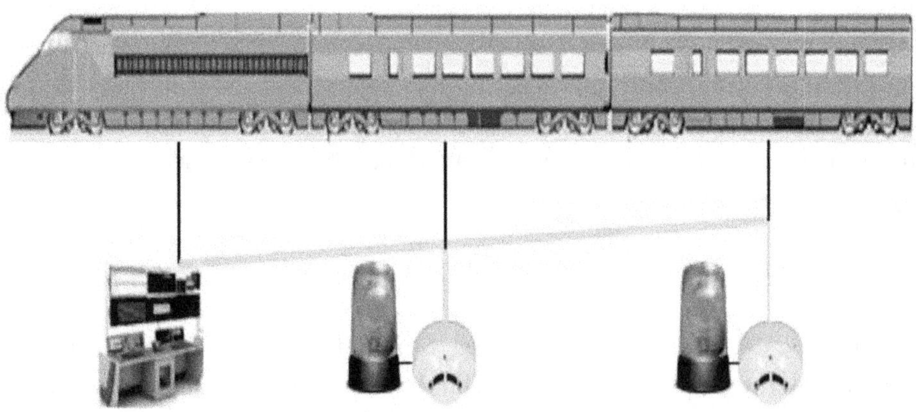

Table 1. On Board LED information display system

Time 02:00AM	Train No. & Train Name		Temperature: 28°C Partly Cloudy Humidity: 25% Wind: 5KM/h	Avg. Speed
Date 12/07/17	18557 BKT VSKP EXPRESS			100KM/h
Next Station	Platform No.	Arrival	Current Status	
Jodhpur	01	04:00AM	Late By 30 Mint.	

Vehicle Tracker, Sensor, Wi-Fi etc. So, that LED display system in every train can provide the information like current status of train, outside weather information, train speed, availability status etc. with audio.

Figure 9 shows PIS working system in this architecture smart train, configure with GPS, which is computed current location, direction and speed of the train and transmit the computed information to the cloud server using high speed connectivity like WiMAX and send to central control room. All these information manages by the control room and share with LED/LCD displays concerned (on-board train, railway stations, and other locations) real time information about arrival and departure of the train with audio announcement. Those with smart mobile devices can download a mobile application or check out the railways information website to find when the train will arrive at their stop. Those who do not have smart phone, can get the information through the control room with the details of train no, route detail and estimated time of arrival. The central control rooms established acts as live hubs to manage and monitor service related data which will be viewable through a centralized web application on PC's and LCD Displays.

Figure 9. PIS working Architecture

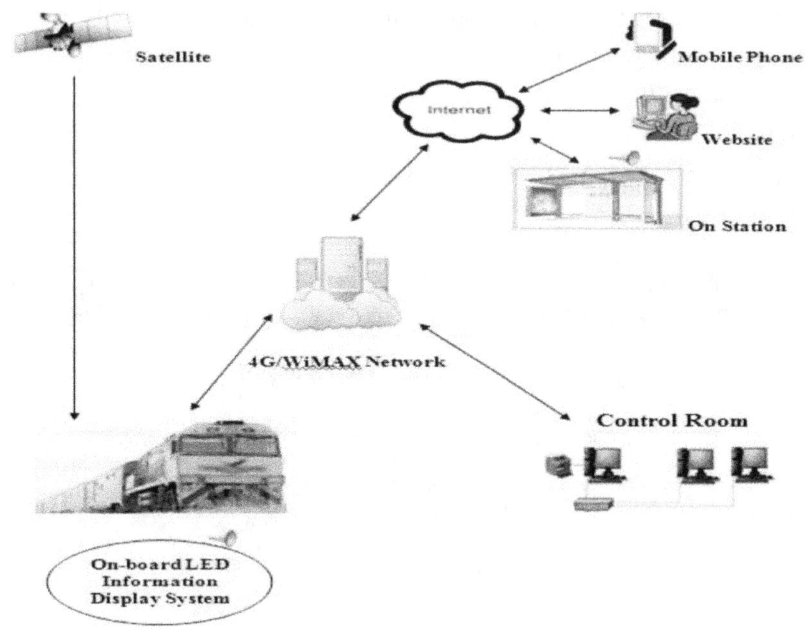

- **Internet Connectivity:** Internet connectivity is most essential part of the smart train because now a day's passengers demanding an Internet connection that is quite enough to quickly search for information, view videos online, email, online chats and connect to their online information. Although many countries around the world are providing some type of Wi-Fi service on board their trains, but most of the time passenger experience is very poor because of unstable or hard to access Wi-Fi connection. This will leave passengers with bad pictures of the service offered by the rail, which becomes the downfall into rail business.

Following challenges need to be solved for a smooth Wi-Fi facility to on-board train:

- Unstable connectivity in high density environment
- Overloaded with single access point
- Safety and privacy from public Wi-Fi system
- Vibration and shock in connectors for on-board environment

Figure 10 shows an architecture of on board train for Internet access by passengers, which incorporates aspects of the train communication management platform (S. Verstichel et al. 2006), uses gateways in each train compartment to make a train-level network. Internet access on the train is provided through the Train Access Terminal (TAT). This terminal, which can support one or many technology types, connects to the access network using an antenna mounted on the outside of train engine or one train compartment. The incoming signal from the TAT is then fed to gateways and wireless access points in the entire rail coach in the train. Within each coach IEEE 802.11 (IEEE Secretary, 2007) is usually offered to provide connectivity to passengers. The access network (Base stations) is close to the train tracks also called Road Side Unit (RSU) which is providing the last hop communications for the TAT. The aggregation network lies between the access network and the service providers' networks, and it forwards data from the access network to the global Internet (Daniel T. Fokum, & Victor S. 2010). Most of the countries using this infrastructure, but some improvement are required for on-board fast and secure Internet access to passengers like:

Figure 10. On-board Wi-Fi connectivity

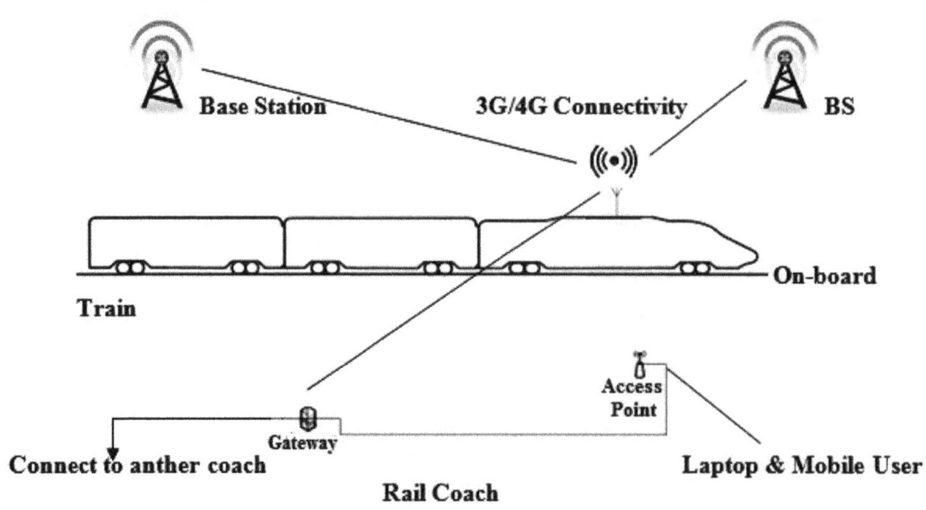

- Best connecters should be designed for on-board application like to deliver can continuously access the Internet under the constant vibration and shock common in on-board environments.
- To ensure stable and concurrent Internet access in high density environments.
- To provide maximum bandwidth for all on-board mobile and other devices.
- Rail maintenance staff constantly adds or remove rail coaches from trains. As a result, it is necessary that communications network to find out these changes automatically.
- Ensure for protection against passengers gaining access to other devices for malicious purposes.

3.2 Automatic Railway Crossing Gate Controller

According to World Health Organization (WHO), 90% of the accident in the world is happening in developing countries and the millions of people around the world die every year because of road and train accidents. Railway transportation is the life line of Indians because it is the cheapest mode of transportation of reaming others. When we go through the daily newspaper we come across many accidents either on rail track or railway crossing gate are more dangerous than other transportation accident in term of severe damage of life and property.

In present scenario large numbers of accidents happen on crossing railway gate due to human error with absence of smart technology. In general, crossing gates are operated manually by a gate keeper or point's men. The gatekeeper receives the information by the telephonic or Red and Blue Signal lights about the train arrived from a nearest station. When the train starts to leave the station, the station in-charge delivers this information to the closest gatekeeper to get ready. But think about if weather disturbance is so high, then the visibility of signal lights very poor and telephonic information also fail due to fault in the cable or may be some wrong information due to human error. In another case where the train is late due to some reason, the gates remain closed for long durations causing dense traffic jam near the gate. So this restriction can be avoided by automating the process.

Now with the help of IoT and Vehicular Ad-hoc Network (VANET) we will propose a model to help automate of rail Gate. Where the gate is automatically opened or closed by detecting the arrival or departing on the train. The scope of VANET application has increased with the recent improvements in technology and development of smart cities across the world. VANET is an infrastructure less network. As the popularity of mobile devices and wireless networks, wireless ad-hoc networks has been now become one of the most active fields of communication and network era. In VANET, nodes are the vehicles which communicate with other vehicles or with the base station which acts as a roadside infrastructure called as RSU (Road Side Unit) for Internet and other services. We can improve the railway transportation system by using the application of VANET where trains can be used as a vehicular node and RSU is rail track side infrastructure. In India, Rail transportation systems are traditionally characterized by how efficient and safely they reached towards their destinations. Improvement in railway transportation system using smart IoT devices such as computing devices, sensors, navigation systems and some advanced information processing tools, all help in realizing this goal of destination-driven.

Here smart train (Vehicular Node) equipped with a wireless device, computing device, On Board Unit (OBU), sensors, digital map, GPS, etc. It is integrated with ad hoc network, cellular technology and WLAN. In which consider V2I (Vehicle to Infrastructure) communication, where infrastructure is a RSU. Standard IEEE 802.11p (WAVE) specially used for wireless access in vehicular domain. It enables V2V and V2I communication in the licensed ITS band of 5.9 GHz (Yaseer Toor et al. 2008). Since the movement of trains is restricted by track and we can deploy fixed infrastructure RSU at critical locations (Railway Crossing Gate) as well as track side also. That provides connectivity support to pass vehicle means both nodes provide the information to each other regarding safety. Every train has two intelligent component OBU and Application Unit (AU) which is working behind OBU and executes program that enable OBU to communicate this unit connects the vehicle with RSU via DSRC radios, and other device holding the train secrete, all the information about the train like, driver identity, trip details, speed, rout, etc. Each vehicle (smart train) has digital maps and positioning technologies (GPS/Wi-Fi/WiMax) as sensing systems to accurately identify the train position and interpret the environment, and also have Unique ID and IP address.

Now, when the train enters the range of the RSU, the GPS device on the train sends its location to the infrastructure because the location information is important to calculation of distance and velocities of a train coming towards to railway crossing gate. RSU which is close to the railway crossing gate send a signal message to smart Bluetooth devices or GSM modem attached to a control circuit. This Bluetooth device receives these signals and transmits them to the microcontroller. Thus, based on the programming, it broadcast the signals to the motor driver to operate the motor. For the operation of the motor in both the clockwise and anti-clockwise directions, a motor driver is used, such as opening and closing of the gate. It can be further improved with a provision of sending an acknowledgment about the status of the gate to the either train operator or near to the station server controlling system (Tarun Agarwal n.d.).

If both trains running on the same tack and suppose both have very nearer to each other than through I2I (Infrastructure to Infrastructure) communication RSU within train range send to all information like speed, location, direction of upcoming train. Therefore, it has helped to remove collision also.

Besides, to detect any accident of the train and then forwarding the corresponding messages in advance to other trains that are approaching the accident are highly important and essential. If an accident takes place on a track, the most important activity is to provide a medical facility and other related help immediately. The time required for information flow from the causality place to a nearby rescue team should be very critical. Because of most of the rail casualty or accident cases, lack of providing quick

Figure 11. Automatic railway crossing gate architecture

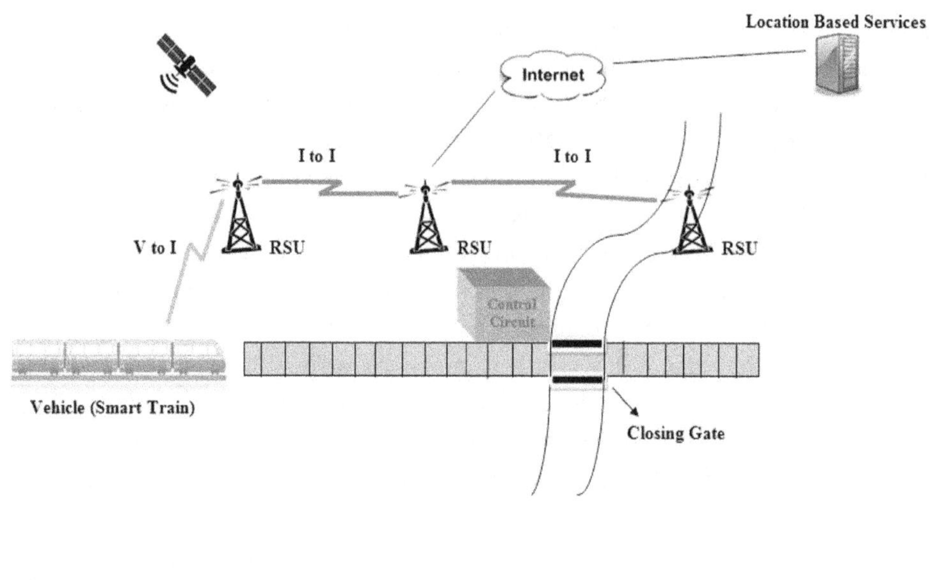

first aid and timely medical service is the main also cause for loss of life. Hence, it is not only important to detect an accident in a timely manner, but it is also important to send the information about the location of the accident to the rescue team immediately (P K Sahoo, M Chiang & S Wu 2014).

This proposed model also helps to improve or saving the lives of the rail accident victims and provides the safety and other useful services to the passengers. VANET technology is used for creating a network with vehicular node (may be train and railway track) that can interact with road or train side units. If any casualty happens in the train or vehicular network, RSU sends emergency message through basic mobile service and internet facility to the nearby smart vehicle that can be used as smart ambulance and sensors with GPS in each vehicle can detect the accident location, they can confirm that the accident has taken place, and the GPS can find the geographical location of the accident. The smart ambulance, then forwarded the message further to the nearby hospital in the smart city which has complete details of the smart ambulances like driver identification number, driver name, and current position of the each ambulance are updated in the main system. The causality message received by the hospital will take decision for saving passenger's lives by dispatching ambulance based on either ambulance, which is near to the causality location or ambulance which was free at the time of emergency and medical personnel to a causality location in a timely fashion.

In July, 2016 Press Information Bureau, Government of India, Ministry of Railways display one report according that, there are total 28607 level crossings in all in Indian Railways. Out of which 19267 level crossings are manned and 9340 level crossing are unmanned. Since unmanned crossings are responsible for the maximum number of train accidents. The reason is that in many sections of rural areas in India, large number of unmanned crossing gates does not have any kind of signaling or alarm system for people with roads vehicle traffic who cross them. During periods of darkness, inclement weather, at night or any condition of reduced visibility, it becomes that much more difficult for the motorist to observe or monitor and then identify the unexpected railroad crossing also one reason of the accident. Thus railway required a light and sound based warning system a pilfer-proof, which can sustain at such typical locations. KHL Chathurange et al. designed model, in this two sensor nodes are placed either side of the railway crossing. These nodes consist of two Ultrasonic sensor devices which is used for measurement of the distance to an object by using sound waves and one vibration sensor which is measuring, displaying, and analyzing linear velocity, displacement and proximity, or acceleration to detect the approaching train. When a

Figure 12. System network

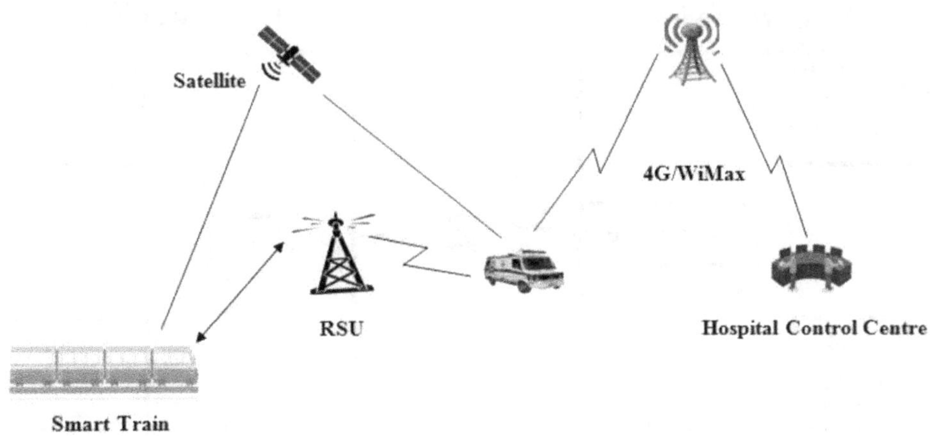

train arrives near the crossing the sensor node which is closed to around 1000m away from the crossing detects the train and transmits to the control node by radio frequency wireless transmission. Then the control node actuates according to the signal that gets from the sensor node. The control node consists of alarm and warning lights. If the train gets near the crossing both these warnings are triggered to inform the public that a train is coming to reduce numbers of accident. The simple block diagram which shows the functionality of the system is shown in Figure 13 (KHL Chathurange et al., 2015).

3.3 Smart Station

In an interesting move, an Indian railway has tied up with the Ministry of Urban Development to ensure that the ambitious, smart cities of India also have smart railway stations. Under an MoU signed between the two ministries railways and urban development, railway stations and surrounding region will be reformulated with an aim to offer easy access to stations, better passenger amenities and also enable optimal utilization of land at railway stations (FE online, 2016). At starting stage the Central Government has approved re-development of 407 railway stations as "world class stations", just over 50 railway stations may undergo the tendering process by the end of 2019, So it is a long process but it should be enabled fully Wi-Fi, display monitor for the live train status, accelerator, smart toilet and smart waiting room.

The main hurdle has been the fact that stations have to be redeveloped without affecting passenger and train movements. Thus selecting the new space for developing the new smart station is a really significant job. Once it is a success, the passengers will be dependable and have a stress free journey.

We have required improvement on following areas for station becoming a smart station.

- Every platform enabled with Internet facility, It should provide high quality free Wi-Fi facility to every passenger.
- Solar panels are the best solution for Zero-net energy consumption. Every station will be installed this infrastructure for power consumption.
- Smart LED Display (Passenger Information System) overcomes the inquiry window passenger crowd.

Figure 13. Block diagram

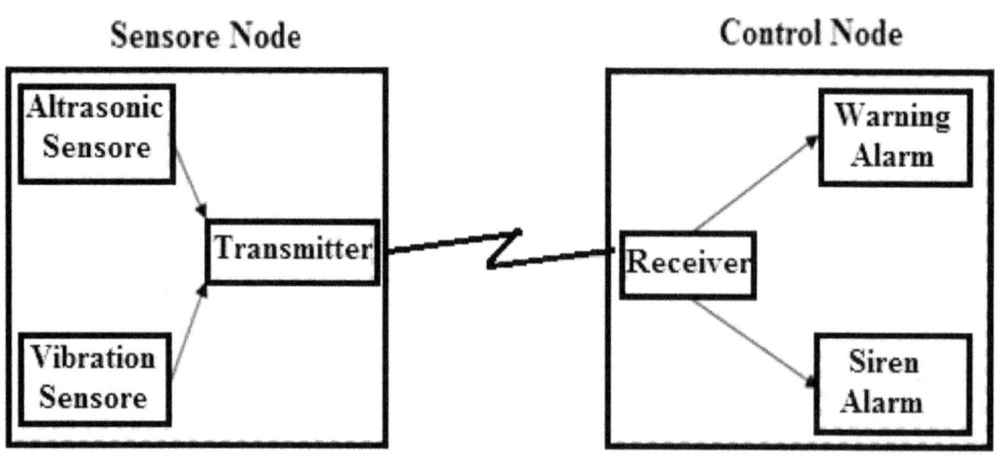

- All the foot over bridge will be replaced with escalators because passengers (especially senior citizens, physically disabled) can cross the platform easily, in less time with lagged.
- Railway platforms can be large, confusing, and intimidating for new travellers and visitors. So, user friendly system providing smart facilities at railway stations should be there.
- Plane to set up "Energy from Waste" plants near to major stations for disposing waste materials in an environment-friendly manner.
- Food and drinks facility can be easily provided to the upcoming train via smart station if data is available in real time regarding the items sold through smart IoT devices.
- The smart stations won't just be locations to grab the train. They will also design for multimodal places where we can access connecting buses, taxis or other services. The most important parking will be available at that, enabled by smart IoT devices.
- Automatic room light controller facility in the waiting room that takes over the task of controlling the lights and fans in order to save power. The sensors are provided at the corners of the seating arrangement to sense the presence of the passengers and accordingly switch the lights and fans over that seating arrangement.
- The condition of toilet facilities on stations very poor condition due to shortage of water and cleanliness. So, first we need to major improvement in this field and also converts existing toilets into Bio-toilets fitted on stations for eco-friendly concern.
- Proposed creation of some new department for keeping stations and trains clean.
- Every Station has a central monitoring system for integrating all IoT devices to provide information to the smart passenger.
- Each platform should configure with highly quality smart IoT camera. Intelligent closed-circuit TV cameras would not only provide a record of events in case of an incident, they would also

Figure 14. Smart railway station with integrated iot devices

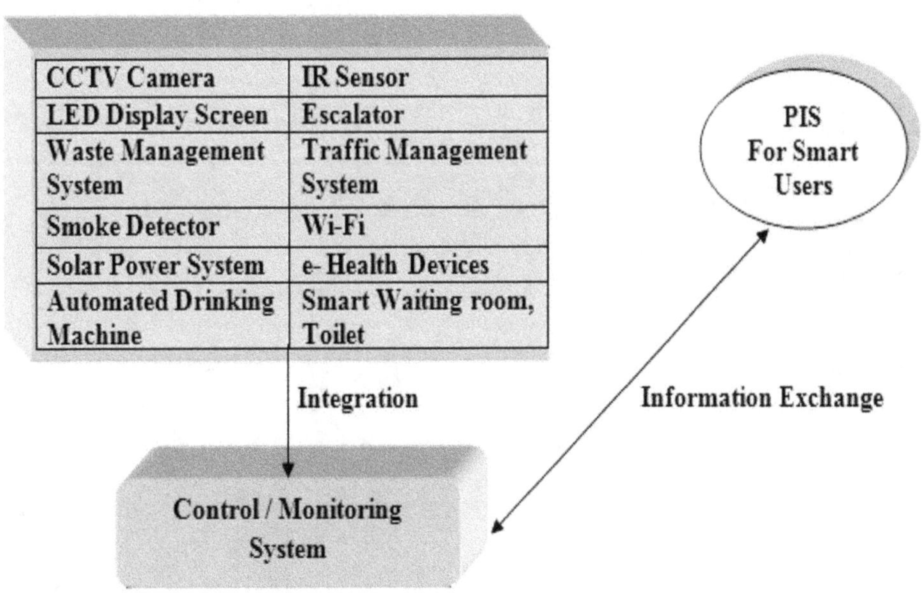

actively provide real-time alarms for potential problems, allowing for more timely intervention responses and potentially reducing service outages.

- Automated ticket vending machines installed at the every big station to reduce burden on ticket windows.

3.4 Track Monitoring

In India, a large number of accidents occurred due to damage of rail track or collision of trains. In recent years, a huge number of research projects are going on in the field of wireless sensor network (WSNs) because the range of sensing technologies has expanded rapidly and also sensor devices have become cheaper. There are a large number of applications of Wireless sensor networks like monitor physical or environmental conditions, such as temperature, sound, pressure, etc. It can be used for monitoring the railway infrastructure such as rail tracks like track beds, and track equipment along with vehicle health monitoring such as bogies and wheels. This can reduce human inspection requirements for maintenance through detecting any defects and improves safety and reliability. Sensor devices are attached to the track or train mechanics. More sensors are attached according to the coverage area. The sensor nodes communicate directly with the server using satellite or GPRS system. The control room accesses the data directly via the cloud server. Infrared Sensor used to monitor the temperature of each wheel in real time when the trains are running and send the data to the central monitoring system.

Figure 15 shows wireless sensor devices are mounted on boards attached to the object being monitored. One or more sensors are mounted on a sensor board (node). The sensor nodes communicate with the base station utilizing a wireless transmission protocol. The base station collects data and transmits it to the central server through satellite or GPRS and monitoring by the system. There may be some variations on this setup. In some systems, the sensor nodes may communicate directly with the server

Figure 15. Sensor information received by operator through GPRS/satellite

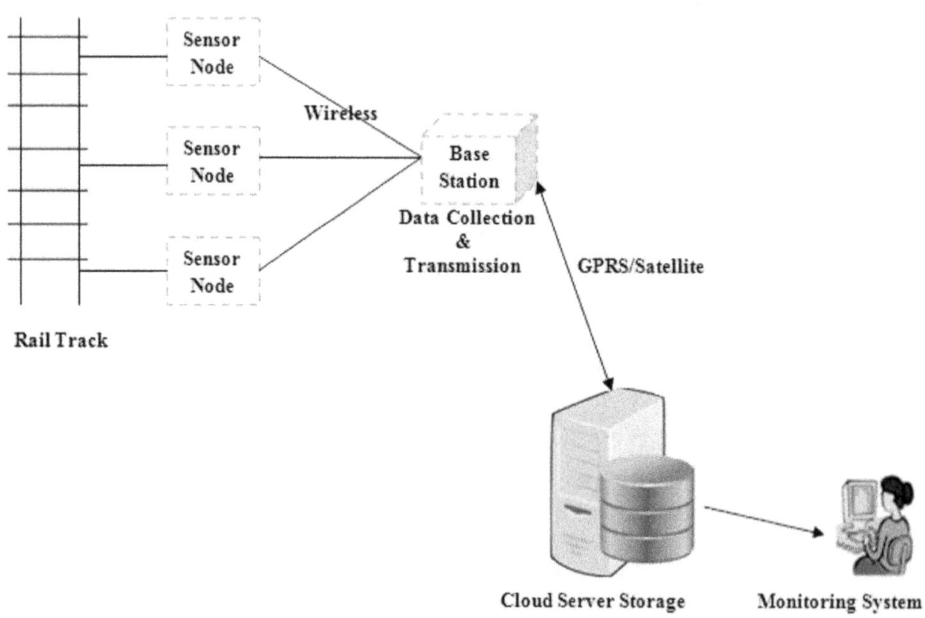

rather than via BS. In other systems, the user accesses the information directly via the BS (Victoria J. Hodge et al. 2015). Wireless Sensor Networks are also able to monitor the moving train. For safety propose it is important that the wagons, containers and their respective contents, train bogies, axle and wheel are also monitored.

3.5 Smart Passenger

IoT system presents the number of smart devices or wearable devices that passengers may have or wear. These devices contain many sensors that could provide specific information related to the journey requirements for the passengers, like location, destination, journey preferences, Seats Availability, Food information on next stoppage etc. (M. H. Eiza et al., 2015). IoT technology will further improve the passengers experience on public transit by offering real time tracking system, indicating exactly how many more minutes their train is away from pulling into the station and which platform it is approaching, also notifications if any unexpected events, and personalized travel news to passengers, So the passenger becomes a smart passenger. By these infrastructure passengers should have some ethics like help to cleanliness station as well as train, do not enter to station or train without any ticket, they should also maintain the rules and regulation imposed by the Govt. of Indian railway.

4. CONCLUSION

In this chapter, authors have introduced the actual use of wireless networking concept VANET and new Internet technology concept IoT. It is environmentally beneficial to switch travelers into rail from other modes of transport when Indian railway provides batter facility to passenger able to make safe, secure and comfort journey. Further, authors have explained and analyzed the utilization of IoT technology is a very promising opportunity to improve Indian Railway Transportation Services and discussed the main components of railway with improvement solutions.

Moreover, authors have introduced a concept to secure and improved passenger's safety by automatic railway gate controlling system and to reduce number of accidents over railway premises. The proposed concept can be further enhanced by implementing of fixed infrastructure RSU at each intersection points in railway premises; this may reduced the train accidents and enhances safety services in rail networks.

REFERENCES

Agarwal, T. (n.d.). *Automatic Railway Gate Control System Alert via SMS*. Retrieved from https://www.elprocus.com/automatic-railway-gate-control-system-projects-using-microcontroller

Ahmad & Habibi. (2011). A Wimax Solution For Real-Time Video Surveillance In Public Transport. *International Journal of Computer Networks & Communications, 3*(2).

Alcaraz, J., Vales Alonso, J., & Garcia Haro, J. (2009). Control-based scheduling with QoS support for vehicle to infrastructure communications. *Wireless Communications*, *16*(6), 32–39. doi:10.1109/MWC.2009.5361176

Ashton, K. (2009). That Internet of Things Thing: In the Real World Things Matter More than Ideas. *RFID Journal*. Retrieved from http://www.rfidjournal.com/articles/view?4986

Blythe, Rackliff, Holland, & Mageean. (2000). ITS applications in public transport: Improving the service to the transport system. *Article in Journal of Advance Transportation*. doi: 10.1002/atr.5670340302

Chathurange, K. H. L., Rathnayaka, R. M. D. P. K., & Wimalasiri, T. S. N. (2015). Railway Warning and Control Systems. In *Proceedings of 8th International Research Conference*. KDU.

Chuck, D., & Chang, J. M. (2010). Bandwidth Recycling in IEEE 802.16 Networks. *IEEE Transactions on Mobile Computing*, *9*(10), 1451–1465. doi:10.1109/TMC.2010.115

Cisco, V. N. I. (2017). *The Zettabyte Era: Trends and Analysis*. White Paper. Cisco Public. Retrieved from http://www.cisco.com/c/en/us/solutions/collateral/service-provider/visual networking-index-vni/vni-hyperconnectivity-wp.html

Deqiang, H., Jain, M., & Xiangyang, L. U. (2008). *Development of Onboard Metro Passenger Information System. Proceeding in ICWMMN*. doi:10.1049/cp:20081022

Eiza, M. H., Randles, M., Johnson, P., Shone, N., Pang, J., & Bhih, A. (2015). Rail Internet of Things: An Architectural Platform and Assured Requirements Model. *Proceedings of 15th IEEE International Conference on Computer and Information Technology*. doi:10.1109/CIT/IUCC/DASC/PICOM.2015.52

Ferreira, N., Meireles, T., & Fonseca, J. A. (2009). An RSU coordination scheme for WAVE safety services support. *Proceedings of the IEEE Conference on Emerging Technologies & Factory Automation*, 1-4. doi:10.1109/ETFA.2009.5347231

Financial Express Online. (2016). Now, smart cities to have redeveloped 'smart' railway stations; 5 things to know. *Financial Express*. Retrieved from http://www.financialexpress.com/economy/indian-railways-smart-cities-railway-station-redevelopment-mou-urban-developmen t-suresh-prabhu-venkaiah-naidu/424492/

Fokum, D. T., & Victor, S. (2010). A Survey on Methods for Broadband Internet Access on Trains. IEEE Communications Surveys & Tutorials, 12(2).

Hodge, V. J., OKeefe, S., Weeks, M., & Moulds, A. (2015). Wireless Sensor Networks For Condition Monitoring In The Railway Industry: A Survey. *IEEE Transactions on Intelligent Transportation Systems*, *16*(3), 1088–1106. doi:10.1109/TITS.2014.2366512

IEEE Secretary. (2007). Wireless LAN Medium Access Control (MAC) and Physical Layer (PHY) Specifications. IEEE Std. 802.11.

Kumar, R. (2015). *IoT, Internet of Things and Indian Railway*. Retrieved from http://www.blog.indianrailways.gov.in /internet-of-things-iot-and-indian-railways/

Lee, Tewolde, & Kwon. (2014). Design and Implementation of Vehicle Tracking System UsingGPS/GSM/GPRS Technology and Smart Phone Application. *IEEE World Forum on Internet of Things (WF-IoT).*

Matsumoto. (2014). Development of On-board Passenger Information Display. Hitachi Review, 63(10).

Mohammeda & Ahmedb. (2017). Internet of Things Applications, Challenges and Related Future Technologies. *WSN, 67*(2), 126-148.

Qureshi, F., & Terzopoulos, D. (2008). Smart Camera Networks in Virtual Reality. *Proceedings of the IEEE, 96*(10), 1640–1656. doi:10.1109/JPROC.2008.928932

Sahoo, Chiang, & Wu. (2014). SVANET: A Smart Vehicular *Ad Hoc* Network for Efficient Data Transmission with Wireless Sensors. *Positioning and Tracking Sensors and Technologies in Road Transport, 14*(12), 22230-22260. Retrieved from https://www.ncbi.nlm.nih.gov/pmc/articles/PMC4299011/

Toor. (2008). Vehicle Ad Hoc Networks: Applications and Related Technical issues. *IEEE Communications Surveys & Tutorials, 10*(3), 74-88.

Vermesan & Fries. (2014). *Internet of Things-From Research and Innovation to Market Deployment.* River Publisher Series in Communication.

Verstichel, S. (2006). On the Design of a Train Communication Management Platform. *Symposium on Communications and Vehicular Technology*, 29–34. doi:10.1109/SCVT.2006.334366

Chapter 9
A Succinct Analysis of Applications and Services Provided by IoT

Sushruta Mishra
C. V. Raman College of Engineering, India

Hrudaya Kumar Tripathy
KIIT University, India

Brojo Kishore Mishra
C. V. Raman College of Engineering, India

Sunil Kumar Mohapatra
C. V. Raman College of Engineering, India

ABSTRACT

The phrase Internet of Things (IoT) heralds a vision of the future Internet where connecting physical things, from banknotes to bicycles, through a network will let them take an active part in the Internet, exchanging information about themselves and their surroundings. This will give immediate access to information about the physical world and the objects in it leading to innovative services and increase in efficiency and productivity. In general, it may be beneficial to incorporate a number of the technologies of IoT with the use of services that can act as the bridge between each technology and the applications that developers wish to implement in IoT. This chapter studies the state-of-the-art of IoT and presents the key potential applications, challenges and future research areas in the domain of IoT. This chapter presents four main categories of services according to technical features. Some major issues of future research in IoT are identified and discussed briefly.

DOI: 10.4018/978-1-5225-5222-2.ch009

Copyright © 2018, IGI Global. Copying or distributing in print or electronic forms without written permission of IGI Global is prohibited.

1. INTRODUCTION

The Internet of Things (IoT) sometimes referred to as the Internet of Objects, will change everything including ourselves. The Internet has an impact on education, communication, business, science, government, and humanity (Ezechina, Okwara,and Ugboaja 2015). Clearly, the Internet is one of the most important and powerful creations in all of human history and now with the concept of the internet of things, internet becomes more favourable to have a smart life in every aspect (Retrieved from http://www.meraevents.com/event/iot-workshop). Internet of Things is a new Technology of the Internet accessing. By the Internet of Things, objects recognize themselves and obtain intelligence behaviour by making or enabling related decisions thinks to the fact that they can communicate information about themselves (Retrieved from http://www.nxp.com/assets).

These objects can access information that has been aggregated by other things, or they can be added to other services (Retrieved from http://www.nxp.com/assets). Figure 1 reviews that with the internet of things, anything's will able to communicate to the internet at any time from any place to provide any services by any network to anyone. this concept will create a new types of applications can involve such as smart vehicle and the smart home, to provide many services such as notifications, security, energy saving, automation, communication, computers and entertainment (Saranya C. M., Nitha K. P. April 2015)(Sapandeep Kaur, I.K.Vinderpal Singh 2016).

In the IoT, the communication language will be based on interoperable protocols, operating in heterogeneous environments and platforms (Retrieved from http://cdn2.hubspot.net/). IoT in this context is a generic term and all objects can play an active role to their connection to the Internet by creating smart environments, where the role of the Internet has changed (Retrieved from http://docplayer.net/). The aim of this chapter is presents the internet of things Applications, Related Future Technologies, and challenges.

2. IOT APPLICATIONS

Internet of things promises many applications in human life, making life easier, safe and smart. There are many applications such as smart cities, homes, transportation, energy and smart environment.

Figure 1. Internet of Things concept

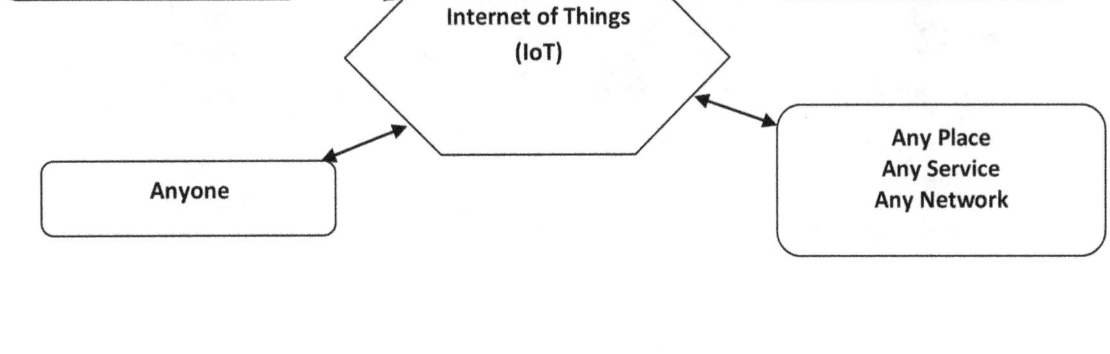

Smart Cities

Many major cities were supported by smart projects, like Seoul, New York, Tokyo, Shanghai, Singapore, Amsterdam, and Dubai. Smart cities may still be viewed as a cities of the future and smart life, and by the innovation rate of creating smart cities today's, it will became very feasible to enter the IoT technology in cities development (Retrieved from https://www.thingworx.com/). Smart cities demand requires careful planning in every stage, with support of agreement from governments, citizens to implement the internet of things technology in every aspect. By the IoT, cities can be improved in many levels, by improving infrastructure, enhancing public transportation reducing traffic congestion, and keeping citizens safe, healthy and more engaged in the community as shown in Figure 2 (Eiman Al Nuaimi1 et al. 2015). By connection all systems in the cities like transportation system, healthcare system, weather monitoring systems and etc., in addition to support people by the internet in every place to accessing the database of airports, railways, transportation tracking operating under

Specified protocols, cities will become smarter by means of the internet of things (Retrieved from http://www.7wdata.be/article-general/) (A. Murray, M. Minevich, and A. Abdoullaev 2011).

Smart Home and Buildings

Wi-Fi's technology in home automation has been used primarily due to the networked nature of deployed electronics where electronic devices such as TVs, mobile devices, etc. are usually supported by Wi-Fi (Farheen Fatima, at el. December 2015). Wi-Fi have started becoming part of the home IP network and due the increasing rate of adoption of mobile computing devices like smart phones, tablets, etc. For example a networking to provide online streaming services or network at homes, may provide a mean to control of the device functionality over the network (Retrieved from http://www.connected-living.org/). At the same time mobile devices ensure that consumers have access to a portable 'controller' for the electronics connected to the network. Both types of devices can be used as gateways for IoT applications (Retrieved

Figure 2. Smart Cities Aspects

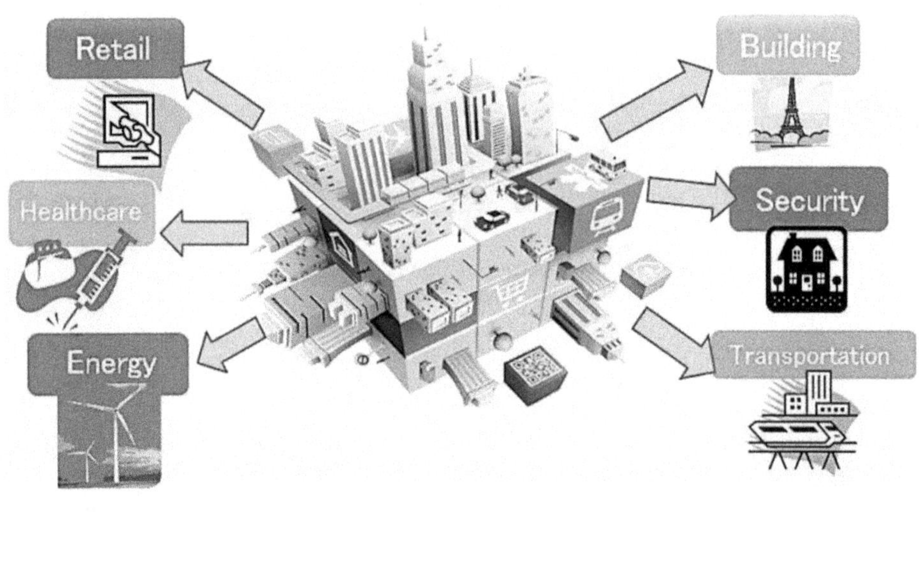

from http://www.gsma.com/). Many companies are considering developing platforms that integrate the building automation with entertainment, healthcare monitoring, energy monitoring and wireless sensor monitoring in the home and building environments (Jukka Suhonen 2013). By the concept of the internet of things, homes and buildings may operate many devices and objects smartly, of the most interesting application of IoT in smart homes and buildings are smart lighting, smart environmental and media, air control and central heating, energy management and security as shown in Figure 3.

Smart Energy and the Smart Grid

A smart grid is related to the information and control and developed to have a smart energy management (Retrieved from http://energy.gov/). A smart grid that integrate the information and communications technologies (ICTs) to the electricity network will enable a real time, two way communication between suppliers and consumers, creating more dynamic interaction on energy flow, which will help deliver electricity more efficiently and sustainable (Retrieved from https://www.gov.uk/government/).The Key elements of information and communications technologies will include sensing and monitoring technologies for power flows; digital communications infrastructure to transmit data across the grid; smart meters with in home display to inform energy usage; coordination, control and automation systems to aggregate and process various data, and to create highly interactive, responsive electricity (Ramyar Rashed Mohassel et al.2014). Many applications can be handling due to the internet of things for smart grids, such as industrial, solar power, nuclear power, vehicles, hospitals and cities power control. Figure 4 shows the most important application may be enabled by the internet of things as in smart grid aspect.

Today's grid is very reliable and can deal with normal electricity fluctuations and it will take a step further towards using a low carbon energy system, by allowing integration between the renewable energy

Figure 3. Smart Home & building applications

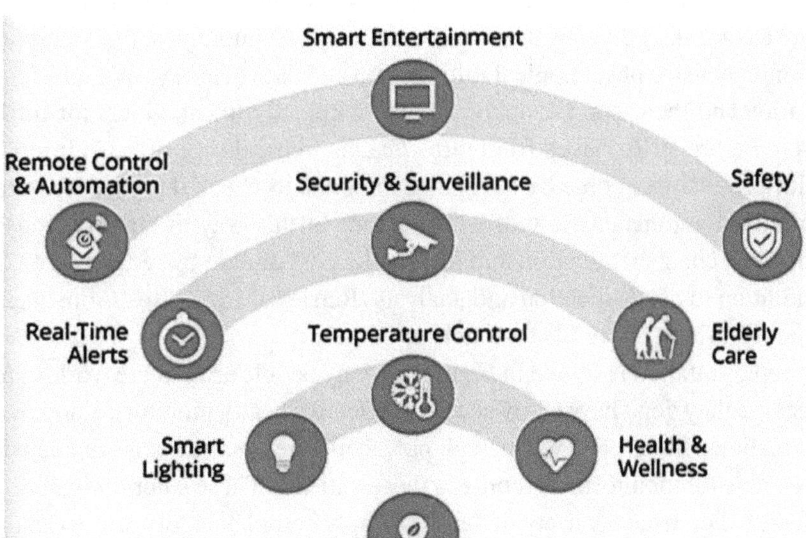

Figure 4. Smart grid applications

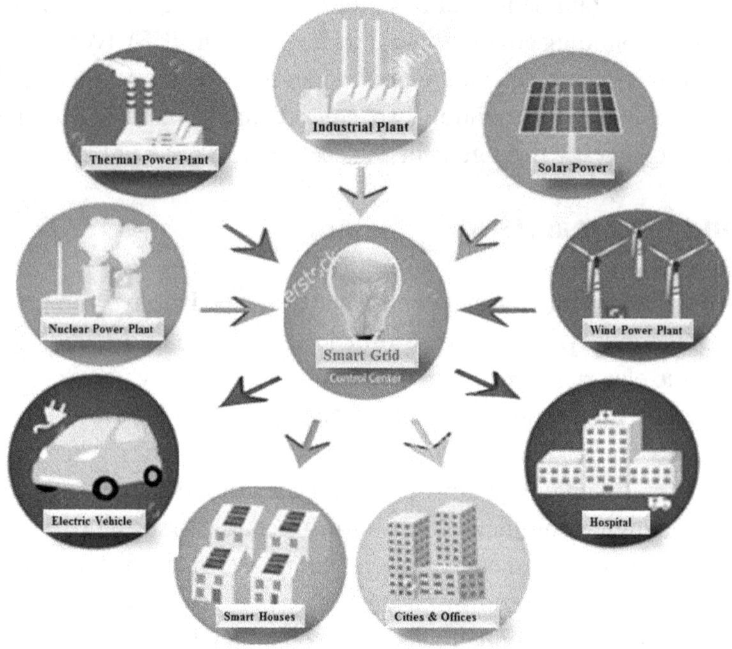

and green technologies, and offering many benefits to customer in cost savings through efficient energy use at home (Rosario Miceli 2013).

Smart Health

A close attention that required to hospitalized patients whose physiological status should be monitored continuously can be constantly done by using IoT monitoring technologies. For smart health sensors are used to collect comprehensive physiological information and uses gateways and the cloud to analyze and store the information and then send the analyzed data wirelessly to caregivers for further analysis and review as shown in Figure 5 (Retrieved from https://cache.freescale.com/files/). It replaces the process of having a health professional come by at regular intervals to check the patient's vital signs, instead providing a continuous automated flow of information. In this way, it simultaneously improves the quality of care through constant attention and lowers the cost of care by reduces the cost of traditional ways of care in addition to data collection and analysis (Retrieved from https://ibmcai.com/2016/03/01/healthcare-internet-of-things-18-trends-to-watch-in-2016/).

Smart Health representation is shown in Figure 5. Many people around the worlds are suffering from the bad health because they don't have ready access to effective health monitoring and may be a suspected to be as critical situation patients. But with small, powerful wireless solutions connected through the IoT is now making possible for monitoring to come to these patients. These solutions can be used to securely capture patient health data from a variety of sensors, apply complex algorithms to analyze the data and then share it through wireless connectivity with medical professionals who can make appropriate health recommendations (Retrieved from https://www.researchgate.net/publication/).

Figure 5. Smart healthcare concept

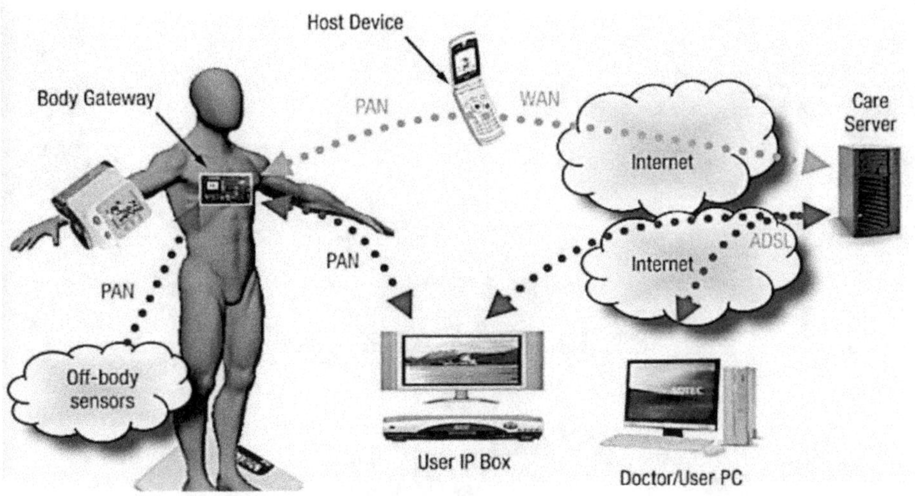

Smart Transportation and Mobility

The development in transportation is one of the factors to indicate the wellbeing of the country. A road condition monitoring and alert application is one of the most important of IoT transformation application (Retrieved from http://www.bth.se/tek/intelligent_gods.nsf/). The main idea of the concept of smart transportation and mobility is to apply the principles of crowd sourcing and participatory sensing. The process began with user identified the route wishes and marked some points as pothole in the smart phone's application (Retrieved from https://web.njit.edu/). The smart transportation is deal with three main conceptions as shown in Figure 6; they are transportation analytic, transportation control, and vehicle connectivity. The transportation analytic represents the analysis of demand prediction and anomaly detection. The routing of vehicles and speed control in addition to traffic management are all known as transportation control which they actually tightly related to the way of the vehicles connectivity (V2X communication), and overall governed by multi-technology dissemination. IoT can also be used in transportation is an electric vehicle, which is an important means to reduce both the fuel cost and the impact of global warming have also gained considerable attention from drivers. Government in many countries has supported researches on systems to monitor performance of Lithium-ion (Li-on) battery for electric vehicle as explored. The system presented was designed to detect the functions of Li-on power battery by deriving the driving situation from the realistic working conditions for driver so that the driver was able to get the idea of the route status. This solution was embedded with many essential functions such as dynamic performance test of the Li-on battery, remote monitoring with on-line debugging and error correction that could significantly reduce the maintenance cost(Georgios Chatzimilioudis, et al. 2011).

Smart Factory and Smart Manufacturing

Smart factory added a new value in manufacturing revolution by integrates artificial intelligence, machine learning, and automation of knowledge work and M2M communication with the manufacturing process (Marc Benioff 2015). The smart factory will fundamentally change how products are invented,

Figure 6. Smart Transportation Aspects

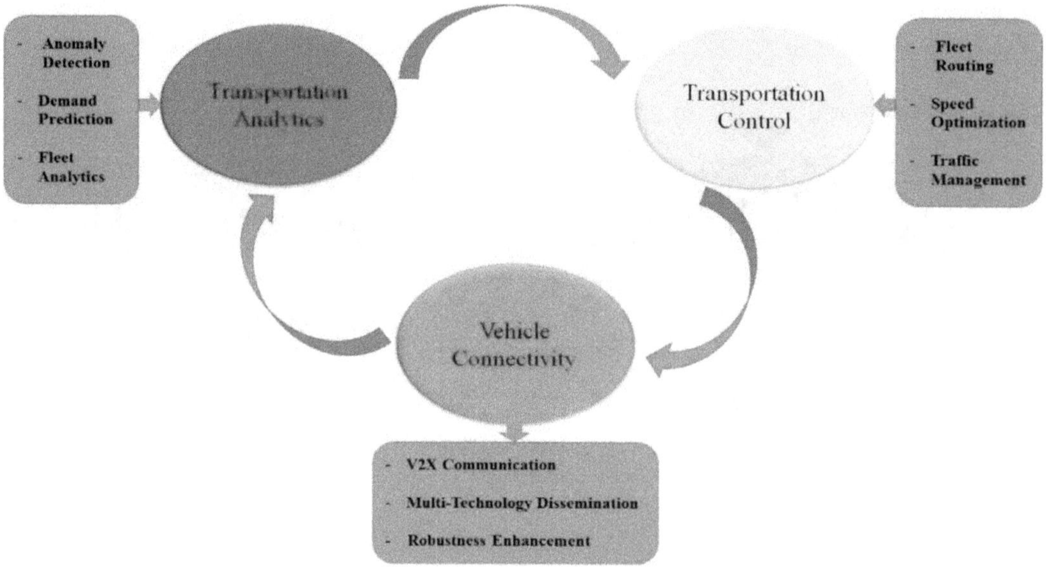

manufactured and shipped. At the same time it will improve worker safety and protect the environment by enabling low emissions and low incident manufacturing. These advances in the way machines and other objects communicate and the resulting way in which decision-making moves from humans to technical systems means that manufacturing becomes "smarter"(Retrieved from http://www3.webforum.org/docs/) new technologies such ; Automation, robotics, and autonomous mobility are all provides a means of smart manufacturing but M2M communications enabled by the "industrial" internet of things will provides a full meaning of smart factory and smart manufacturing by the way of Big Data concept which in this context, refers to the analytical possibilities offered by the volume and variety of data that is generated by a networked economy to optimize the industrial processes to implying less maintenance downtime, fewer outages and much reduced energy consumption (Retrieved from https://www.munichre.com/). Industries and manufacturing revolution became one of the most developed technologies nowadays, the growth of the industry evolution taken many generations. The first generation related to the mechanical machines in addition to water and stream power. The second industry generation deal with mass production, assembly lines and electricity. In the end of the last century, industries operated under control of computers and automation which recognized as third generation of industries. The smart industry as a fourth generation known as industry 4.0 is based on cypher physical systems which can able to connect with the internet. The industry 4.0 concept with the internet of things can achieve great expectations for industries resolution deals with many aspects a shown in Figure 7. By introducing the high-tech strategy 2020 initiative focusing the country's research and innovation policy on selected forward-looking projects related to scientific and technological developments.

Smart Environment

Environment plays a major effect in human life. People, even animals, birds, fishes and plants may be affected in unhealthy environment. There were many researches efforts has been paid to solve the prob-

Figure 7. Smart Factory

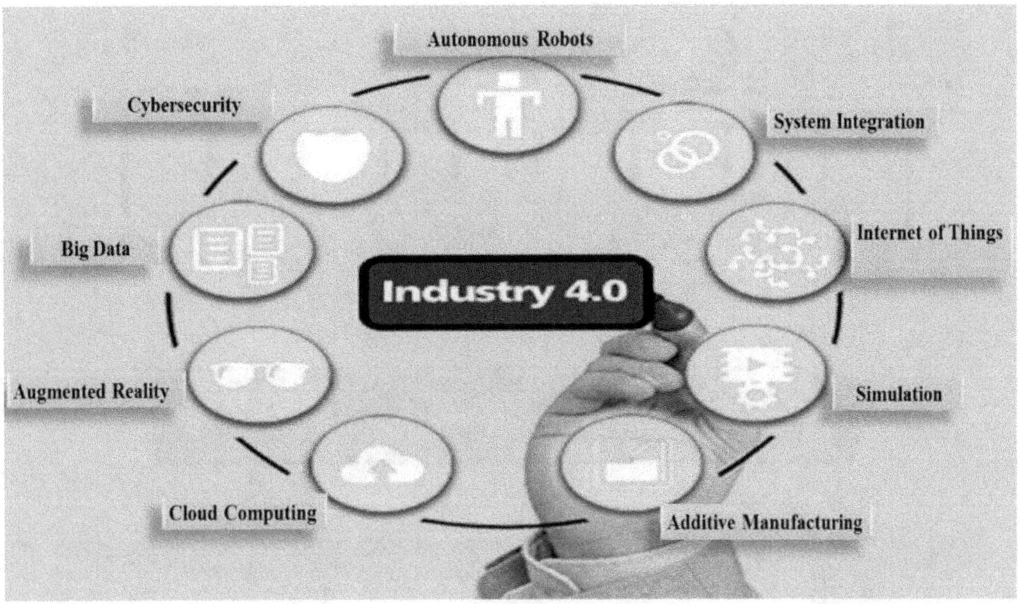

lems of environmental pollution and waste resources (Retrieved from https://atos.net/content/). Creating of a healthy environment is not easy because of industries and transportations wastes, with irresponsible human activities are daily factors that make the environment damaged (Arko Djajadi, Member 2016). The environment needs a smart ways and new technologies for monitoring and management. Monitoring the environment is important in order to assess the current condition of the environment to takes correct life decision according to collected data from monitoring systems, and management is needed to have an efficient resources consuming and use in addition to decrease the factories and vehicles wastes. Both monitoring and waste management provide a large amount of data to force the health standard by governments or healthy environment organizations to protect people and environment, and to mitigate or to avoid natural disaster that might occur (D. Bhattacharjee and R. Bera 2014). Smart environment is an important technology in our everyday life which provides many facilities and solutions for many environmental applications such as water and air pollution, weather and radiation monitoring, waste management, natural disaster, and many other environment indicators as shown in Figure 8 and all may connected to each person through home area network. Smart environment devices integration with Internet of Things (IoT) technology is developed for tracking, sensing and monitoring objects of environment which provide potential benefits to achieve a green world and sustainable life (Peng Jiang, Hongbo Xia, Zhiye He and Zheming Wang 2009).

There are many applications of internet of things in environment and that can be divided to two main categories environmental resources management, and environmental quality and protection management (Nomusa Dlodlo 2012). The resources management relates to all natural resources include animals, planets and forests, birds and fishes, coal, petroleum, land, freshwater, air and heavy metals including gold, copper and iron. All these resources are likely to decrease significantly or affected by several factors, including pollution, waste, and abuse. IoT can provides an effective way to communicate between each of these resources sensors with research and monitoring centres to make appropriate decisions in

Figure 8. Smart Environment based internet of things

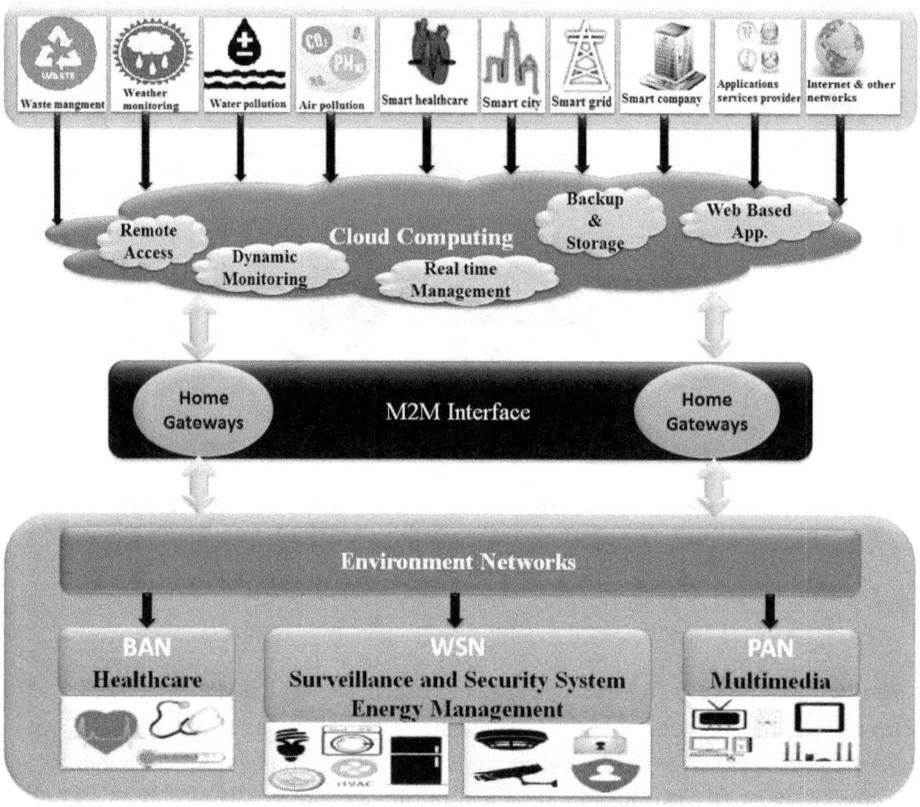

the consumption of these sources. Renewable resources include sunlight, and wind also can be managed and sensed to Ideal use in several uses, such as the provision of renewable energy sources. IoT can control these sources and their use in a number of important applications in the environment (Retrieved from http://www.ti5.tu-harburg.de/events/). The IoT technology is able to monitoring and managing the air quality by to collectingdata from remote sensor across the city, and providing full-time geographic coverage to achieve a way of better managing urban traffic in major cities (Retrieved from http://www.gov.uk/government/). The IoT also can be used to measure the levels of pollution in water in order to inform decisions on water usage and treatment. Waste management is also one of the most important environment issues (Retrieved from http://senseable.mit.edu/papers/). The various types of waste material chemical or elements can pollute the environment and threaten life in a number of ways in ground effect on animals, peoples and plants and in addition to air and water. IoT provides an environmental protection means by control the industrial pollution by real time monitoring and management systems integrated to supervision and decision-making networks to reduce waste, and improved environment (Retrieved from http://auskogroup.com/how-iot-is-changing-the-waste-industry). Other environment aspect is a weather forecast and monitoring. IoT can provide a high resolution, and accuracy for weather monitoring by data exchange and information sharing.

It's enabling weather systems to collect data from various vehicles on the road, and wirelessly communicate to the weather stations to support data that is inclusive of air temperature, barometric pressure, visibility or light, motion and other data needed. Sensors equipped in many buildings, vehicles integration with IoT help in collecting weather data which is further stored in clouds for analysis (P. Susmitha, G. Sowmyabala 2014). Radiation of course is one of the most serious problems facing the safety of the environment. The radiation produced by nuclear power plants and some industries negatively affected safety of an environmental and human health, animal and agricultural productivity (Retrieved from http://iotworm.com/internet-of-things-technology-weather-forecasting/). For nuclear radiations, radiation control IoT sensor network is able to continuous monitoring of radiation levels around nuclear facilities for leakage detection and propagation prevention (Retrieved from https://indico.cern.ch/event/). A natural disaster is a major adverse event resulting from natural processes of the earth include floods, volcanic eruptions, earthquakes, hurricanes, wildfires, blizzards and, and other geologic processes. IoT can avoid or reduce the impact of a large number of natural disasters that affect in many aspects of life through the distribution of a number of sensor systems for many types of natural disasters and linking these systems with research and rescue announcement stations, also for declaration of emergency networking with hospitals and police stations. IoT will provides a means of smart agriculture and adding great potential in resource saving. By using sensors networks, and scientific research databases, growing of plants and other agriculture productions needed by humans like vegetables and fruits can monitored and save their production processes based on managing many resources such as weather, water and sunlight. In addition, the IoT for environmental monitoring can aid in measuring emissions from factories detect forest fires or aid in agriculture.

3. CHALLENGES OF IOT

The fact that Internet of things applications and scenarios outlined above are very interesting which provides technologies for smart everything., but there are some challenges to the application of the Internet of Things concept in cost of implementation. IoT are also faced with many other challenges (M. Dragusin, D. Stanga, D. Gurau, E. Ionescu 2014) (Ron Davies 2015), such as:

- **Scalability:** Internet of Things has a big concept than the conventional Internet of computers, because of things are cooperated within an open environment. Basic functionality such as communication and service discovery therefore need to function equally efficiently in both small scale and large scale environments. The IoT requires a new functions and methods in order to gain an efficient operation for scalability.
- **Self-Organizing:** Smart things should not be managed as computers that require their users to configure and adapt them to particular situations. Mobile things, which are often only sporadically used, need to establish connections spontaneously, and able to be organize and configure themselves to suit their particular environment.
- **Data Volumes:** Some application scenarios of the internet of things will involve to infrequent communication, and gathering information's form sensor networks, or form logistics and large scale networks, will collect a huge volumes of data on central network nodes or servers. The term represent this phenomena is big data which is requires many operational mechanism in addition to new technologies for storing, processing and management.
- **Data interpretation:** To support the users of smart things, there is a need to interpret the local context determined by sensors as accurately as possible. For service providers to profit from the

disparate data that will be generated, needs to be able to draw some generalizable conclusions from the interpreted sensor data.

- **Interoperability:** Each type of smart objects in Internet of Things has different information, processing and communication capabilities. Different smart objects would also be subjected to different conditions such as the energy availability and the communications bandwidth requirements. To facilitate communication and cooperation of these objects, common standards are required.
- **Automatic Discovery:** In dynamic environments, suitable services for things must be automatically identified, which requires appropriate semantic means of describing their functionality.
- **Software Complexity:** A more extensive software infrastructure will be needed on the network and on background servers in order to manage the smart objects and provide services to support them. That because the software systems in smart objects will have to function with minimal resources, as in conventional embedded systems.
- **Security and Privacy:** In addition to the security and protection aspects of the Internet such in communications confidentiality, the authenticity and trustworthiness of communication partners, and message integrity, other requirements would also be important in an Internet of Things. There is a need to access certain services or prevent from communicating with other things in IoT and also business transactions involving smart objects would need to be protected from competitors' prying eyes.
- **Fault Tolerance:** Objects in internet of things is much more dynamic and mobile than the internet computers, and they are in changing rapidly in unexpected ways. Structuring an Internet of Things in a robust and trustworthy manner would require redundancy on several levels and an ability to automatically adapt to changed conditions.
- **Power Supply:** Things typically move around and are not connected to a power supply, so their smartness needs to be powered from a self-sufficient energy source. Although passive RFID transponders do not need their own energy source, their functionality and communications range are very limited. Hopes are pinned on future low power processors and communications units for embedded systems that can function with significantly less energy. Energy saving is a factor not only in hardware and system architecture, but also in software, for example the implementation of protocol stacks, where every single transmission byte will have to justify its existence.
- **Wireless Communications:** From an energy point of view, established wireless technologies such as GSM, UMTS, Wi-Fi and Bluetooth are far less suitable; more recent WPAN standards such as ZigBee and others still under development may have a narrower bandwidth, but they do use significantly less power.

4. SERVICES PROVIDED BY IOT

There are a large number of applications and services provided by Internet of Things and these can be classified according to different criteria (Saranya C. M., Nitha K. P. 2015).According to technical features, Internet of Things services can be divided into 4 types: identity-related services (Sapandeep Kaur, I.k. vinderpal Singh 2016), information aggregation services, collaborative-aware services, and ubiquitous services(Retrieved from http://cdn2.hubspot.net/hubfs/).For each application, a particular IoT service can be applied in order to optimize application development and speed up application implementation. Figure 9 illustrates the IoT stack.

Figure 9. The IOT Stack

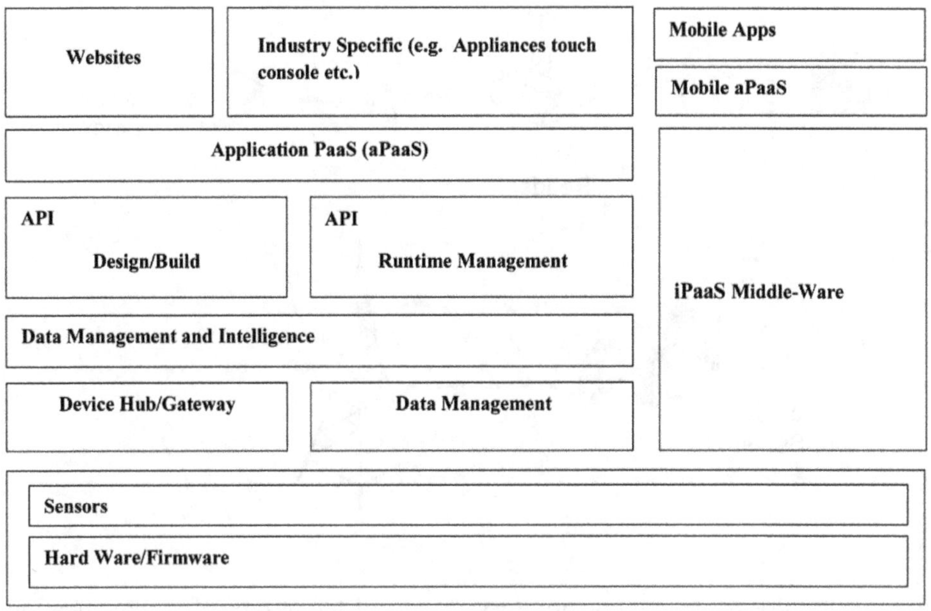

Identity-Related Services

The Identity-related services can be basically used in RFID, bar Code and two-dimensional code. Identity-related services can be basically divided into two categories active and passive and used either in individuals or enterprise purpose, which can lead to different kinds of applications. In general identity-related service consists of two major components: first the devices, which are equipped with some kind of identification identifier, such as an RFID tag; and second the read device(s), which read the identity of the device(s) based on its label. In this case reading the information encoded into the RFID tag and thenthe read device makes a request to the name resolution server of the Internet of Things and obtains the Uniform Resource Identifier (URI) of the thing. Finally, the read device obtains further information from the URI.

Active identity-related services are associated with broadcast information and having constant power source. Passive identity-related services have no power source and require some external device or mechanism in order to pass on its identity. For example as shown n Figure 10, an active RFID tag is battery powered and can transmit signals once an external source has been identified. A passive RFID tag, has no batteries, and requires an external electromagnetic field in order to initiate a signal transmission. In general, active identity services can transmit or actively send their information to another device, whereas passive services must be read from.

Information Aggregation Services

Information Aggregation Service based on some service collecting or acquiring data from different sensors. Then process the data, transmitting and reporting that data via IoT devices to the user application. SomeSpecific applications include automatic meter reading, elevator management, logistics, and

Figure 10. RFID network example

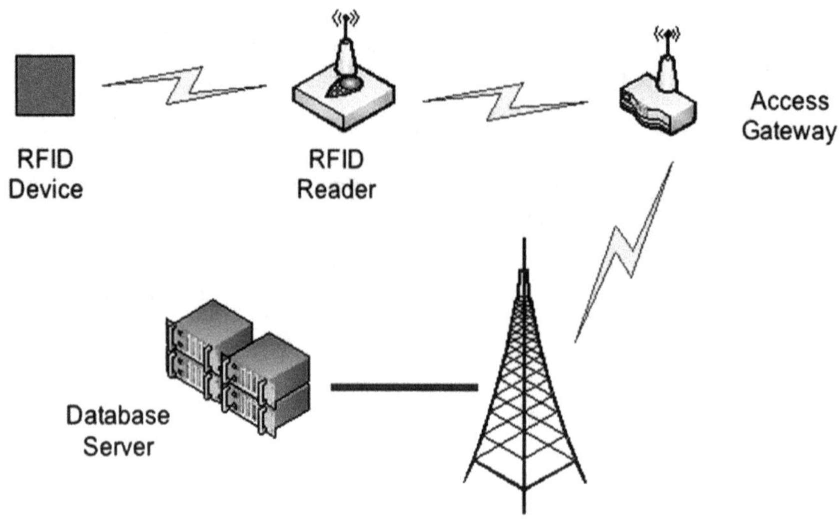

traffic management. Information aggregation services use different type of communication channel in order to work together. This service provides access gateways to make use of different types of sensors and network devices and share their data via common service to the application. For example, an application could make use of RFID tags to be aware of the identity of some devices, while also using a ZigBee network to collect data from sensors, and then use a gateway device to relay this information to the application under the same service, say a Web Service such as JSON (JavaScript Object Notation) or XML.In this regard, the WSN can be a powerful tool for collecting and communicating data between terminals and the platform (host of application), as long as the platform is within range of the WSN.

Information aggregation services are useful in monitoring situations, such as energy monitoring in the house and in the enterprise, or, if the Internet of Things has been realized, monitoring of anything, anywhere as depicted in Figure 11. For example, Shen et al. (Retrieved from http://docplayer.net/1073234-Internet-of-things-converging-technologies-for-smart-environments-and-integrated-ecosystems.html) introduces a monitoring and control system for use in an agriculture greenhouse production environment. The system measures and records critical temperature, humidity and soil signals which is then transmitted through the network to the platform for processing. Another application; Zhao et al. (Retrieved from https://www.thingworx.com/) uses a ZigBee WSN to monitor physiological data of patients that automatically generates electronic medical records. In Shen (Retrieved from http://docplayer.net/1073234-Internet-of-things-converging-technologies-for-smart-environments-and-integrated-ecosystems.html) research, the importance of extending the information aggregation service to beyond the WSN is proposed by using a cellular network (CN) to extend the range of the WSN. The idea is that if a terminal is outside of the WSN of interest, it uses CN resources to access that information with an "IoT gateway," which essentially implements both WSN and CN resources.

Collaborative-Aware Services

The development of the Internet of Things should bring about the delivery of more important and complicated services. (Saranya C. M., Nitha K. P. 2015) such services often require terminal-to-terminal

Figure 11. Aggregate Network diagram with sensor network and access gateways

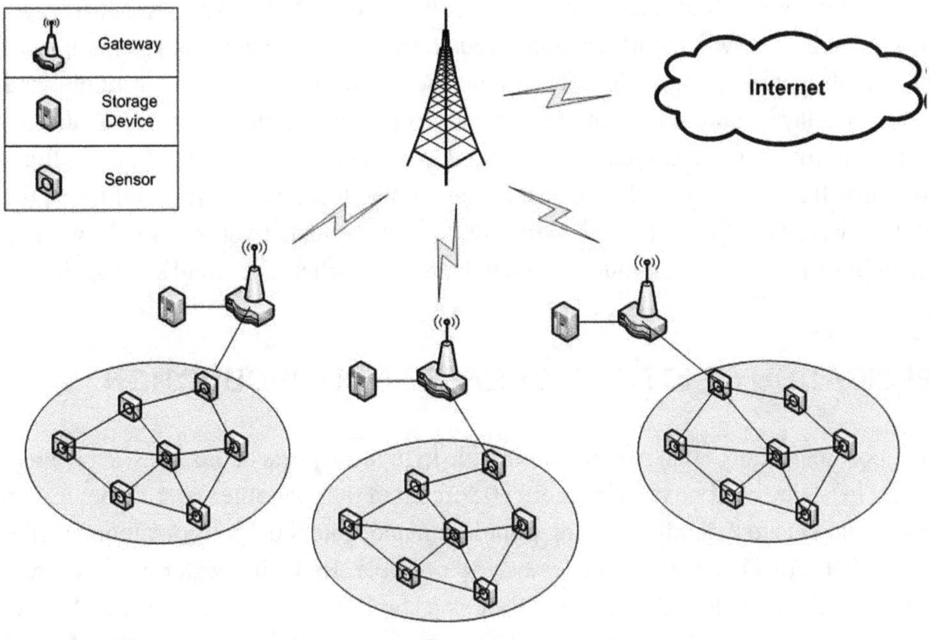

and terminal-to-person communication. Moreover, these communication capabilities impose higher requirements on reliability and delay, and require terminals to be smarter. Only in this way, can collaborative processing be done. (Eiman Al Nuaimi1 et al. 2015) Collaborative aware services are services that use aggregated data to make decisions, and based on those decisions perform an action. There are fewer applications published in terms of IoT and collaborative-aware services. An example of a new technology that will help shape the way the Internet of Things grows is IPv6. By providing collaborative aware services, the IoT infrastructure naturally requires greater reliability and speed, and will require the terminals to either have more processing power or be linked with some other device that does. A network is there where three types of nodes, all of which can be reprogrammed to function as any of the three types. These three types basically a base station node (IPv6 router), a mobile node (wireless dongle that allows WSN connectivity to a standard laptop) and specialized nodes, which are used for specialized tasks.

This becomes a collaborative-aware service because it incorporates terminal-terminal and terminal-person communication, which is accomplished due to the use of the IPv6 protocol (Saranya C. M., Nitha K. P. 2015) (Retrieved http://www.7wdata.be/article-general/).

Ubiquitous Services

Ubiquitous services are the ultimate goal of the Internet of Things, taking collaborative-aware services to the next level by providing complete access and control of everything around us, whether it is through a computer or a mobile phone or something else. (Saranya C. M., Nitha K. P. 2015) So far, little research has been carried out into the research of ubiquitous services from the perspective of telecom networks. In

September 2009, the Telecommunication Standardization Sector of the International Telecommunication Union (ITU-T) released the draft recommendation Y.2002 (Y.NGN-UbiNet) (A. Murray, M. Minevich, and A. Abdoullaev 2011), which outlines ubiquitous networks and their visions.(Saranya C. M., Nitha K. P. 2015) The ubiquitous network is generally defined as a fully connected, reliable, and intelligent network at the sub layer, and containing integrated content technology, micro technology, and bio-technology. Its communication services are extended into fields such as education, intelligent building, supply chain, health care, everyday life, disaster management, safety service, and transport to provide people with better services. The ultimate objective of ubiquitous networks is to allow people to enjoy convenience in information and communication, to better serve their lives, and even to change their lives.

5. AN APPLICATION OF IOT TO INCREASE FOOD PRODUCTION

Water is an important resource that plays a crucial role in many aspects of our lives, especially in growing the food we eat. In Malaysia, for example, about 70 percent of the available water resources are consumed for rice production. Due to a rapidly growing population and water competition among different sectors, it is imperative that farms use water as efficiently as possible. Reducing water usage in rice production makes more water available for other sectors. Rice is a staple food of Malaysians, and the country produces enough to meet about 80 percent of the need and imports the rest. Recently, Malaysian farmers started taking advantage of Internet of Things (IoT) technologies to boost rice production, with the goals of doubling yields and becoming a rice exporter. Providing technical assistance, Abbaco Controls, an automation systems integrator since 2009, deployed IoT technologies from Intel and Kontron to help farmers control irrigation water in real time, optimize water usage, lower system cost, and ultimately, increase rice production. The IoT solution replaced a SCADA-based control system.

Key Business Objective

Boost rice production by implementing a water management system that allows farmers and the Malaysian Ministry of Agriculture (MOA) to monitor water resource status and remotely control the water distribution to their farms.

Business Challenges

Rice is grown under various conditions, and typically the best case is to continuously submerge the crops in five to seven centimetres of water. This makes the irrigation infrastructure vital to rice production. Most areas do not have water dams to create reservoirs of stored water, so irrigation water is sourced directly from rivers. In Malaysia, the MOA governmental agency had centralized control over the water gates that delivered water to the country's agricultural fields. This meant farmers had to call the MOA to request changes to the irrigation schedule in cases such as recent rainfall reducing the need for irrigation or warmer weather necessitating more watering. Farmers found contacting the MOA to be time-consuming or even impossible during off hours, like nights and weekends. The inflexibility of the manually steered system led to suboptimal use of water resources, and in turn, negatively impacted rice production.

Solution Benefits

Abbaco Controls, with help from Intel and Kontron, designed and deployed an IoT-based irrigation system that decentralized management of water gates, allowing farmers to control water supplies to their fields. In addition, this highly automated system makes real-time watering decisions based on a comprehensive analysis of sensor data (e.g., temperature, current water levels). The system uses IoT technologies to enable secure and cost-effective communications throughout the irrigation infrastructure, thus producing many benefits, including:

Real-Time Irrigation Control

In the event of any emergency situation or on-demand controlling of water level, the solution enables users to initiate immediate action by controlling a series of water gates. Furthermore, the solution can automatically trigger an alarm to alert users about any abnormal event (e.g., water levels too high from strong rains or too low from a lack of rainfall).

Optimized Irrigation Water Usage

The water management solution helps farmers determine the minimal amount of irrigation water needed for crops by generating recommendations based on water level trend charts, rain patterns, and temperature over months and years.

Lower System Cost

The previous system used SCADA to connect to devices, which was expensive due to SCADA software license fees. The new IoT-based system uses Modbus TCP protocol instead, allowing it to be about half the overall cost of the prior system.

Increased Rice Yield

Early data shows the new water management system is increasing rice yields, with the expectation it will help double production.

Solution Overview

The Abbaco Controls water management system presents farmers, the MOA, and other users with useful information from hundreds of sensors attached to water gates in the rice fields across Malaysia. This information includes water level, water flow rate, temperature, acidity, etc. Figure 12 illustrates how IoT technology is used to collect sensor data and send it securely to a back-end cloud server, where it is processed by Abbaco Control's data mining and analytic infrastructure. End users can view the results on user-friendly interfaces on PCs or cell phones. Figure 12 also shows the architectural differences between the previous water management system and the new one based on IoT technology. The previous system was based on SCADA, whereas the new IoT-based system from Abbaco Controls connects to field devices using the open Modbus TCP protocol, which is a lower cost alternative. In addition, the

Figure 12. Simplified Architectural Diagrams (Before and After)

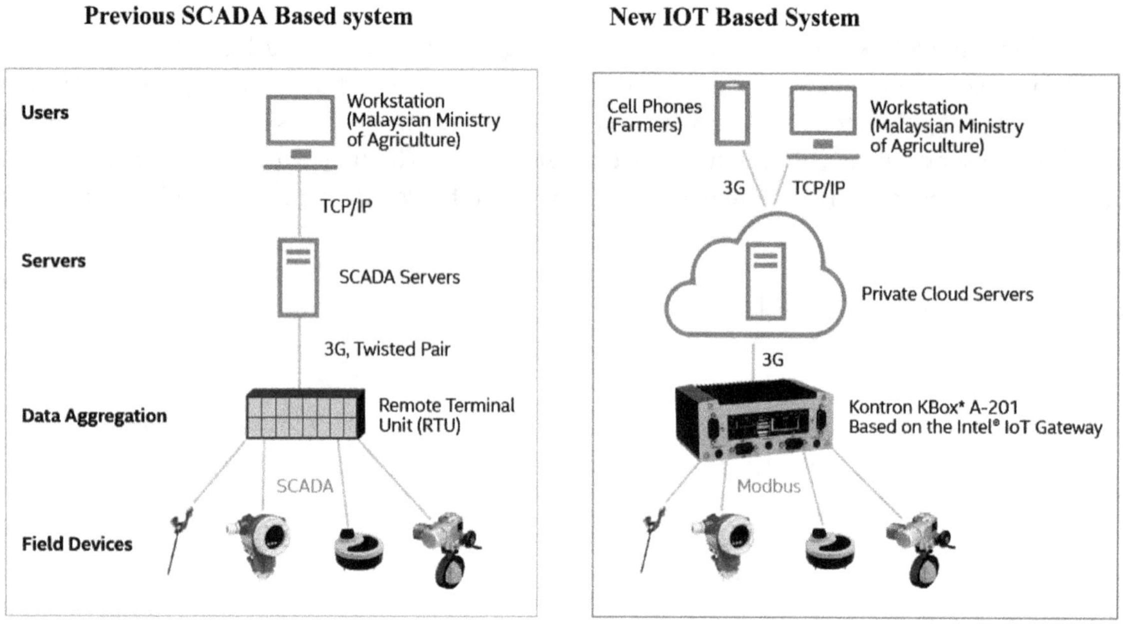

new cloud-based system makes it easier to deploy data analytics software and develop interfaces for a multitude of wireless user devices.

The Abbaco Controls water management solution has many advantages, including the following:

Remote Control

Users can remotely monitor and control the system from anywhere and at any time. This is a big step forward over the prior system that required MOA personnel to drive to each water gate in vast open fields, which was time-consuming, expensive, and schedule dependent.

Low Maintenance

The solution requires minimal or no on-going service since it employs a robust, industrial-rated IoT gateway designed to be maintenance-free.

Fast Deployment and Scalability

The use of Intel IoT building blocks allows the solution to be deployed quickly and easily expanded by adding I/O modules, which may be sourced from different vendors.

Data and System Security

The solution protects user data and software updates with security features such as whitelisting and integrity monitoring.

Technological Architecture of IoT

Technology ingredients from Intel and Kontron are available to deploy a water management solution like the one previously described. Such a solution can also be used whenever there are distributed field devices, as in water recycling, aqua-agriculture, and flood management applications. Figure 13 shows a detailed view of the IoT architecture utilized by the Abbaco Controls water management solution. In the bottom right quadrant, field devices connect to the Kontron Industrial Computer Platform A-201* IoT gateway via the Modbus TCP protocol, as previously described. The Abbaco Controls solution uses the protocol for reading and controlling sensors and devices.The Industrial Computer Platform A-201 also runs an Intel® IoT Gateway software stack that supports device management and configuration, and an MQTT client as a data agent, as shown in the bottom left quadrant. MQTT is a publish-and-subscribe protocol built on top of TCP/ IP protocol and is commonly used for machine-to-machine (M2M) communications. The two main components of MQTT are the MQTT clients and the MQTT broker. The MQTT clients publish messages to a particular topic, or subscribe and listen to a particular topic. The MQTT broker receives all published messages from MQTT publishers and forwards the relevant messages to all MQTT subscribers. The Industrial Computer Platform A-201 communicates over a TCP/ IP connection (wired or wireless) to a private cloud (upper left quadrant) running the Intel® Broker Module, which includes an MQTT broker server responsible for subscribing the data coming from all

Figure 13. Detailed IoT Architecture

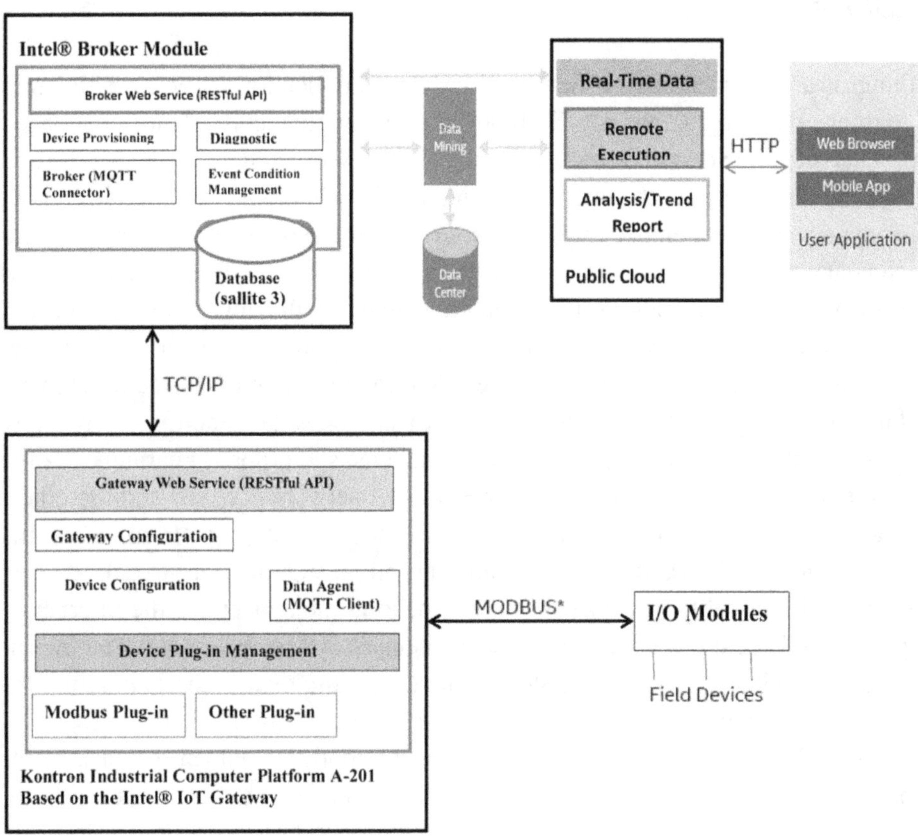

gateways. It sorts the data before storing it in a data warehouse, making it available for data mining and data analytics by applications running in a public cloud. The module also performs device provisioning, diagnostics, event management, and broker web services. In the upper right quadrant, the public cloud (web application servers) performs real-time data analysis, generates trend reports, and pushes information to user applications over the Internet via HTTP. Abbaco Controls does not host the servers, but instead uses a renowned cloud service provider to provide reliable and consistent service. The web application server hosts Abbaco Controls' IoT solution portal, which is powered by ASP, .NET, and HTML5. The portal supports all the user-accessible functionalities, including the ability to remotely control the water gate (e.g., open gate), check the water gate and alarm status, and view historical data.

With the goals of doubling rice production and transitioning from a rice importer to exporter, the Malaysian government found it necessary to revamp its agricultural water management system to make better use of the country's water resources. It selected the Abbaco Controls solution because it gives farmers more control over how their farms are irrigated while also making the process more cost-effective and time-efficient for everyone involved. In collaboration with Intel and Kontron, Abbaco Controls provides a secure and scalable solution that allows farmers to control water gates in real time, optimize water usage, lower system cost, and increase rice production. By partnering with systems integrators like Abbaco Controls, Intel and Kontron are enabling scalable IoT solutions across the world in support of truly transformational ideas. The possibilities are endless, and Intel looks forward to working with partners like Kontron to drive economic value and social change with the IoT.

6. CONCLUSION

Internet of things is a new technology which provides many applications to connect the things to things and human to things through the internet. Each object in the world can be identified, connected to each other through internet taking decisions independently. All networks and technologies of communication are used in building the concept of the internet of things such technologies are mobile computing, RFID, wireless sensors networks, and embedded systems, in addition to many algorithms and methodologies to get management processes, storing data, and security issues. IoT requires standardized approach for architectures, identification schemes, protocols and frequencies will happen parallels, each one targeted for a particular and specific use. by the internet of things many smart applications becomes real in our life, which enable us to reach and contact with every things in addition to facilities many important aspects for human life such as smart healthcare, smart homes, smart energy, smart cities and smart environments. Internet of things may face two major challenges in order to guarantee seamless network access; the first issue relates to the fact that today different networks coexist and the other issue is related to the big data size of the IoT. Other current issues, such as address restriction, automatic address setup, security functions such as authentication and encryption, and functions to deliver voice and video signals efficiently will probably be affected in implementing the concept of the internet of things but by on-going in technological developments these challenges will be overcome. The internet of things promises future new technologies when related to cloud, fog and distributed computing, big data, and security issues. By integrating all these issues with the internet of things, smarter applications will be developed as soon. This paper surveyed some of the most important applications of IoT with particular focus on what is being actually done in addition to the challenges that facing the implementation the internet of things concept, and the other future technologies make the concept of IoT feasible.

REFERENCES

Ahmed, Björkman, Čaušsević, Fotouhi, & Linden. (n.d.). *An Overview on the Internet of Things for Health Monitoring Systems*. Retrieved from https://www.researchgate.net/publication/281062554

Benioff. (2015). *Industrial Internet of Things: Unleashing the Potential of Connected Products and Services*. Academic Press.

Bhattacharjee & Bera. (2014). Development of smart detachable wireless sensing system for environmental monitoring. *International Journal on Smart Sensing and Intelligent Systems*, *7*(3).

Chamberlin, B. (n.d.). *Healthcare Internet of Things: 18 trends to watch in 2016*. IBM Center for Applied Insights. Retrieved from https://ibmcai.com/2016/03/01/healthcare-internet-of-things-18-trends-to-watch-in-2016/

Chatzimilioudis, G. (2011). Crowdsourcing with Smartphones. *IEEE Internet Computing*.

Christin, Reinhardt, Mogre, & Steinmetz. (n.d.). *Wireless Sensor Networks and the Internet of Things: Selected Challenges*. Retrieved from http://www.ti5.tu-harburg.de/events/fgsn09/proceedings/fgsn_031.pdf

Curioni, Murtas, & Silari. (n.d.). *Internet of Sensors*. Politecnico di Milano. Retrieved from https://indico.cern.ch/event/470460/attachments/1303283/1948255/P10_TWD2016_Cur ioni.pdf

Davies, R. (2015). *The Internet of Things Opportunities and challenges*. Retrieved from http://www.europarl.europa.eu/RegData/etudes/BRIE/2015/557012/EPRS_BRI(2015)557012_EN.pdf

Djajadi. (2016). Ambient Environment quality monitoring Using IoT Sensor Network. Interworking Indonesia Journal, 8(1).

Dlodlo, N. (2012). Adopting the internet of things technologies in environmental management in South Africa. In *International Conference on Environment Science and Engineering* (vol. 3). IACSIT Press.

Dragusin, M., Stanga, D., Gurau, D., & Ionescu, E. (2014). Radiation monitoring under emergency conditions. *Rom. Journal. Phys.*, *59*(9-10), 891–903.

Ezechina, Okwara, & Ugboaja. (2015). The Internet of Things (Iot): A Scalable Approach to Connecting Everything. *The International Journal of Engineering and Science, 4*(1), 9-12.

Fatima. (2015). Internet of things: A Survey on Architecture, Applications, Security, Enabling Technologies, Advantages & Disadvantages. *International Journal of Advanced Research in Computer and Communication Engineering*, *4*(12).

Jiang, P., Xia, H., He, Z., & Wang, Z. (2009). Design of a Water Environment Monitoring System Based on Wireless Sensor Networks. *Sensors (Basel, Switzerland)*, *9*(9), 6411–6434. doi:10.3390/s90806411 PMID:22454592

Kaur & Singh. (2016). A Survey Report on Internet of Things Applications. *International Journal of Computer Science Trends and Technology*, *4*(2).

Mattern & Floerkemeier. (n.d.). *From the Internet of Computers to the Internet of Things*. Academic Press.

Miceli. (2013). *Energy Management and Smart Grids Energies*. Academic Press.

Mirzabeiki. (n.d.). *An Overview of the Freight Intelligent Transportation Systems*. Division of Logistics and Transportation, Chalmers University of Technology. Retrieved from http://www.bth.se/tek/intelligent_gods.nsf/bilagor/Mirzabeiki,2010,ITS%20World%20Busan_pdf/$file/Mirzabeiki,2010,ITS%20World%20Busan.pdf

Mohassel, R. R. (2014). A survey on Advanced Metering Infrastructure. *International Journal of Electrical Power & Energy Systems*, *63*, 473–484. doi:10.1016/j.ijepes.2014.06.025

Murray, Minevich, & Abdoullaev. (2011). Being smart about smart cities. *KM World*.

Niewolny, D. (n.d.). *How the Internet of Things Is Revolutionizing Healthcare*. Retrieved from https://cache.freescale.com/files/corporate/doc/white_paper/IOTREVHEALCARWP.pdf

Nuaimi. (2015). Applications of big data to smart cities. *Journal of Internet Services and Applications*.

Saranya, C. M., & Nitha, K. P. (2015). Analysis of Security methods in Internet of Things. *International Journal on Recent and Innovation Trends in Computing and Communication, 3*(4).

Smart Grid enabling energy efficiency and low-carbon transition. (n.d.). Retrieved from https://www.gov.uk/government/uploads/system/uploads/attachment_data/file/321852/Policy_Factsheet_-_Smart_Grid_Final__BCG_.pdf

Suhonen, J. (2013). *Experiences and Future Plans for WSN-enabled Service Development in Home Environment*. Realin white paper.

Susmitha, P., & Sowmyabala, G. (2014). Design and Implementation of Weather Monitoring and Controlling System. *International Journal of Computers and Applications*, *97*(3).

Talasila, Curtmola, & Borcea. (n.d.). *Mobile Crowd Sensing*. New Jersey Institute of Technology. Retrieved from https://web.njit.edu/~mt57/publications/Chapter4.pdf

Chapter 10
Secured Optimal Cost Approach for Bimodal Deep Face Recognition in IoT and Its Applications

Madhavi Gudavalli
JNTUK–UCEN, India

Vidaysree P
Stanley Women's Engineering College, India

S Viswanadha Raju
JNTUH CEJ, India

Surekha Borra
K.S. Institute of Technology, India

ABSTRACT

This chapter proposes an optimal cost security approach for the current and emerging trends in the Engineering centric IoT applications that offer an optimized infrastructure and human safety through bimodal deep face recognition. Human face determines the person identity that reveals information like age, gender, emotions, attractiveness and others. Face recognition attracted researchers to enhance its performance because of its potential usage in several commercial, law enforcement, government and video surveillance applications in which individuals perceive each other. In this chapter, authors propose a new secured optimal cost approach for deep face recognition based on feature level fusion of bi-features extracted through unsupervised deep learner, Autoencoder and Local Binary Patterns (LBP) respectively. The dimensionality of fused feature map is reduced and protected through Forward Error Correction (FEC) technique. An efficient optimal cost region matcher (OCRM) is accomplished with Canny edge detector to maximize the face recognition accuracy. OCRM uses north-west corner rule of the transportation problem that fulfills the Monge property. The experimental results demonstrate the superiority of the proposed face recognition system over unimodal systems (Autoencoder and LBP alone) when tested on ORL and Real face datasets with OCRM matcher which is interfaced through diverse IoT applications.

DOI: 10.4018/978-1-5225-5222-2.ch010

Copyright © 2018, IGI Global. Copying or distributing in print or electronic forms without written permission of IGI Global is prohibited.

1. INTRODUCTION

A biometric system is fundamentally a pattern recognition system that automatically identifies individuals based on their physiological and behavioral characteristics. (Jain, A. K.et al.2007) demonstrated that physiological biometrics use measurements from the human body, like face, fingerprint, iris and retina, while behavioral biometrics use dynamic measurements based on human action, like signature, voice, keystroke and gait. The striking feature of face biometric considered in this work when compared with diversified biometric traits is that facial images can be acquired from a distance without user cooperation. This feature is particularly beneficial for security and surveillance purposes. Furthermore, data obtained from hand and finger images will be inoperative if the skin is injured. Correspondingly, the data acquisition from retina, iris modalities necessitates costly devices which are easily susceptible to body motion. Voice recognition is vulnerable to environmental conditions and sound-related variations on a telephone line or tape recording while signatures can be easily spurious and alterable. However, facial data can be captured with an ease through low cost rigid cameras. The various approaches to extract face features are grouped into three categories, namely, geometric, holistic and hybrid approaches. A few researchers in the literature like (Xie, J et al. 2012; Boureau, Y. L., and Cun, Y. L. 2008; Glorot, X et al. 2011; Krizhevsky et al. 2012) proposed various machine learning feature extractors such as deep neural networks, deep belief networks, deep convolution neural networks, learning deep face are tested and illustrated by (Taigman et al. 2014; Fan, H.et al. 2014) and Zhu, Z. et al. 2013) explained how to preserve face space with deep learner. The features extracted from these learning algorithms reduce the input dimensionality and reconstruct the feature vector to minimize the intra-class variations in face biometrics is well explained by (Bengio, Y. et al. 2013). (Bronstein, A. M. et al. 2007) demonstrated an expression invariant representation of a face can also be used for recognition through canonical form. (Besides, Abaza, A. et al. 2014) illustrates that the image quality factors like brightness, focus, illumination, contrast and sharpness are significant in face recognition systems. Further, face recognition is absolutely non-invasive and does not convey any health hazards. It has turned out to be progressively vital owing to quick advances in image acquisition gadgets (surveillance cameras, camera in mobile phones), accessibility of extensive face images on the Web, and raise in demand for higher security is explained by (Jain, A. K., and Li, S. Z. 2011).

Motivation: The motivation behind developing face recognition system is because of its pervasiveness in contrast with other biometric traits as any human cannot exist with its absence. Also, there may be variations in faces due to aging and distractions like beard, glasses or change of hairstyles which may affect the recognition accuracy. An ideal biometric system should give the correct decision when a biometric identifier sample is submitted. The accuracy estimate of biometric systems depends on the number of test conditions including the sensor employed, acquisition protocol used, subject disposition, number of subjects, number of biometric samples per subject, demographic profile of test subjects, subject habituation, time lapse between data acquisition and matcher selection. The results of these evaluations clearly indicate that biometric systems have non-zero error rates and that there is a possibility to enhance the recognition accuracy. Hence, it is significant to enhance the accuracy of biometric recognition system by executing appropriate feature extractor and classifier. Therefore, in this paper, we propose a face recognition system that integrates the holistic (global) and geometric (local) features extracted from autoencoder, a basic deep learner and LBP respectively at feature level in which template selection and protection is accomplished through FEC. A novel similarity matcher called optimal cost region matcher

(OCRM) is incorporated to maximize the accuracy of face recognition system and expanding its usage in real time applications of border crossings, mass surveillance, e-commerce, banking, military sites, law enforcement and digital entertainment. The paper is organized as follows. Section 2 describes the proposed system, while Section 3 validates the efficient performance through a set of experiments on ORL and real face datasets. Section 4 gives conclusions and future work.

2. PROPOSED SYSTEM

The facial recognition systems measure and analyze the overall structure, shape and propositions of face which are stored in database for recognition purpose. An edge detection method, Canny operator is employed in preprocessing phase that emphasizes regions of high spatial gradients corresponding to edges. The holistic face features (global) are then extracted with an artificial neural network known as autoencoder. This autoencoder method not only reduces the dimensionality of the image, but also denoises the input and retains some of the variations in the image data there by providing compact representation of facial image. The global features are cascaded with geometric features extracted from LBP at feature level. The Forward Error Correction (FEC) method generates the template from the concatenated feature vector to strengthen the security for stored templates. A novel and optimal similarity matcher, known as optimal cost region matcher (OCRM) is proposed to establish an efficient face recognition system that augments the identification accuracy. The following steps demonstrate the process of proposed face recognition.

Step 1: Face images are acquired from built-in laptop web camera. The obtained color images are converted into gray scale images.

Step 2 - Preprocessing: The purpose of the preprocessing is to eliminate the variations in face due to illumination. An edge detection Canny operator is employed to find high spatial gradients at each point in a facial image, while preserving its important structural properties.

Step 3(i) - Feature Extraction Using Autoencoder: An autoencoder which is a feed forward non-recurrent neural network suitable for efficient deep representation of data is used to extract global face features. It trains the large input data to small representation at hidden layers and decodes it to reconstruct the encoded information as output which is demonstrated in "Figure 1". This forces the input into smaller dimensions that represents the compressed data which is the basis training for the auto encoder. It sends the input $\vec{r}$ to the feed forward neural network and obtains $\vec{o}$ as output after training. The neural network contains N layers and is represented by weight and bias matrices ($\vec{b}^p, W^p$) where 'p' represents the layer to which (w,b) belongs to. The activation of $\vec{g}^p$ of each layer depends on the activation of its preceding layer and it is calculated using "(1)".

$$g^{\vec{p}+1}\left(b^{\vec{p}}, W^p, g^{\vec{p}}\right) = \tanh\left(b^{\vec{p}} + W^p g^{\vec{p}}\right) \tag{1}$$

The output activation layer is represented with $g^{\vec{p}+1}$ and tanh makes the neural network to be nonlinear. The output pattern is reconstructed from the input pattern using mathematical statement "(2)"

Figure 1. Global face feature extraction with autoencoder

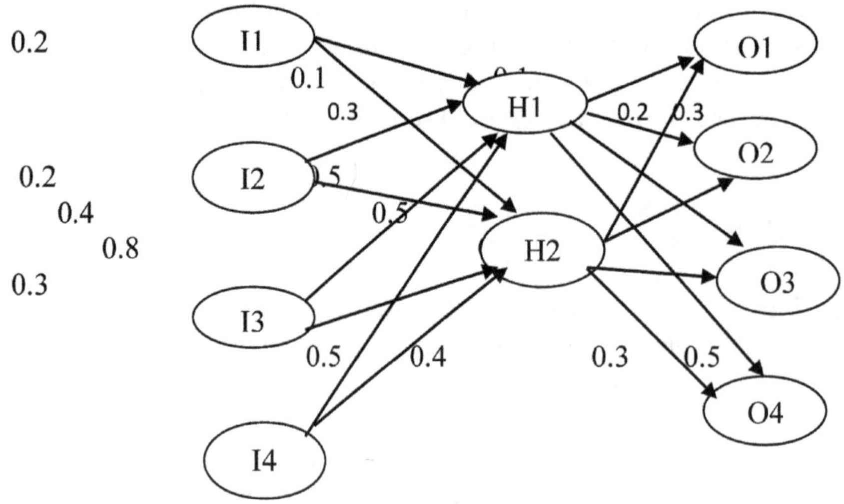

and the minimum error between the desired and actual output is indicated in "(3)". Table 1 illustrates the reconstructed output of a sample face image trained with autoencoder and "Figure 2" exemplifies its best training performance at epoch 689.

$$g_q^{p^{\rightarrow}+1}\left(b_q^{\rightarrow p}, W_q^p, g^{\rightarrow p}\right) = \tanh\left(b_q^{\rightarrow p} + W_q^p g^{\rightarrow p}\right) \tag{2}$$

$$\left[\min\right]_{\top\theta}\left[Er\left(s^{\rightarrow}, r^{\rightarrow}, \theta\right)\right] \tag{3}$$

where

$$Er\left(s^{\rightarrow}, r^{\rightarrow}, \theta\right) = \frac{1}{2}\left\| f\left(r^{\rightarrow}, \theta\right) - s^{\rightarrow}\right\|^2$$

and

Table 1. Reconstructed output of a trained face image

Input	Hidden Layer Output	Actual Output	Reconstructed Output
I1=1	H1=5.5	O1=1.21	O1=1.2238
I1=2		O2=2.75	O2=1.7762
I1=4	H2=3.3	O3=4.07	O3=3.7762
I1=3		O4=3.74	O4=3.2238

Figure 2. Best Training performance at echo 689

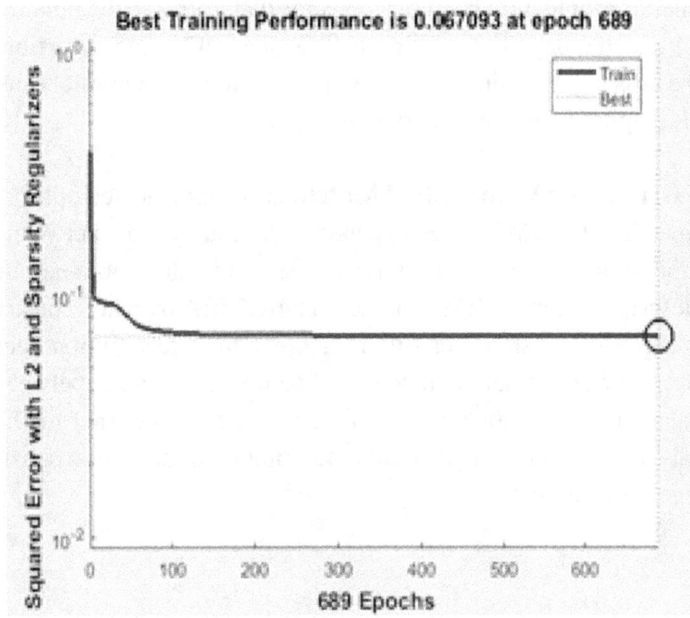

$$\theta = \left\{ W^{0\ldots M-1} b^{\rightarrow 0\ldots M-1} \right\}$$

Step 3(ii) - Feature Extraction With Local Binary Patterns (LBP): The Local binary patterns are retrieved from small regions of the face image which labels the image pixels by thresholding the 3x3-neighbourhood of each pixel with the center value resulting in binary number and then converted to decimal values. The local textures are labeled into histograms which are consolidated to recover the whole face feature. The LBP feature extraction is illustrated in "Figure 3".

Step 4 - Feature Level Fusion: Heterogeneous feature concatenation is used as the holistic and geometric feature sets are originating from different feature extraction algorithms. The extracted global and local face features are fused with horizontal concatenation method.

Step 5 - FEC as Template Generator: The vulnerable storage may lead to an attacker stealing biometric templates and impersonating the legitimate user.

Figure 3. Feature extraction using LBP

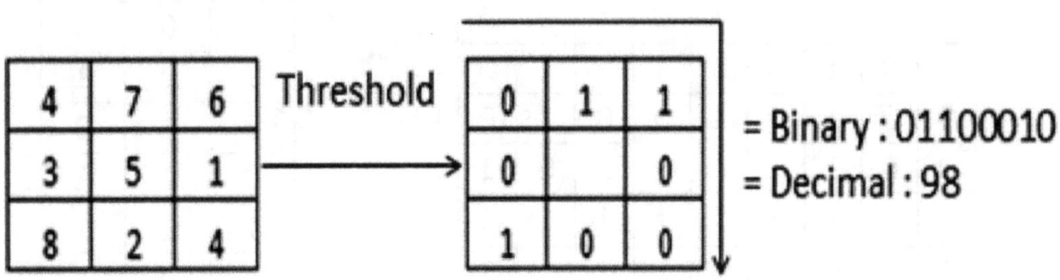

To prevent unauthorized access against stored biometric templates, Forward Error Correction (FEC) is used as template generator for feature level fused vector that averages the noise and reduces the image dimensionality by 30% which is depicted in "Figure 4". Since FEC is non-invertible, it is difficult for the intruders to remove the noise and obtain original template with in polynomial time. Thus it strengthens the security for stored templates even on network storage devices.

Step 6 - Match Score Generation With OCRM Matcher: A sophisticated optimal matcher called optimal cost region matcher (OCRM) is used to generate similarity score between set of query (claimed identity) and enrolled images (training dataset). The pixel values obtained in template generation are the region descriptors for OCRM matcher. The OCRM matcher constructs Monge distance matrix and uses the north-west corner rule to achieve high recognition accuracy in comparison with other similarity or dissimilarity matchers. The distance matrix between query and enrolled face images is calculated using statement "(4)". The north-west corner method is a transportation problem which always yields results that are both computationally inexpensive and optimal when applied for Monge distance matrix,

$$d_{i,j} = \left|q_i - t_j\right| \tag{4}$$

where $d_{i,j}$ is the distance between pixel values (region descriptors) of query and enrolled projection matrices, q_i is the ith pixel value of query projection matrix and t_j is the jth pixel value of enrolled projection matrices.

Step 7 - Recognition Performance: A reference threshold 'r_t' is calculated from distance matrix, where FAR and FRR becomes equal. This decision threshold identifies the genuine user with less number of iterations at low cost. The recognition accuracy of the proposed system based on OCRM matcher

Figure 4. FEC generated biometric template

Input Image Size: 9X9

1	0	1	0	0	1	1	1	0
0	0	1	1	1	0	1	1	1
0	0	0	0	0	1	1	0	1
1	1	1	0	1	0	1	0	0
1	0	1	0	0	1	1	1	0
0	0	1	1	1	0	0	1	0
0	0	1	1	0	1	1	0	1
1	1	1	1	1	1	1	1	1
0	0	0	0	0	1	1	1	1

FEC →

Output Image Size: 9X3

1	0	1
0	1	1
0	0	1
1	0	0
1	0	1
0	1	0
0	1	1
1	1	1
0	0	1

is tested using ORL and JNTUK UCEV real face datasets. The performance of proposed system is compared with recognition accuracy of unimodal face recognition systems employing autoencoder and LBP feature extractors respectively.

3. EXPERIMENTAL RESULTS AND DISCUSSIONS

The proposed face recognition system performance is analysed using ORL face database which is tested at (AT&T Laboratories Cambridge 2002) and real face dataset captured using Sony and Dell laptops' web camera. The ORL (OLIVETTI RESEARCH LABORATORY) face dataset consists of 400 images of 40 persons, 10 images per each person are acquired in BMP format with the size of 112 x 92 pixels, while real dataset consists of 200 face images acquired from 40 students of JNTUK UCEV, 5 images per student with different facial expressions. All the students of JNTUK UCEV are in the age group of 20 to 25 years and the captured image sizes are 120 x 160 pixels stored in JPEG format. The performance of secured face recognition system is measured in terms of accuracy [7] expressed in math statements "(5)" and "(6)".

$$\text{accuracy} = 100 - \text{EER} \quad (5)$$

$$\text{EER} = \frac{FAR + FRR}{2} \quad (6)$$

"Figure 5(a) and 5(b)" depicts the enrolled and query face images of proposed system using ORL and JNTUK UCEV face datasets. The preprocessed query and enrolled images of these datasets with Canny edge detection are shown in "Figure6 (a) and 6(b)". The holistic and geometric features extracted using autoencoder and LBP are depicted in "Figure 7 (a) & 7(b)" and "Figure 8 (a) & 8(b)" respectively.

Figure 5. Query and Enrolled face images of ORL and real datasets

5(a)

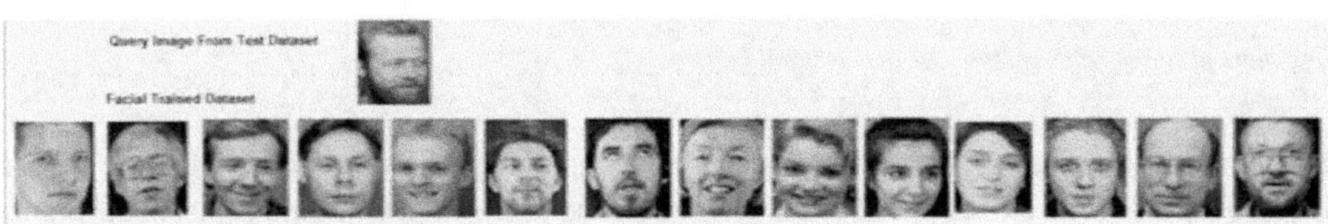

5(b)

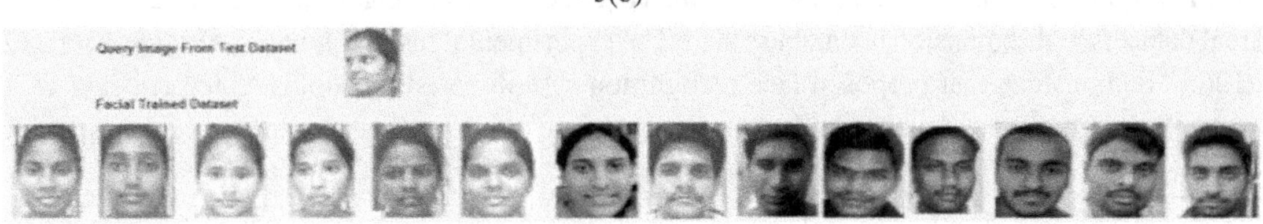

**For a more accurate representation see the electronic version.*

Figure 6. Preprocessed query and enrolled face images of ORL and real datasets using canny edge detection method

6(a)

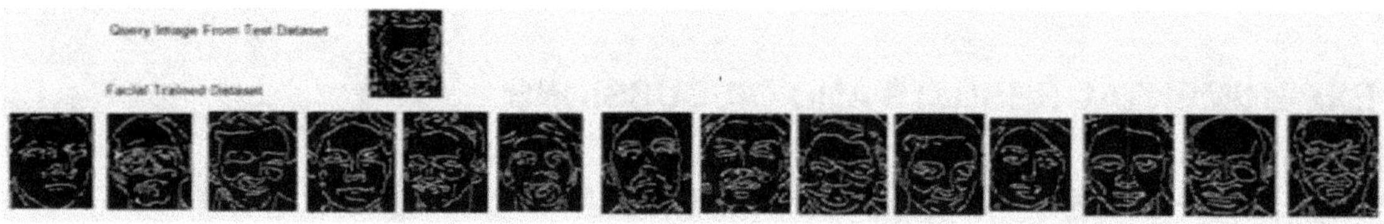

6(b)

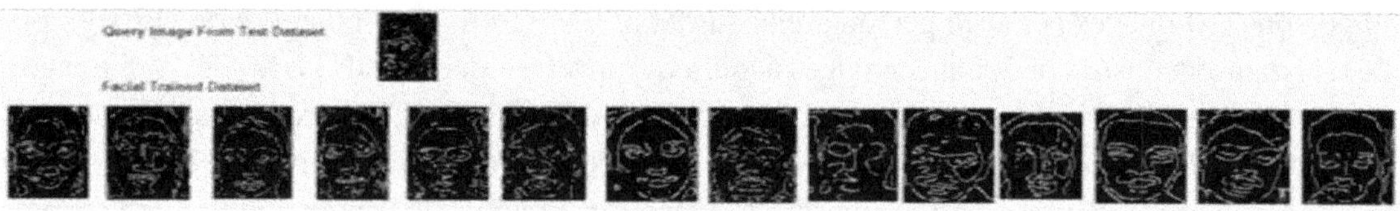

**For a more accurate representation see the electronic version.*

Figure 7. Holistic features extracted from query and enrolled face images of ORL and real datasets with autoencoder

7(a)

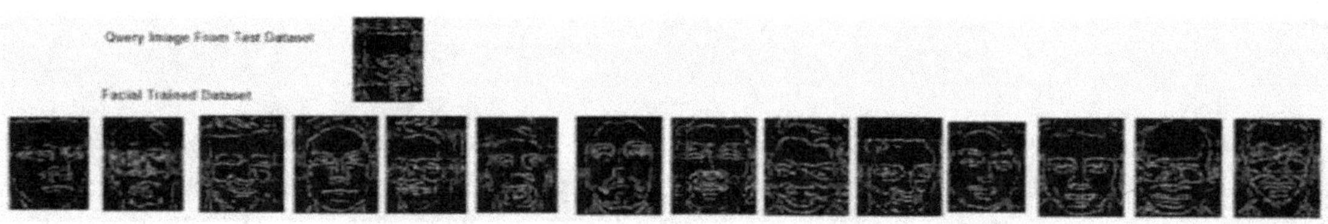

7(b)

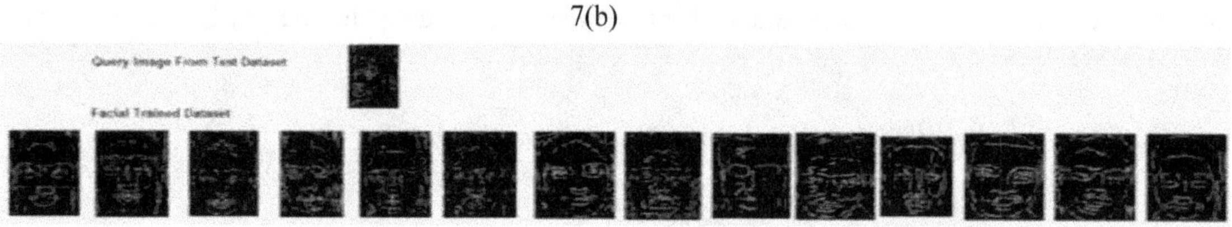

**For a more accurate representation see the electronic version.*

The fused features and templates generated using FEC method are shown in “Figure 9 (a) & 9(b)” and “Figure10 (a) & 10(b)” respectively. The match scores generated with OCRM are depicted in “Figure11 (a) & 11(b)”.

From “Figure 12”, it is evident that OCRM matcher accomplishes higher performance for both ORL and real datasets with expansion in database size. The experimental results shown in “Figure 12(a), 12(b) and 12(c)” demonstrate that proposed face recognition system based on sophisticated matcher OCRM maximizes recognition accuracy with less number of computations there by making the system more

Figure 8. Geometric features extracted from query and enrolled face images of ORL and real datasets with Local Binary Patterns (LBP)

8(a)

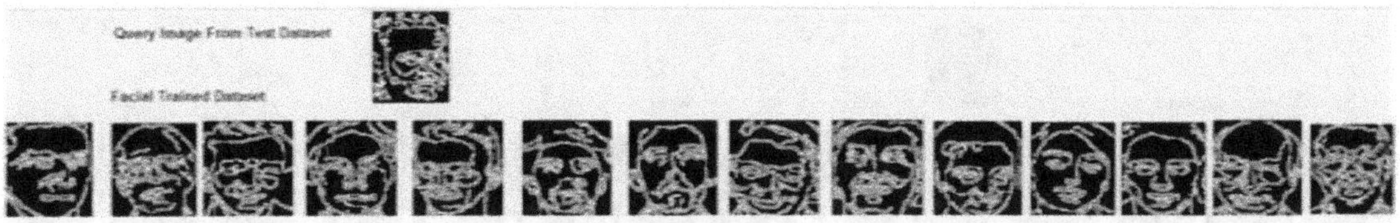

8(b)

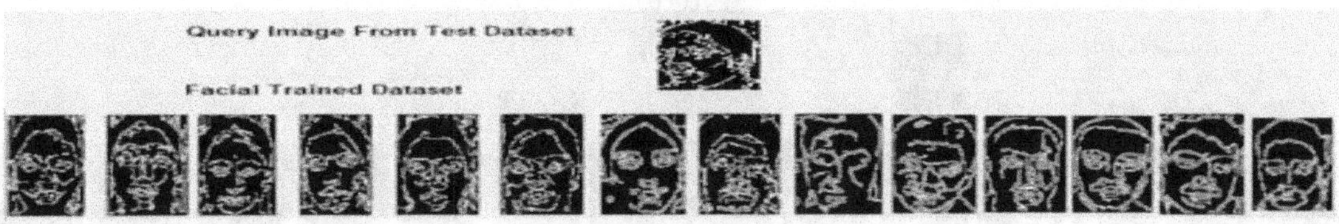

**For a more accurate representation see the electronic version.*

Figure 9. Feature level fusion of holistic and geometric features extracted from query and enrolled face images of ORL and real datasets

9(a)

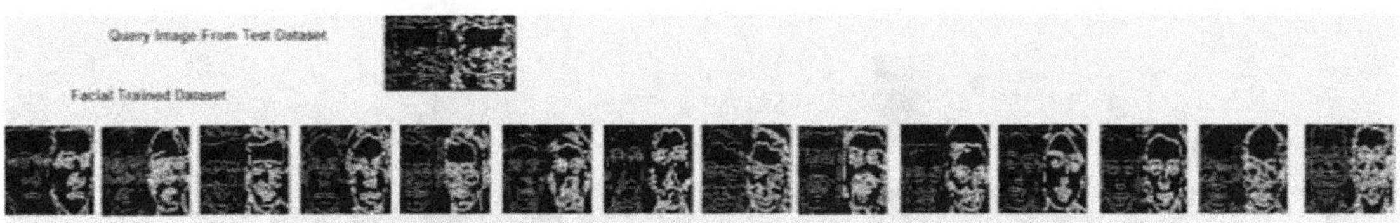

9(b)

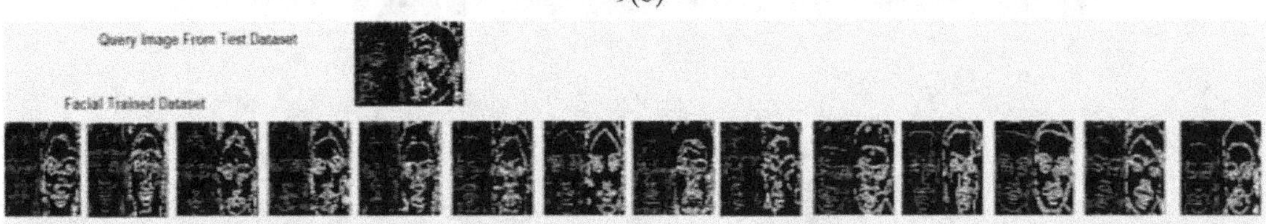

**For a more accurate representation see the electronic version.*

efficient and cost effective. It is evident from the results that FEC template generator outperforms when compared with several methods and provides better security for face recognition systems in order to use them in high security areas or applications.

4. CONCLUSION AND FUTURE WORK

IOT confluences various technologies, efficient wireless protocols, interoperable communication protocols and productive secured strategies to construct a smart environment applications. Security concern

Figure 10. Template generation for fused features of query and enrolled face images of ORL and real datasets using Forward Error Correction(FEC)

10(a)

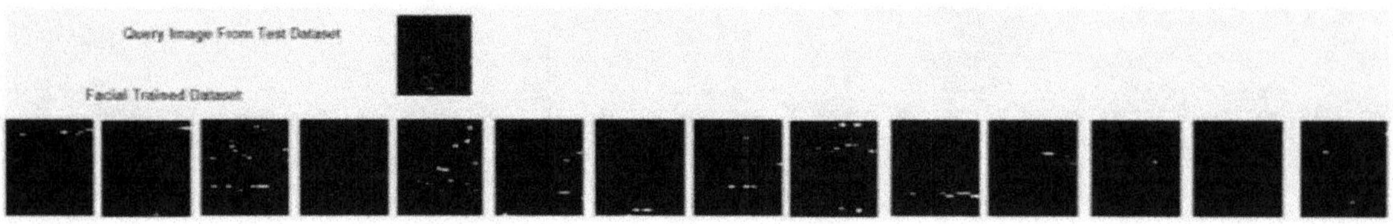

10(b)

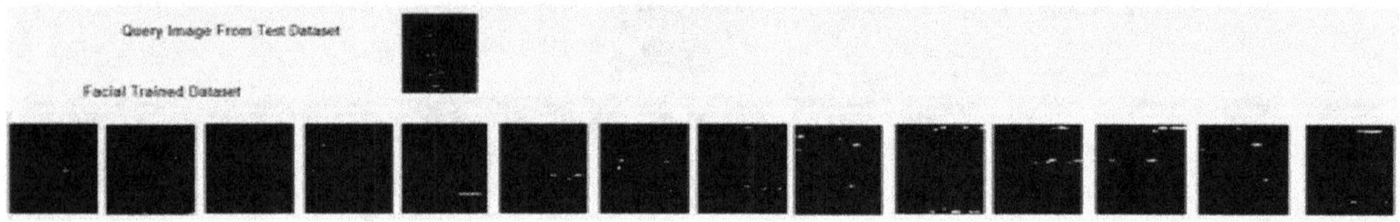

**For a more accurate representation see the electronic version.*

Figure 11. Match score generated for fused biometric templates of ORL and real datasets with OCRM matcher

(a)

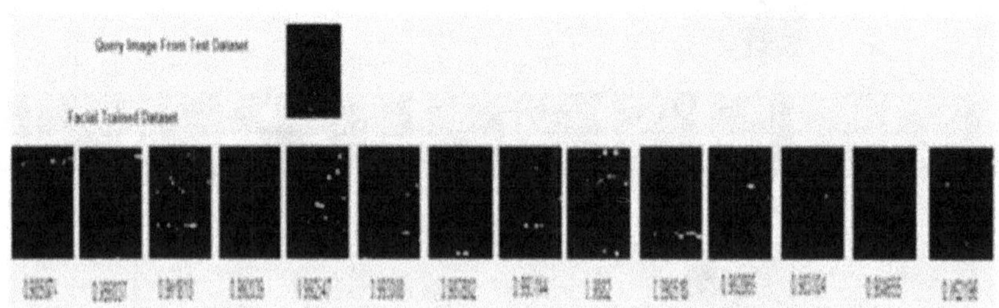

(b)

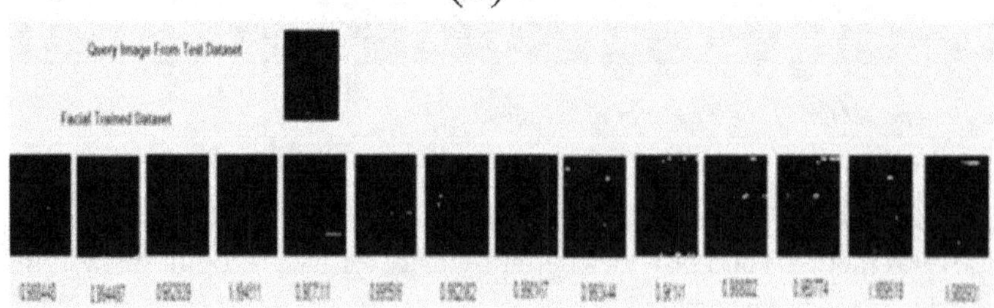

**For a more accurate representation see the electronic version.*

is expanded with expansion of the internet. High end security is needed from the primary layer of the IOT to perform the transactions, confidential data exchange through internet to the connected computers. This chapter proposed an optimal cost security approach for IOT applications that enhances the security through bimodal face recognition. It is necessary to develop good computing techniques for

Figure 12. ROC curves depicting the performance comparison of proposed face recognition system with unimodal systems using ORL and real datasets

12(a)

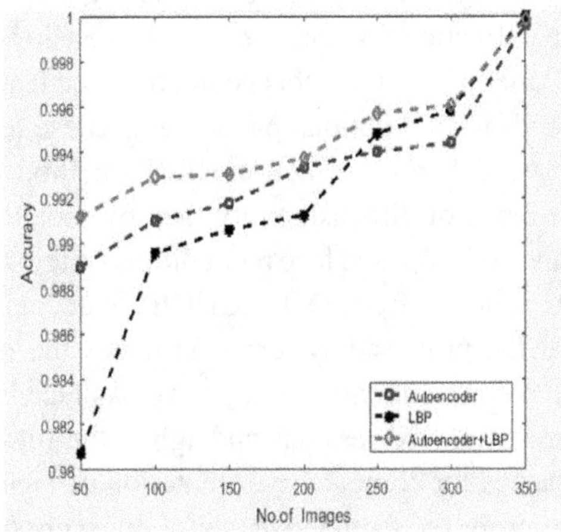

12(b)

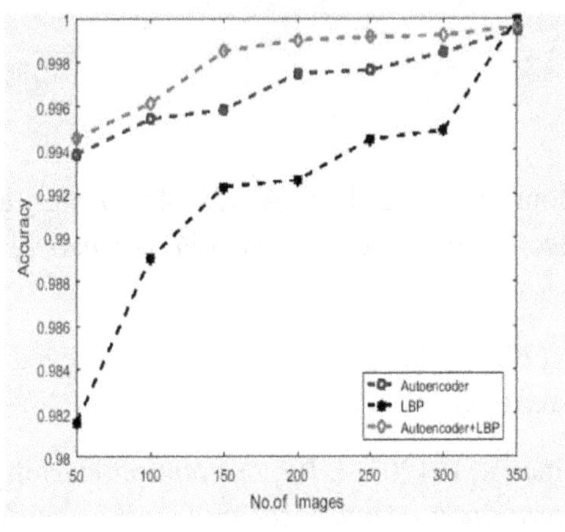

12(c)

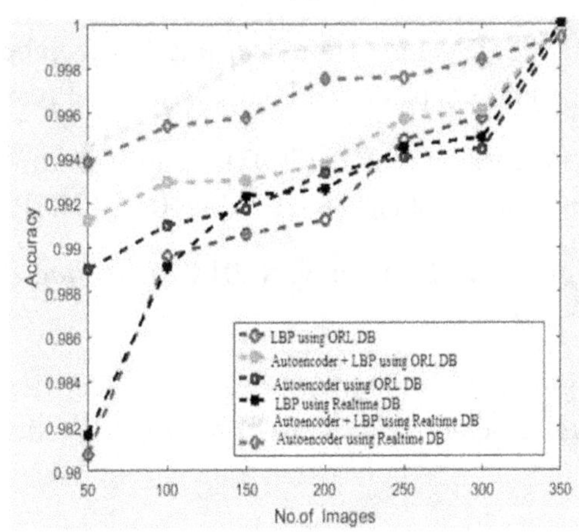

**For a more accurate representation see the electronic version.*

face recognition due to its multidimensional structure. The slight reduction in accuracy can compromise the biometric system performance, therefore, an efficient novel approach is proposed to maximize the recognition accuracy and strengthen the security provided by face biometric systems. The gray scale face images captured from the biometric sensors are filtered through Canny edge detection operator and the autoencoder used for feature extraction reduces the large dimensions of facial feature space to low intrinsic feature vector. The LBP method that extracts geometric face features requires simple computations in contrast with other methods to find optimal parameters. These feature vectors are concatenated and then transformed using Forward Error Correction (FEC) method that achieves cancelability by adding noise and minimizes the curse of dimensionality thereby protecting stored templates from the intruders hacking. The performance of proposed face recognition system accomplishing OCRM matcher are tested with real time datasets acquired from JNTUK UCEV students as well as ORL database. The experimental results proved that the proposed system maximizes the recognition accuracy with less number of iterations resulting in computationally inexpensive. As face biometrics are more vulnerable to spoofing with respect to illumination, expressions and aging, the future work involves investigating supervised deep learning approaches for compact representation of face templates so that they can be reconstructed and revoked if compromised from the database. Incorporating the proposed bimodal face recognition system into IOT addresses the some of the security issues and aids to enhance the high end authentication of user recognition when it is integrated within the smart device with a minimum cost.

REFERENCES

Abaza, A., Harrison, M. A., Bourlai, T., & Ross, A. (2014). Design and evaluation of photometric image quality measures for effective face recognition. *IET Biometrics*, *3*(4), 314–324. doi:10.1049/iet-bmt.2014.0022

AT&T Laboratories Cambridge. (2002). *The database of faces*. Retrieved from http://www.cl.cam.ac.uk/research/dtg/attarchive/facedatabase.html

Bengio, Y., Courville, A., & Vincent, P. (2013). Representation learning: A review and new perspectives. *IEEE Transactions on Pattern Analysis and Machine Intelligence*, *35*(8), 1798–1828. doi:10.1109/TPAMI.2013.50 PMID:23787338

Boureau, Y. L., & Cun, Y. L. (2008). Sparse feature learning for deep belief networks. In Advances in neural information processing systems (pp. 1185-1192). Academic Press.

Bronstein, A. M., Bronstein, M. M., & Kimmel, R. (2007). Expression-invariant representations of faces. *IEEE Transactions on Image Processing*, *16*(1), 188–197. doi:10.1109/TIP.2006.884940 PMID:17283777

Fan, H., Cao, Z., Jiang, Y., Yin, Q., & Doudou, C. (2014). *Learning deep face representation*. arXiv:1403.2802

Glorot, X., Bordes, A., & Bengio, Y. (2011, June). Deep sparse rectifier neural networks. In *Proceedings of the Fourteenth International Conference on Artificial Intelligence and Statistics* (pp. 315-323). Academic Press.

Jain, A. K., Flynn, P., & Ross, A. A. (2007). *Handbook of biometrics*. Secaucus.

Jain, A. K., & Li, S. Z. (2011). Handbook of face recognition. New York: Springer.

Krizhevsky, A., Sutskever, I., & Hinton, G. E. (2012). Imagenet classification with deep convolutional neural networks. In Advances in neural information processing systems (pp. 1097-1105). Academic Press.

Taigman, Y., Yang, M., Ranzato, M. A., & Wolf, L. (2014). Deepface: Closing the gap to human-level performance in face verification. In *Proceedings of the IEEE conference on computer vision and pattern recognition* (pp. 1701-1708). doi:10.1109/CVPR.2014.220

Xie, J., Xu, L., & Chen, E. (2012). Image denoising and inpainting with deep neural networks. In Advances in Neural Information Processing Systems (pp. 341-349). Academic Press.

Zhu, Z., Luo, P., Wang, X., & Tang, X. (2013). Deep learning identity-preserving face space. In *Proceedings of the IEEE International Conference on Computer Vision* (pp. 113-120). Academic Press.

Chapter 11

Diabetes Preventive Knowledge Management System for Recommending an Ice Cream to University Grads Based on Their Life Style and Eating Habits

Preeti Mulay
Symbiosis Institute of Technology (SIT), India

Rahul Raghvendra Joshi
Symbiosis Institute of Technology (SIT), India

Akash Rameshwar Laddha
Symbiosis Institute of Technology (SIT), India

ABSTRACT

Lifestyle and eating habits with the special focus on young university grads are considered to design and develop a Knowledge Management System (KMS). An appropriate ice cream is suggested via KMS to university grads, which keeps blood glucose level in control and acts as a diabetes preventive KMS. Designed KMS is based on effective Data Science (DS), Big Data techniques considering standalone and proposed distributed versions of Analytical Hierarchy Process (AHP), Monte Carlo AHP (MC-AHP), Goal Programming (GP), K-Means and Artificial Neural Network (ANN) Clustering and Collaborative Filtering (CF). Incremental-learning gains and updates knowledge at each level of applied DS techniques. Developed KMS analyzed ice cream consumption pattern, lifestyle & health condition attributes of university students to promote a novel KM strategy in terms of ice cream recommendation and can give altogether novel trigger to health-conscious students. The confluence of health, students, ice creams and DS is achieved and discussed in this chapter.

DOI: 10.4018/978-1-5225-5222-2.ch011

Copyright © 2018, IGI Global. Copying or distributing in print or electronic forms without written permission of IGI Global is prohibited.

INTRODUCTION

According to article on *Express.co.uk* website, Sunlight, Vitamins and regular exercise can prevent and cure diabetes. In relation to thoughts portrayed by *Express.co.uk*, Robert J. Hastings, Tinyburg Tales quoted that:

...stop pacing the aisles and counting the miles. Instead, climb more mountains, eat more ice cream, go barefoot oftener, swim more rivers, watch more sunsets, laugh more and cry less. Life must be lived as we go along.

Life at University is a key instance point in an individual's life. It represents a stage of increased responsibility about food choices and healthy lifestyle practices. Young adults often lack the experience of food shopping, meals planning etc. The changes in living arrangements determine food choices of university grads. It may also depend on the type of stream in which they are studying. Medical students are aware of healthy eating habits. There are possible chances that they will bring those in their daily routine. It is likely impossible in the case of engineering students, the other stream students. Deficit knowledge about healthy food choices affects eating habits of university grads.

Home away eating, snacking, frequent consumption of ice cream is unhealthy. Figure 1 presents ABCD framework of unhealthy eating habits introduced in this research. Healthy eating does not become routine in sudden. It takes a time to become a part of a daily schedule. Good or awful habits can twist in anything, including eating. No contemplation is set to where, when, and what is to eat. Eating habits is a major worry among university grads. It is the determinant of their health status. Unhealthy eating habits may lead to metabolism disorders like diabetes, over the years. So, accurate eating habits in young adults are useful for future health and well-being.

Figure 1. "ABCD framework of unhealthy eating habits introduced in this research" ™

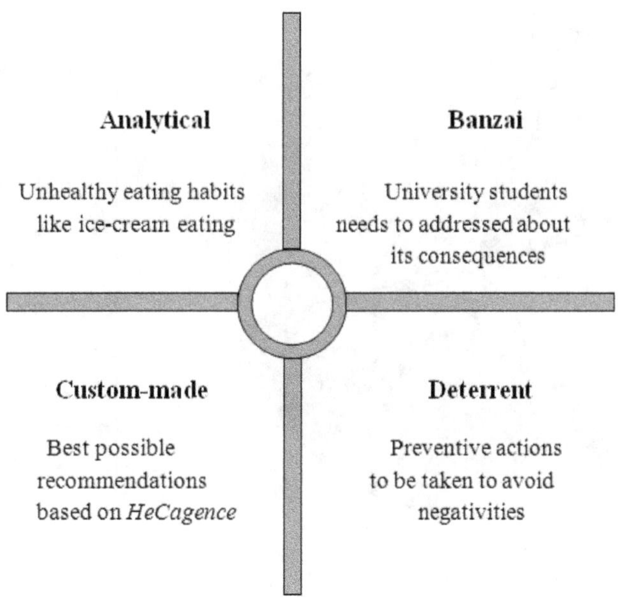

It is imperative to get insight into factors influencing eating behaviors of university grads. There are of four types of factors viz.

1. Intra and interpersonal (lack of time, self-will),
2. Community settings (communal support),
3. Large-scale environment (product costs, inadequate budgets) and
4. University characteristics (accessibility and access to unhealthy food).

The report of global flavor industry (2011) shows ice cream contributes to 2% of flavored products (Figure 2). Also, the study of VanderMey (2014) shows average ice cream consumption tops over the other types of frozen products (Figure 3). The ice cream survey report on *StatCrunch* shows ice cream eating frequency over a period of two weeks (Figure 4).

Taste is an influential parameter which may lead to temptation like eating ice cream. There are daily consumers also, for ice cream. Ice cream contains real fruits, milk, dry fruits and is available in small quantities. These days even bite-size ice creams is picking up as the new term. Churning and chilling of high-fat milk and glucose based sweeteners prepares ice cream. More often it is in the form of corn syrup, and flavorings such as vanilla or chocolate (Marie, & Media, 2012). After keeping this combo into freeze rich, uniform and smooth ice cream is available. Ice cream eating can influence health in both positive and negative ways (Marie, & Media, 2012). In the university canteen, ice creams are generally available in all seasons to students. They are available in the form of milkshakes, flavored sherbets, and toppings in fruit salads. Ice cream with high sugar can contribute to carbohydrates (Marie, & Media, 2012).

Figure 2. Global consumption of flavors according to product category (The Global Flavor Industry, 2011) (https://www.gov.mb.ca/agriculture/market-prices-and-statistics/food-and-value-added-agriculture-statistics/pubs/ma_global_flavours_industry_en.pdf)

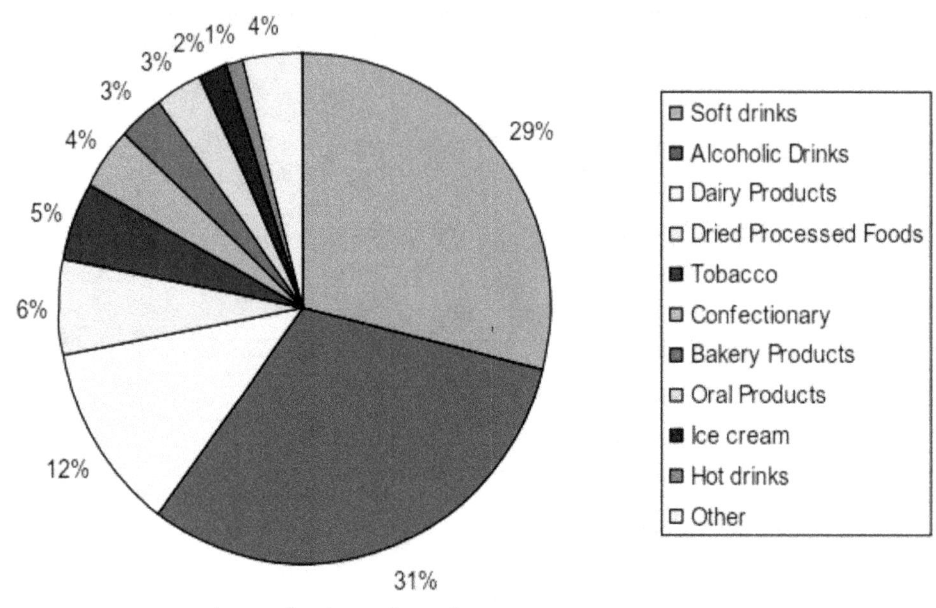

**For a more accurate representation see the electronic version.*

Figure 3. Ice cream consumption is at top as compared to other frozen treats (VanderMey, 2014) (http://fortune.com/2014/07/24/icecream-sales/)

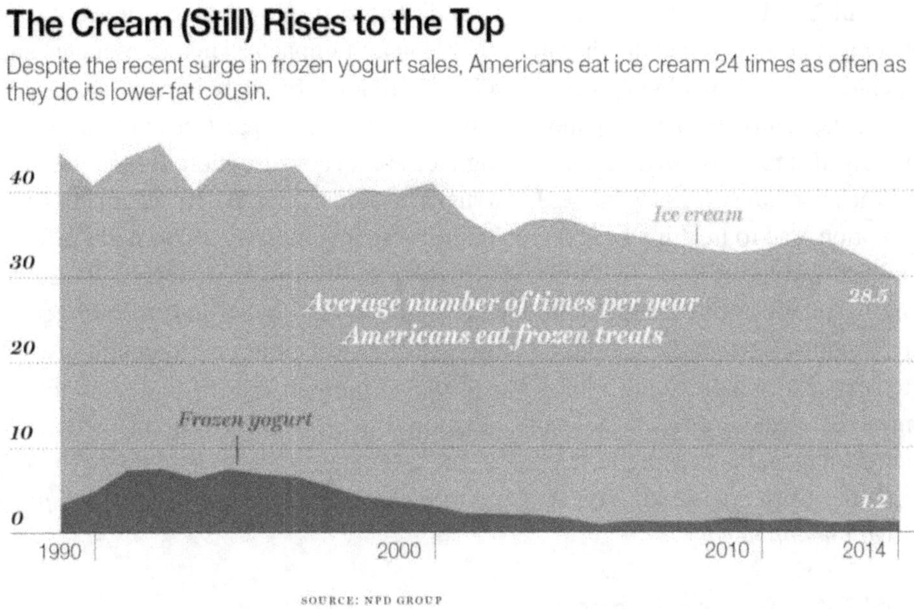

Figure 4. Ice cream consumption frequency over a two week period (http://www.statcrunch.com/5.0/viewreport.php?reportid=25427)

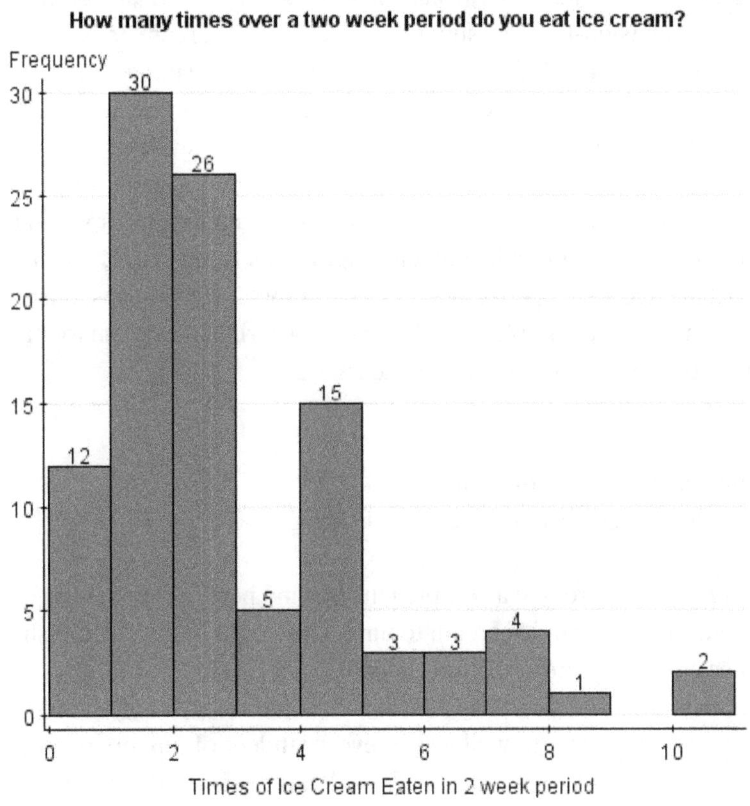

According to the research document of *britishcouncil.org* titled *Word_on_the_Street_Farming _Ice cream_Transcript*, ice cream in general is a favorite treat irrespective of age, gender whose roots can be found in early childhood days which was filled up milk-based sweet products. Hence it is hard to get a thought that consumption of ice cream has undesirable health impacts. This necessitates analysis of ice creams composition impact on blood glucose levels of individual living being across age-groups, health conditions etc. This, in turn, triggers one momentous question "Are sugar-free ice creams free of sugar?" This analysis may also focus on sugar intake through ice cream consumption. It is a good move as out of total daily calories in regular diets 5% comes from sugar (Siddique, 2015), (Revelant, 2014). Frequent ice cream consumption lead to health problems including weight gain, cavities, to name a few, which may shoot up an unhealthy type of fat called as blood triglycerides (Marie, & Media, 2012). Eating ice cream in small quantity can lower down risks of high cholesterol & sugar risks and add feel good factor too.

The study conducted by Andrew Hough (2012) says that ice cream is as addictive as the drug. He had conducted experiments on young adults. The results of his study shows that brain responses during excess eating of ice cream are similar to drug addiction. Mudur acknowledged ice cream related AHP work of Preeti Mulay and according to his article on Telegraph India website in 2015, he had quoted that Mulay and her team are working on an *"App to pick right ice cream - Engineers propose tool to match tastes with health needs"*.

Summary of Introduction Section

The integrated research discussed in this chapter comprises of different domains viz., Machine Learning, Big Data Mining, Internet of Things (IoT) and Data Discovery. Decision support is a fundamental and decisive task in healthcare because of multi-part processes and data dealings, tough to mold, indeed. This chapter develops "decision-making support model for ice cream intake". This study develops taxonomy of ice cream eating knowledge for improving decision-making about diabetes. "Confluence of technology-based study" explained in this chapter, constructs knowledge related to diabetes, fitness, university student behavior, food intake, time management skill of students etc., to name a few.

Designed KMS captures and distributes the knowledge related to diabetes preventative ingestion habits. It has both social and business values. It enables the transformation of captured Big Data into useful knowledge assets for iterative and incremental learning. Inputs to this KMS are attributes of university student, ice cream details and CF is performed based on inputs. KMS maps clusters of university student's data and ice creams compositions to recommend appropriate ice cream for prevention of diabetic.

KMS framework proposed in this chapter considers

1. Problem context,
2. Selection of applicable interventions and
3. Validation of designed KMS through relevant findings.

The aim of this chapter is to provide a comprehensible and perceptive view of DS, Big Data and IoT techniques for recommending an apt ice cream to university grads. This chapter shows that DS can dig out knowledge from available data/information. Till date various entities of university might be working with isolation but with this IT-healthcare system it is feasible to have a system to achieve the journey from health to fitness and ultimately to wellness of every student of university. Figure 5 shows process flow diagram of undertaken study. This process flow diagram shows database1 i.e. db1 for university

Figure 5. Process flow diagram

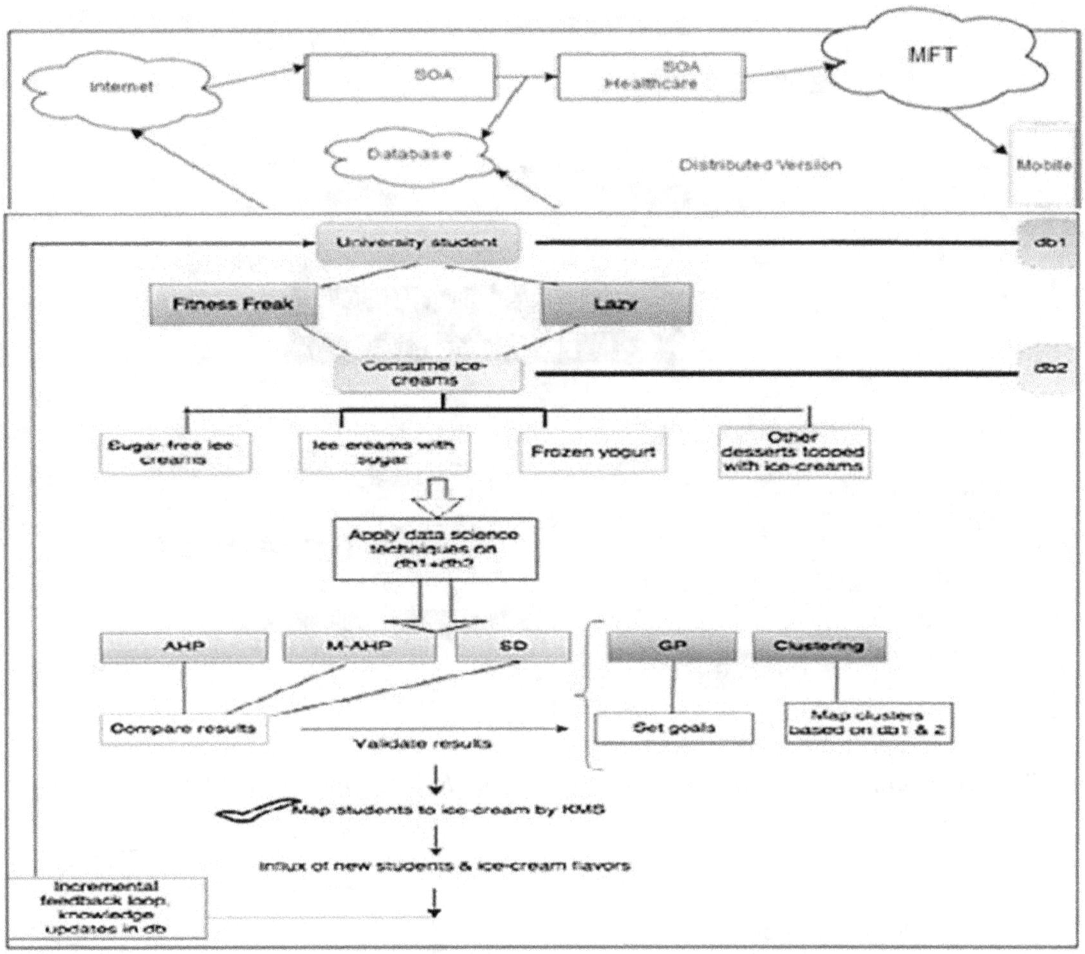

student, database2 i.e. db2 for ice cream consumed by students, DS techniques to be applied on db1 and db2 and knowledge update in db. Figure 6 shows the mind map of this research having three portions. In the center of this mind map is the name of integrated research (black colored rectangle). Inputs to this system are university students and ice cream details (shown in blue and green color respectively). DS techniques applied on Big Data and IoT to generate knowledge and learning is visible in orange color. Knowledge management based on various inputs and DS techniques are relevantly useful to upcoming entrepreneurs, employees of industries shown in red color blocks. All these blocks together make a system which is a learning system that generates the healthcare related useful knowledge. Figure 7 shows system architecture of carried out research in standalone and in distributed form.

BACKGROUND

DS is a versatile field and retrieves useful information from facts in different formats. DS use techniques from Information Science, Computer Science, Data Engineering and uncertainty modeling. Healthcare

Figure 6. Mind map for undertaken study

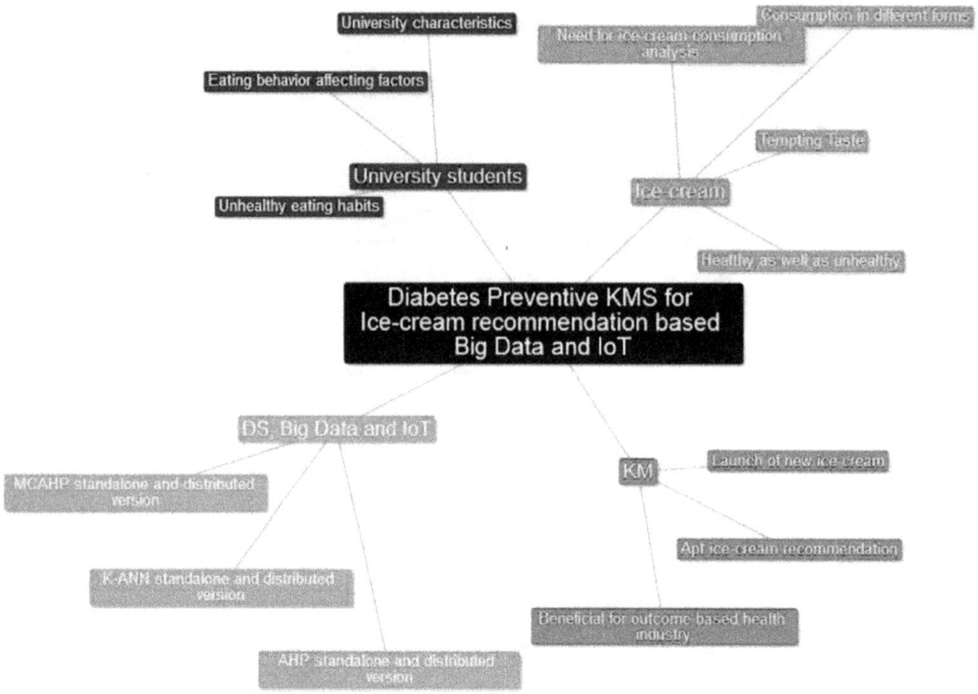

Figure 7. Architectural overview of DS techniques used in diabetes preventive KMS

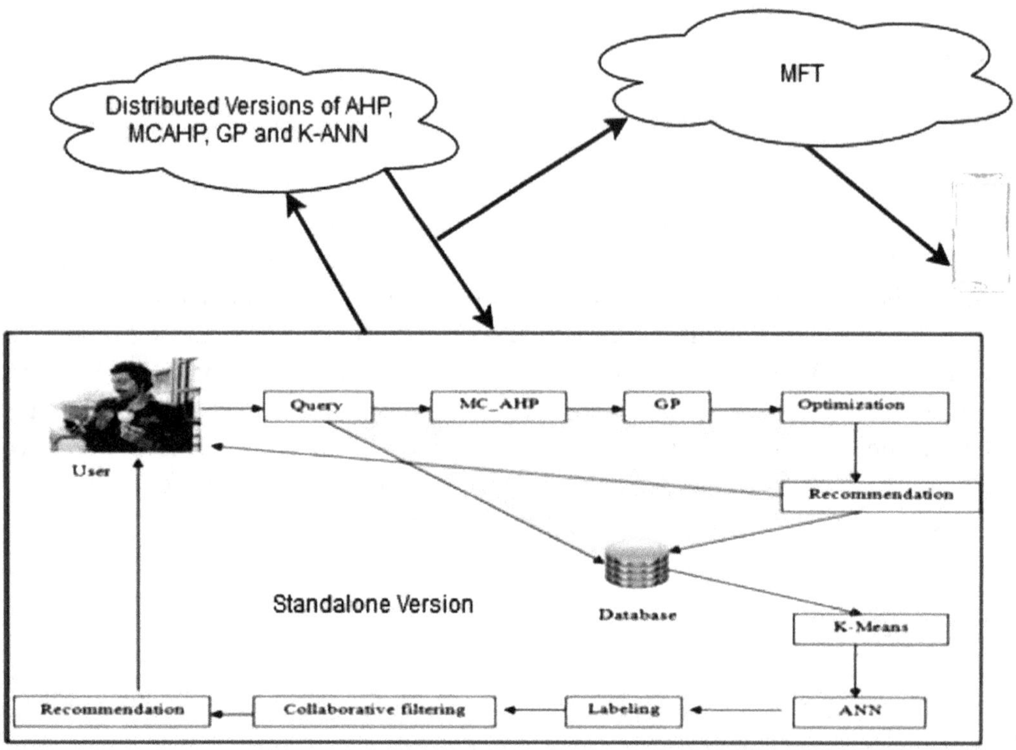

industry has innovative data formats like Electronic Health Records (EHRs), Heath-Claims. This type of data can add insight and smog of visibility to healthcare industry. Knowledge head of IT-Healthcare is increasing with linkages to Information Technology & Communication Technologies. "*Digital is critical for life*", "*Players reward for lower cost, higher quality care*" becomes true. The backbone factors for IT-healthcare are different ways of using innovative data and accessibility to innovative data. The researchers derive sensible information through IT-healthcare innovative data for outcome-based payment business. This in a way it triggers the digital economy (O'Reilly, Loukides, Steele, & Hill 2012). So, DS is not discretionary in health care amendments; it is the key player of IT-healthcare process.

IT-healthcare systems provide an efficient and improvised environment for better decision making (Nagaraj, 2016). Information Management System (IMS) in IT-healthcare does continuous monitoring and recording of frequent activities. The IMS based diagnostic helps to reduce the complexity of the diagnosis process. Process mining approach is useful in such diagnostic. Process mining has three phases' viz., discovery, conformance analysis and enhancement (Nagaraj, 2016). Important events in process mining are play-in, play-out and reply (Nagaraj, 2016). These aspects and characteristics of IT-healthcare IMS are taken into account while deploying DS techniques for underway problem.

Healthcare data is rich in information due to its varied nature. It has accountability, choice, efficiency, user satisfaction, innovation and outcomes. Healthcare data generation undergoes three processes viz., creation, sharing and collaborative filtering. Health data from different sources when mixed together becomes more influential. DS techniques can identify and check all hypotheses from such influential data. Identified hypotheses can extract useful and actionable information from data. These features of healthcare data are considered while applying DS technique on university grads health attributes dataset in order to obtain apt sugar-free ice cream recommendations for them.

The novel, appropriate use of analytics is a key feature to understand and use healthcare data. Effective uses of DS processes provide serviceable insights for undertaken problem. Rosen (2016) proposed a following framework for DS processes and underway research is aligned to this framework:

1. Collection,
2. Curation,
3. Analysis &
4. Explanation.

Now-a-days major challenge in front of health care industry is to understand the problem. With the aid of effective strategies, DS methodologies can verify problems in healthcare industry. Life cycle of IT-healthcare solutions follows following five distinct phases and solution to underway problem is designed by taking into account these phases (Rosen, 2016):

1. Insight,
2. Strategy,
3. Recommendations,
4. Capabilities development and
5. Deployment.

Following factors play important role in developed KMS for underway scenario.

1. Data Sharing,
2. Life style of university grads,
3. Statutory compliance about ice cream compositions,
4. Repeat-ability of applied DS techniques,
5. Archives and history of university grads preferences about ice cream,
6. Decision support system (DSS) for apt ice cream recommendations,
7. Convergence of recommendations and,
8. Efficiency of designed system on the basis of developed knowledge.

To develop IT-healthcare system, there is a need of appropriate data model. Barlow (2014) discussed about best data models for healthcare. Such a data model for IT-healthcare takes data from, many sources as a preliminary input. It is then given to Data Warehouse (DW). DW's output is then given as an input to disease profile alerting engine. It takes into account available health attribute profiles and suggests associated interventions in terms of ice cream recommendations.

Data processed through DS approaches and techniques generate new kind of metadata. It may change common perspective of looking towards a particular disease like diabetes. Also it may changes or develops new practices to administer diabetes. The future of everybody will change if IT-healthcare has full-fledged DS hold. The game of DS ends when decision-makers are able to convert available intellect into action. DS transforms data and information into HeCagence™ which is combo of Healthcare and Intelligence (Figure 8). The HeCagence™ developed through underway study can provide sensory milieu for ice cream recommendations to diabetic.

One of the imperative predicaments is to recommend an apt ice cream to young university adults, who are upcoming entrepreneurs, employers, technocrats and the like. Table 1 shows the list of few research papers who have analyzed this problem through innovative data driven techniques, by using Big Data and IoT.

Figure 8. HeCagence ™ term introduced in this research

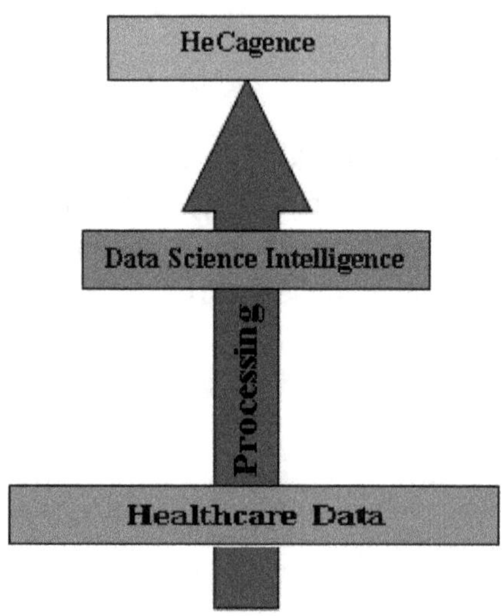

Table 1. Papers who had analyzed problem of recommending an ice cream to diabetic and Big Data, IoT in Healthcare

Sr. No.	Title of Paper	Tools and Techniques used	Name of Journal, Indexing	Publication Year
1	Enriching Process of Ice cream Recommendation using Combinatorial Ranking of AHP and Monte Carlo AHP	Analytical Hierarchy Process, Monte Carlo Analytical Hierarchy Process	Journal of Theoretical and Applied Information Technology, SCOPUS	2016
2	Modified Analytical Hierarchy Process to Recommend an Ice cream to a Diabetic Patient	Modified Analytical Hierarchy Process	Association for Computing Machinery	2016
3	Cohort Intelligence and Genetic Algorithm along with Modified Analytical Hierarchy Process to Recommend an Ice cream to a Diabetic Patient	Cohort Intelligence and Genetic Algorithm, Modified Analytical Hierarchy Process	Advances in Intelligent Systems and Computing SPRINGER	2016
4	Cohort Intelligence and Genetic Algorithm along with AHP to recommend an Ice cream to a Diabetic Patient	Cohort Intelligence and Genetic Algorithm, Analytical Hierarchy Process	Lecture Notes in Computer Science	2016
5	System Dynamics Modelling for Analyzing Recovery Rate of Diabetic Patients by Mapping Sugar Content in Ice cream and Sugar Intake for the Day	System Dynamics Modelling	Advances in Intelligent Systems and Computing SPRINGER	2015
6	Cluster Mapping with the help of New Extended MCF Algorithm and MCF Algorithm to Recommend an Ice cream to the Diabetic Patient	New MCF Clustering Algorithm	International Journal of Computer Applications	2015
7	Analytical Network Process (ANP) to Recommend an Ice cream to a Diabetic Patient	Analytical Network Process	International Journal of Computer Applications	2015
8	Analytical Hierarchy Process to Recommend an Ice cream to a Diabetic Patient Based on Sugar Content in it	Analytical Hierarchy Process	Procedia Computer Science	2015

DATA SCIENCES FOR DIABETES PREVENTIVE KMS

In 2016, Akash et al. carried out implementation of AHP & MC-AHP to recommend an ice cream to diabetic person. The propose KMS is an extension of that work and is thoughtfully designed with new set of DS techniques including GP, K-Means & ANN, CF etc. The following section discusses all these techniques in details, with results.

Standalone Analytical Hierarchical Process (S-AHP) Results and Proposed Distributed AHP (D-AHP)

The AHP based mining allows mixing of data from different levels and provides a successful data model. It in turn also provides ease in mining of relevant ice cream recommendations to university grads. That's why AHP is used as a first DS technique in this study. This section elaborates results of standalone version of AHP and proposed distributed AHP. AHP takes three sugar-free ice creams as alternatives and their different tangible and intangible criteria. AHP analyzed underway problem by using arithmetic and psychology. AHP obtains subjective preferences for getting a preferred ice cream. AHP is the most cherished and reliable prioritization technique due to its analytical aspect. It has enormous applications in literature. It has found acceptance in fields like the business (Hsu, Lin, & Tsai, 2016), Medicine (Balubaid, & Basheikh, 2016), Engineering (Chen, Wang, Liu, Zeng, & Chen, 2016) and Politics (Rahul, Kalyani, Maya, & Vrashali, 2015).

Akash et al (2016) presented AHP on sugar-free ice creams. Figure 9 presents pseudo code for this AHP (Akash, Rahul, & Preeti, 2016). In this AHP at initial level, sugar-free ice cream recommendations orchestrated its entities into a progressive hierarchical system as shown in Figure 10. No firm rules are available for creating these hierarchies. Hierarchies are flexible and can be altered with the addition of new ice cream or an ingredient in ice cream.

In Table 2, ingredient details about following sugar-free ice creams mentioned (Akash, Rahul, & Preeti, 2016).

1. Brayers Vanilla,
2. Butterscotch Ripple
3. Blue Bunny

Figure 9. AHP Pseudo code (Akash et al, 2016)

Step 1: Calculate column sum of weighted values as CS_1, CS_2... CSn where 'n' is the number of elements.

Step 2: Divide each weight in column by its column sum

i.e. divide every weighted value in n_{th} column by CS_n and store as $temp_n$

to get n*n temp values

Step 3: Calculate normalised Principal Eigen Vector matrix (Priority Vector Matrix)

$\frac{1}{n}$ * [temp1+temp2+...+temp n]

Step 4: Calculate Eigen value i.e. λ_{max} which is a single value

for i=1 to n

do addition of

(CS_i * value of Principal Eigen Vector from i_{th} row of Eigen Vector matrix)

Step 5: Calculate Consistency Index (C.I.)

C.I. = (λ_{max}-n) / (n-1)

Step 6: Random Consistency Index (RI)

if n=4 RI=0.9

Step 7: Calculate Consistency Ratio (CR)

CR= CI/RI where CR<=0.1

= CI/0.9

Figure 10. Analytical hierarchy structure for sugar-free ice cream recommendation to diabetic and non diabetic (Akash et al, 2016)

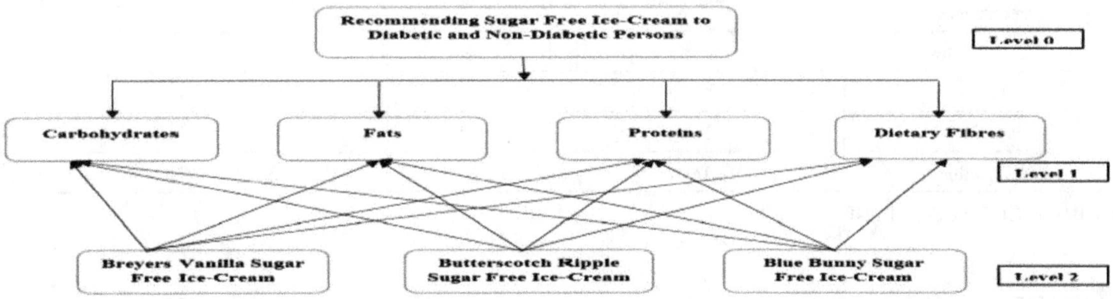

Table 2. Details about attributes of alternatives to carry out AHP (Akash et al, 2016)

Attributes (in milligrams)	Brayers Vanilla	Butterscotch Ripple	Blue Bunny
Carbohydrates	13	16	15.086
Fats	4	6	4.526
Proteins	2	1	3.017
Dietary Fibers	4	0	2.011

The nine point relativity scale developed by Saaty et al. (2008) converts semantic description into weighted matrices for considered ice creams and their ingredients as shown in Table 3 and 4 (Akash et al, 2016). AHP never requires absolute judgments or assessment. Local and global priorities can be computed using relativity between ice creams and their ingredients. Eigen vectors and Eigen values are computed for obtained weighted matrices (Saaty, 2008). Consistency Index (CI) and Consistency Ratio (CR) of the weighted matrices confirm obtained ice cream recommendations. CI and CR values are to be consistent if they are less than ten percent (Saaty, 2008). The rankings of ice cream recommendations obtained on the basis of consist weighted matrices is shown in Figure 11. Cost-Benefit Analysis of ice cream recommendations is shown in Figure 12. Figure 12 shows Brayers Vanilla is the most preferred ice cream. Figure 13 shows input dialogue for AHP implementation. Through this input dialogue user can submit relative values for ice cream ingredients for e.g. 7 (very strong) for carbohydrates with protein. The systemic implementation obtained through AHP is shown in Figure 14. It shows AHP implementation is consistent as CI and CR are below ten percent. Figure 15 shows proposed distributed version of AHP. AHP is run individually on each node and cluster database is created. Data obtained from different nodes is then combined or merged. The rankings for university grads and ice cream data sets are obtained through distributed AHP and then mapped for recommending ice cream to university grads.

In addition to ice creams mentioned in Table 2 for AHP and following five more ice creams are considered during MC_AHP implementation of this study.

1. Brayer Neopolitan
2. Chocolate Fudge Pops
3. Sugar-free Creamsicle

Table 3. Weighted matrix for considered ice creams on the basis of their attributes (Akash et al, 2016)

Criteria Preferences	Carbohydrates	Fats	Proteins	Dietary Fibres
Carbohydrates	1	3	7	9
Fats	1/3	1	5	7
Proteins	1/7	1/5	1	3
Dietary Fibres	1/9	1/7	1/3	1

CI: 0.0549 CR: 0.0617 λ: 4.1648

Table 4.Weighted matrix for considered ice creams on the basis of their attributes (Akash et al, 2016)

Carbohydrate	Brayers Vanilla	Butterscotch Ripple	Blue Bunny
Brayers Vanilla	1	5	3
Butterscotch Ripple	1/5	1	¼
Blue Bunny	1/3	4	1

CI: 0.0428 CR: 0.0824 λ: 3.085

Figure 11. Ranking obtained for considered sugar free ice creams (Akash et al, 2016)

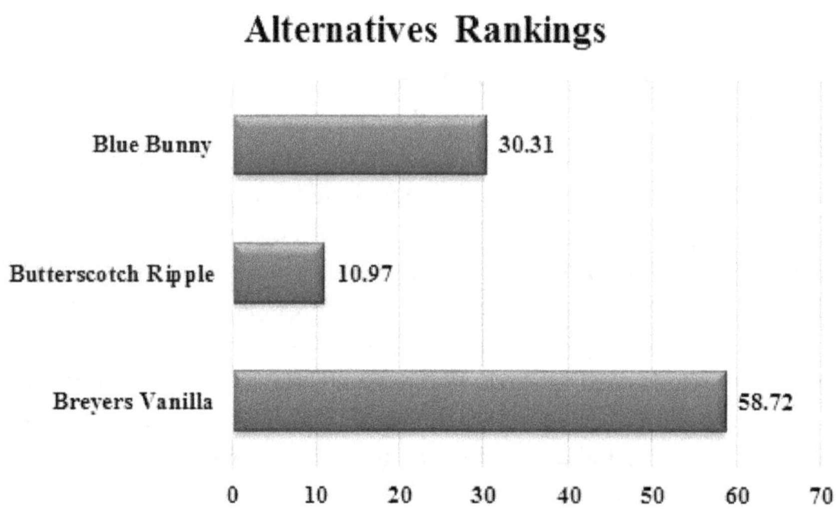

4. Almond Lites
5. Brownie Yogurt

Principle Components Analysis (PCA) applied at pre-clustering stage of K-ANN implementation of this study gives a list of impactful attributes in ice creams. These impactful attributes of PCA are once again confirmed at post-clustering stage after clusters formation. The research carried out about ice creams by this study validates following attributes as impactful one.

Figure 12. Cost-benefit analysis of considered sugar-free ice creams (Akash et al, 2016)

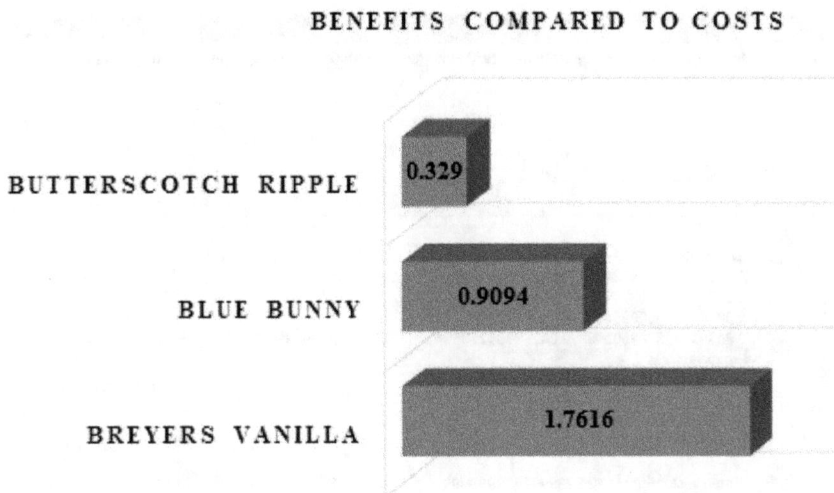

Figure 13. AHP input dialogue screen

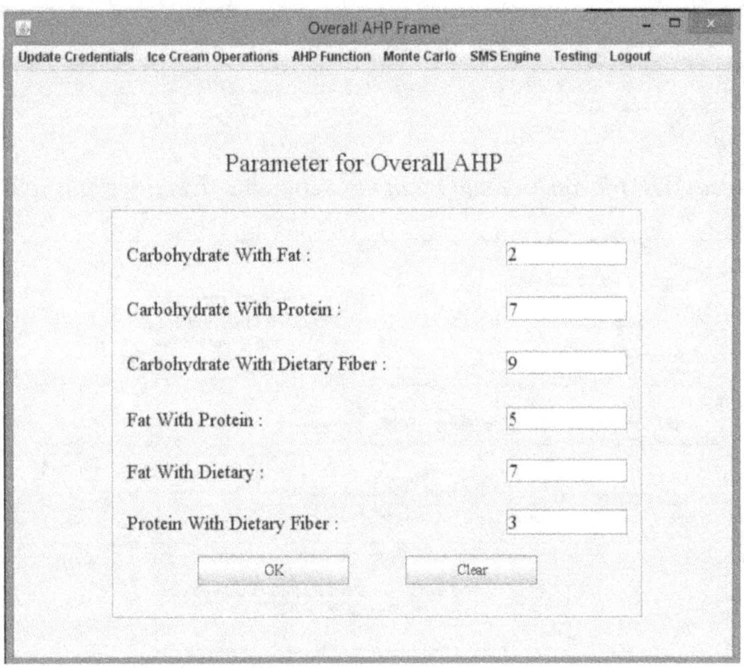

1. Carbohydrates is more impactful attribute,
2. Second impactful attribute is fats,
3. Third is proteins and
4. The least impactful attribute is dietary fibers (Suhas, & Rahul, & Preeti, 2015).

Figure 14. AHP systemic results show consistency checks

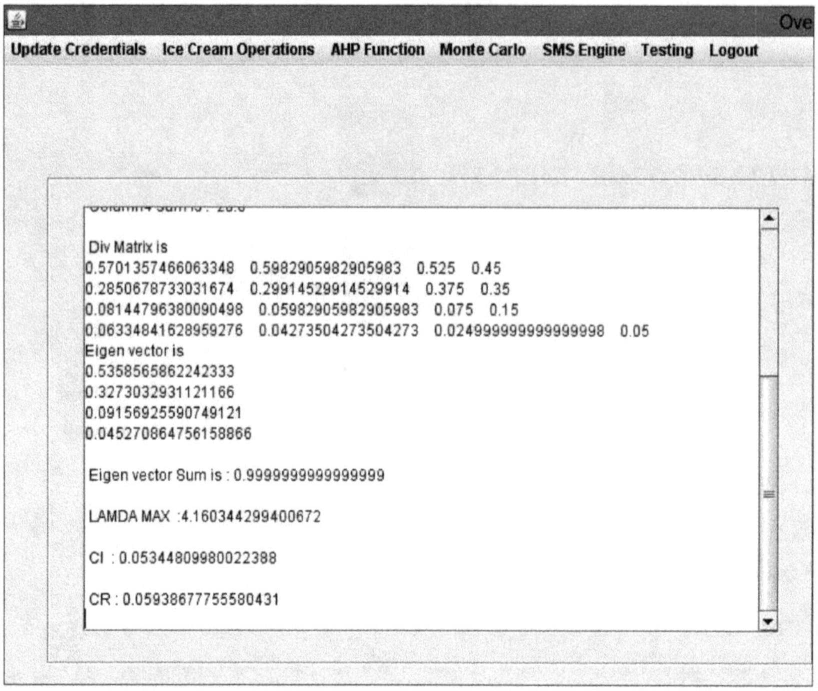

Figure 15. Distributed AHP for ranking and mapping between university grads and ice cream datasets

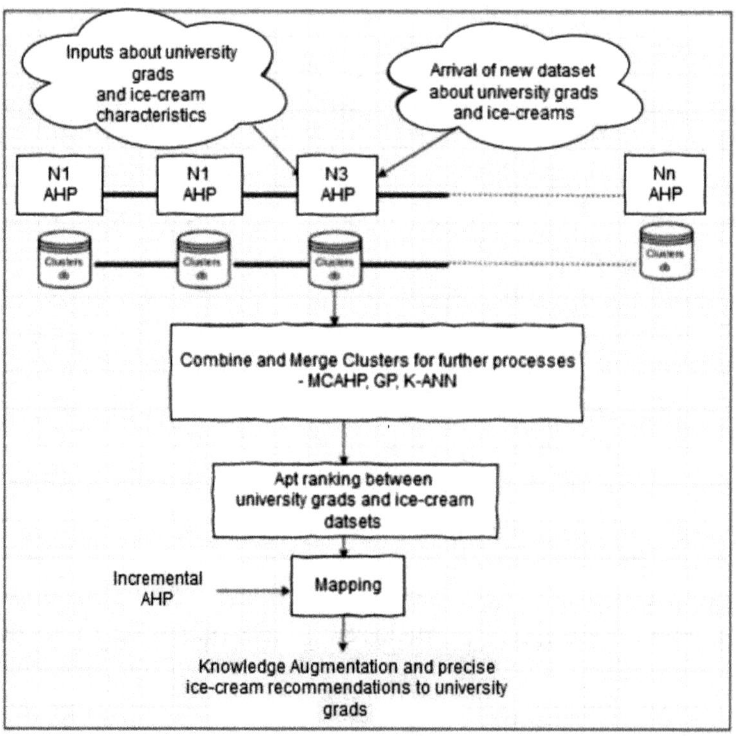

When more than four ice creams to be ranked, it is impossible to convert them into AHP or into a hierarchical format. It in a way makes difficult to analyze interaction between the same levels deceive attributes or feedback among two different levels of AHP (Kou, Ergu, Peng, &Shi, 2012). In AHP, obtained recommendations are conceivable if and only if they pass consistency checks. So, in a way it is difficult to prepare weighted matrices for a complex problem where eight ice creams to be ranked (Kou, Ergu, Peng, &Shi, 2012). To overcome these pitfalls of AHP, a complementary method called Monte Carlo AHP (MCAHP) is used in the next section of this study (Kou, Ergu, Peng, &Shi, 2012).

Standalone Monte Carlo AHP (SMC-AHP) and Proposed Distributed MC-AHP (DMC-AHP)

In literature MC-AHP has applications in variety of fields like in ranking of dental quality attributes (Hsu, & Pan, 2009), to select best mining method, for selection of material handling equipment selection (Momani, &Ahmed, 2011), for system reliability evaluation (Huseby, Naustdal, & Varli, 2004). Simulation tool offers tests and experiments to real life alternatives like ranking of ice creams in undertaken study. Simulation offers a better projection to the problem underway. A probabilistic simulation like Monte Carlo Simulation (MCS) is useful for the random behavior of considered eight ice creams and their ingredients. MCS uses repetitive sampling and obtains same probabilities for recommending ice cream to university grads (Gutierrz, 2013). MCS in turn facilitates incremental advancement for underway ice cream research.

In this study MC-AHP is applied after AHP due to below-mentioned attractive features (Yaraghi, Tabesh, Guan, & Zhuang, 2015) viz;

1. Effective mining through major criterions like Carbohydrates in sugar free ice cream
2. Uncertainty inclusion i.e. runtime addition of new ice cream or any of its ingredient
3. Free from compounded complexity
4. Each added extra ice cream or any of its ingredients is computed linearly
5. Preference structure distribution from university grads and ice cream point of view
6. Probabilistic distribution avoids instability
7. An appropriate convergence of ice cream ingredients assures accuracy
8. Not an analytical perturbation like AHP that's why not cumbersome
9. Proliferation of AHP through random values of MC-AHP
10. Combinatorial model decreases risk of improper ice cream recommendations
11. Automates majority of mechanism behind building models
12. Can construct composite decision support models in a simple way

This study makes use of following four steps for MC-AHP implementation (Raychaudhuri, 2008) viz;

1. Static model generation for ice cream recommendations,
2. Distribution ice creams and their ingredients using Mean, Mode, Key Percentiles and Standard deviations (Figure 19),
3. Generation of random values for ice creams, their ingredients and
4. Analysis and ice cream recommendations through generated results.

Figure 16 presents flow chart for MC-AHP approach for undertaken study (Akash et al, 2016). It shows that it is applied on ice creams composition vector. Figure 17 shows MC-AHP process initialization where ice creams get compared with each other for e.g. Sugar-free creamsicle with Breyers Neopiltan. Figure 18 shows MC-AHP's consistency checks as CR is ten percent. Then, Mean, Standard Deviation (SD) for each ingredient of sugar-free of ice creams are computed (Figure 19 & Figure 20). Normal distribution applied on generated values for ice creams and their ingredients. Identified weights for ice cream compositions are sorted. Ice creams are ranked on the basis of these weights (Figure 21). Likewise proposed distributed version AHP, Figure 22 shows proposed distributed version of MC-AHP. In distributed MC-AHP, MC-AHP is run on each node. The out of each node is then considered for ranking which is based on standard deviation. This ranking is then in turn helpful for mapping between considered datasets.

The Brayers Vanilla ice cream has highest precedence in AHP and MCAHP implementation (Akash et al, 2016). Thus, AHP and MCAHP rakings for considered sugar-free ice creams are same (Akash et al, 2016). These empirical results confirmed capabilities of developed model for sugar-free ice cream recommendations. These kinds of capabilities of the final developed model used to rank eight sugar-free ice creams.

Figure 16. Flow chart for MC-AHP implementation (Akash et al, 2016)

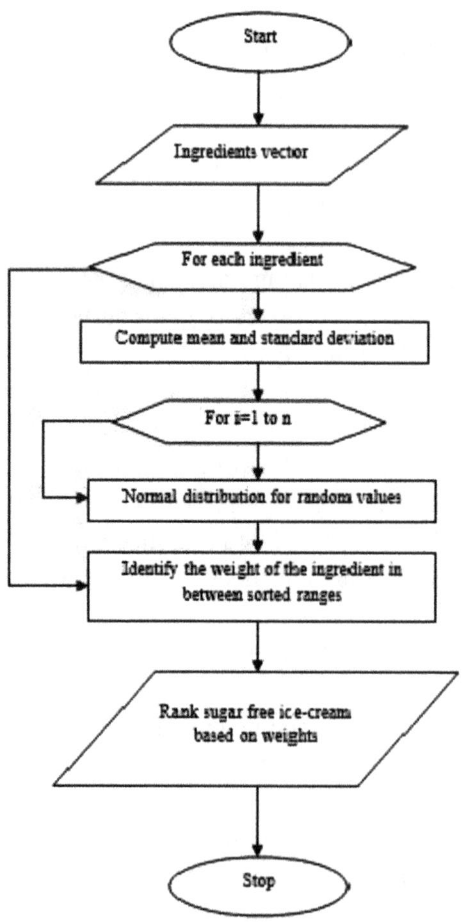

Figure 17. MC-AHP process initiation (Akash et al, 2016)

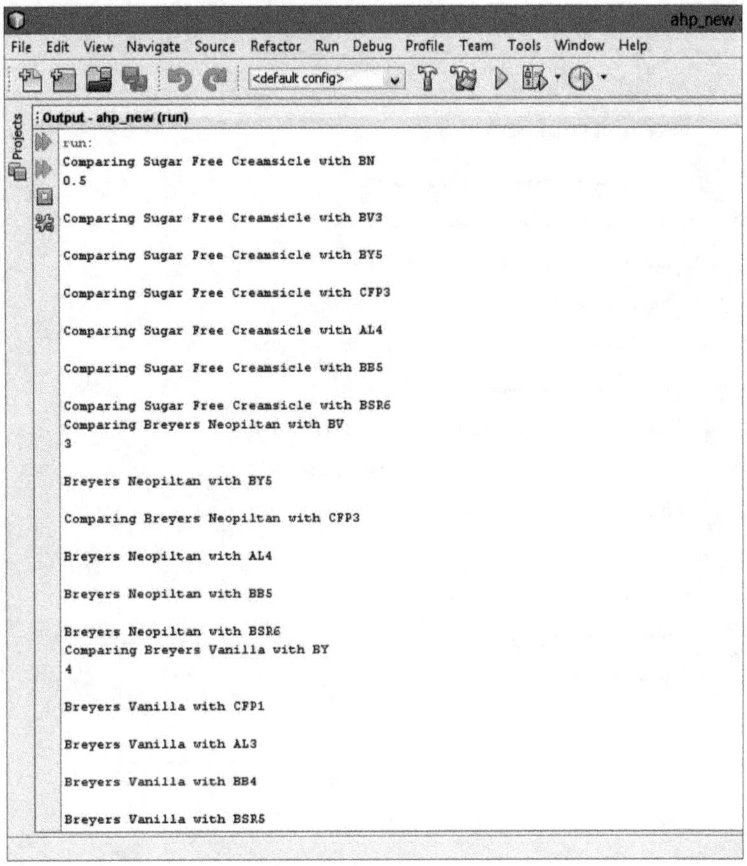

Figure 18. MC-AHP's Consistency Cheks (Akash et al, 2016)

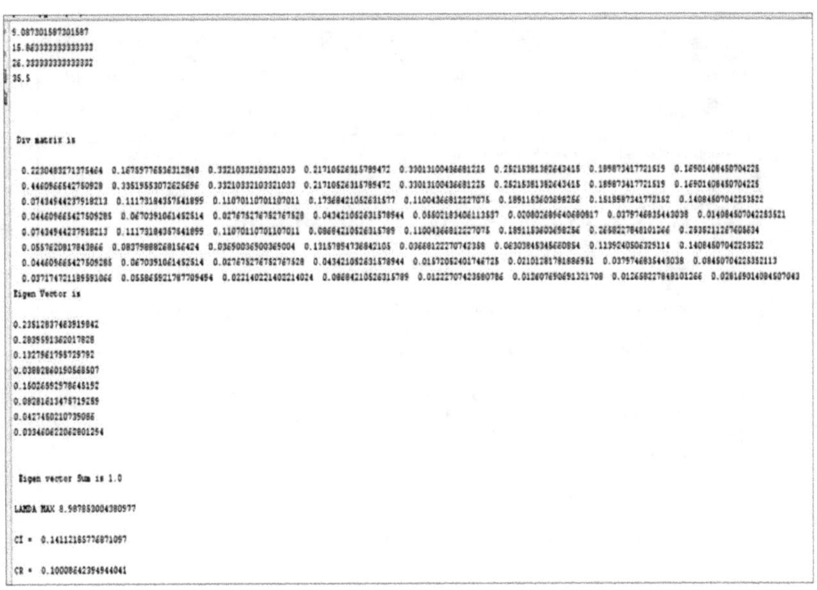

Figure 19. MC-AHP's Mean and Standard Devation calculations for ice creams (Akash et al, 2016)

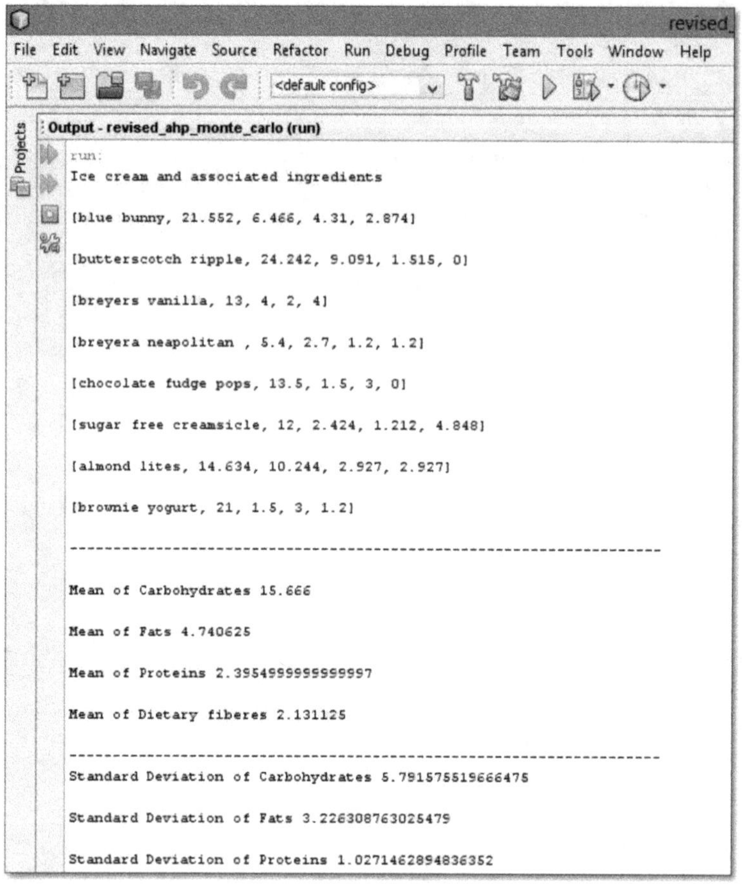

Figure 20. Validation of results of AHP and MCAHP (Akash et al, 2016)

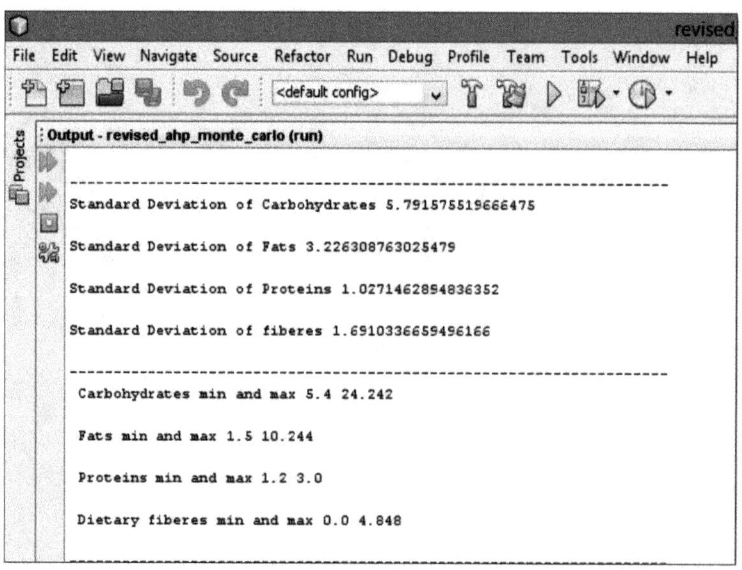

GOAL PROGRAMMING (GP)

GP is an optimization technique which was first used by Charles et al. in 1995. GP is of two categories viz., (a) Preemptive GP (PGP) and (b) Non Preemptive GP (NPGP).

PGP vs. NPGP

PGP forces decision makers to rank goals into different priority levels. Each individual level contains one or more goals. Scrutinizing levels into different priorities allow selection of best priority for achieving goals. Less attention is to be given to goals at low levels than those which are at high level. In NPGP weights assigned at different priority levels. The useful thing about NPGP is that one can convert the given GP problem into linear programming problem (LPP) by using these weights. The undertaken study makes use of NPGP approach to convert considered ice creams into LPP by doing weight assignment from university grads dietary habits point of view.

In real word scenario, there is not a single apt solution. The main motto of NPGP is in this study to find out optimal solutions which in turn reduce health cost to university grads. Here, NPGP makes use of achievement function to cut unwanted ice cream recommendation to university grads.

GP settles down Multi Objective Decision Making (MODM) issues to fulfilling solutions by treating objectives as goals. In this study GP settles MODM of recommending an apt ice cream to university grads by considering earlier developed AHP's and MC-AHP's analytical framework.

Implementation of GP

In this study, GP provides deviances from nutritional ingredients of ice creams. Figure 23 shows the systemic standalone implementation of GP. It shows that GP is to be applied on Carbohydrates, Fat, Protein and Dietary Fiber and then positive and negative deviations are to be obtained for each of them. Figure 24 shows start of mining engine to query database. Figure 25 shows ice cream recommendation as per user query for e.g. for a person with age 25, weight 65, food status "after meal" and nd i.e. Non Diabetic. Then ice creams get ranked by MC-AHP process (Figure 24). Figure 25 shows goal achievement for each nutritional ingredient of ice cream for e.g. Goal achievement for Carbohydrates is 5.4. Figure 28 shows ice cream recommendation through GP for a user query as sugar free creamsicle and breyers vanilla for a person with age 25, weight 65, "after meal" food status and non diabetic. Figure 29 shows proposed distributed version of GP. Distributed GP shows that it takes distributed MC-AHP's output as input. The advantage of distributed GP is that due to incremental GP, apt ranges for attributes of newly arrived data along with the existing datasets can be obtained. The deviations through GP for ingredients of each ice cream are further used in K- ANN. From Higher and lower limits of ice cream ingredients, their optimal values computed by using below mentioned formula viz.,

Optimal Value = Lower Limit + [(Higher Limit – Lower Limit)/2].

These optimal values are further used to get their positive and negative deviations.

There are different ways of obtaining solutions to GP. Graphical programming and Excel solver are the two techniques used to solve GP. In excel solver, manual addition of constraints carried out at the different priority level. In graphical GP graphs used to do the said tasks. This study makes use of Excel solver approach.

Advantages of using GP are ease in obtaining deviational values of ice cream ingredients. It has disadvantages like difficult to set appropriate weights at different levels of its implementation.

GP Results for Ice Creams and Associated Ingredients

[Ice cream name, Carbohydrate Content, Fats Content, Proteins Content, Dietary Fibers Content]
[Blue Bunny, 21.552, 6.466, 4.31, 2.874]
[Butterscotch Ripple, 24.242, 9.091, 1.515, 0]
[Brayers' Vanilla, 13, 4, 2, 4]
[Brayers' Neapolitan, 5.4, 2.7, 1.2, 1.2]
[Chocolate Fudge Pops, 13.5, 1.5, 3, 0]
[Sugar-free Creamsicle, 12, 2.424, 1.212, 4.848]
[Almond Lites, 14.634, 10.244, 2.927, 2.927]
[Brownie Yogurt, 21, 1.5, 3, 1.2]

Goal Achievement for Carbohydrates in Terms of Positive and Negative Deviations (Figure 25)

Ideal value for carbohydrate is [GOAL]: 5.4
Goal constraint deviations [Ice cream name, carbohydrate value, deviation from GOAL]

Figure 21. Research Outcome: System diagram of GP implementation

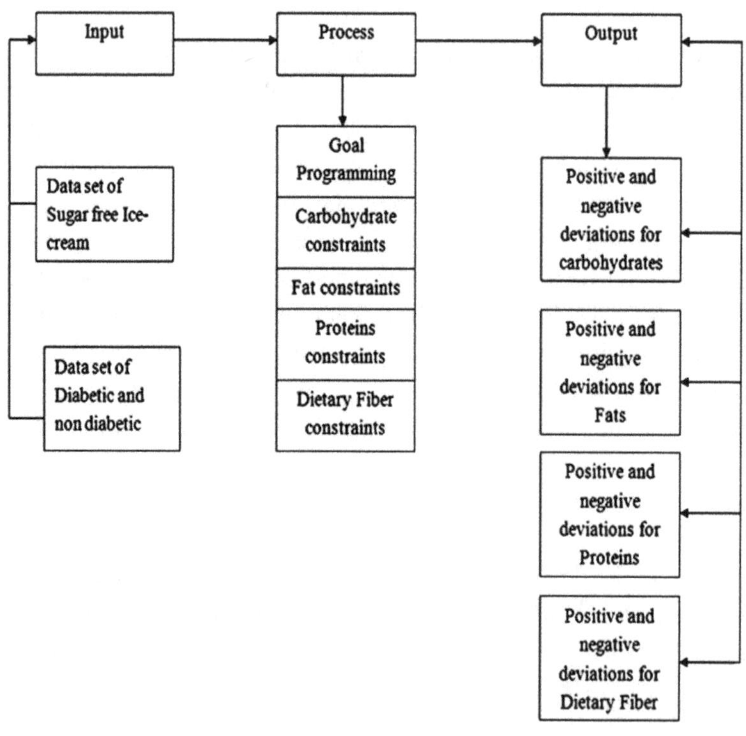

Figure 22. Start of mining engine to query database (Akash et al, 2016)

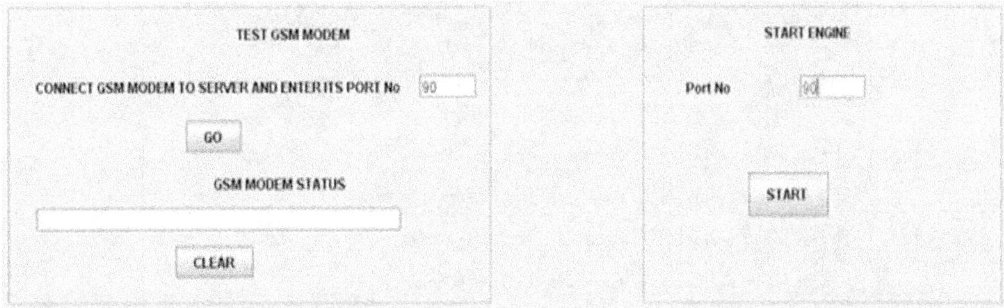

Figure 23. Screenshot of ice cream recommendation research (Akash et al, 2016)

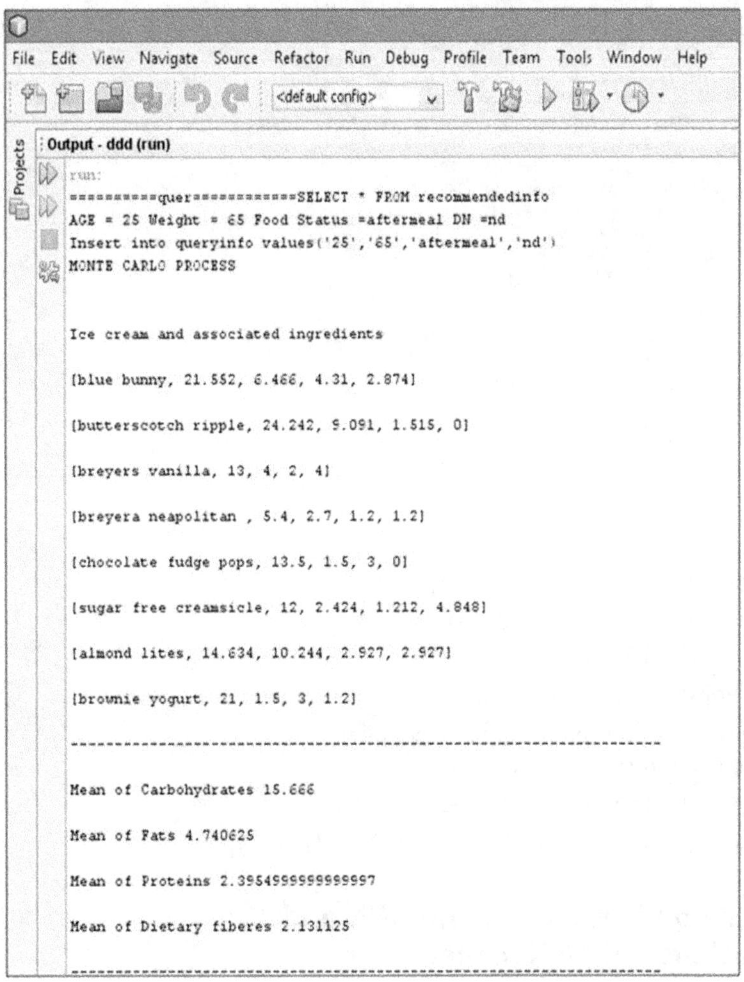

Figure 24. MCAHP's rankings for ice creams (Akash et al, 2016)

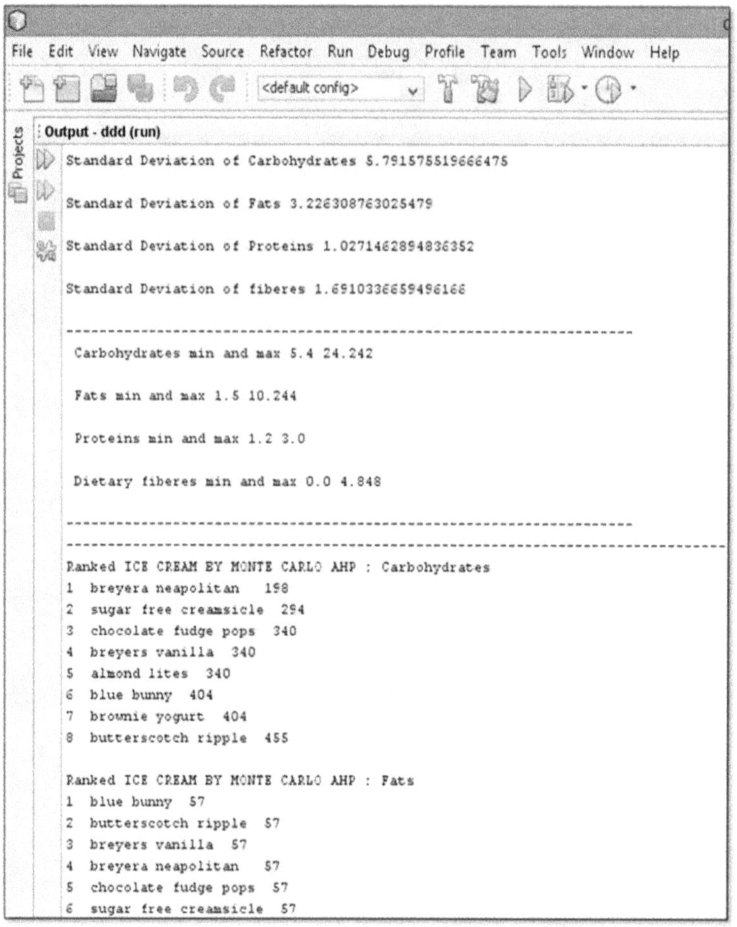

[Brayers' Neapolitan, 5.4, 0.0 (5.4-5.4 = 0.0)]
[Sugar-free Creamsicle, 12, -6.6 (5.4-12 = -6.6)]
[Brayers' Vanilla, 13, -7.6 (5.4-13 = -7.6)]
[Chocolate Fudge Pops, 13.5, -8.1 (5.4-13.5 = -8.1)]
[Almond Lites, 14.634, -9.234 (5.4-14.634 = -9.234)]
[Brownie Yogurt, 21, -15.6 (5.4-21 = -15.6)]
[Blue Bunny, 21.552, -16.152 (5.4 -21.552 = -16.152)]
[Butterscotch Ripple, 24.242, -18.842 (5.4 - 24.242 = -18.842)]

Cluster Computing via K-Means and ANN and Proposed Distributed K-ANN Model

Data mining through clustering can distinguish and expect patterns from available data series. The acquired results can then be accepted with the aid of new tactics. Clustering falls under unsubstantiated

Figure 25. Goal programming process for underway research (Akash et al, 2016)

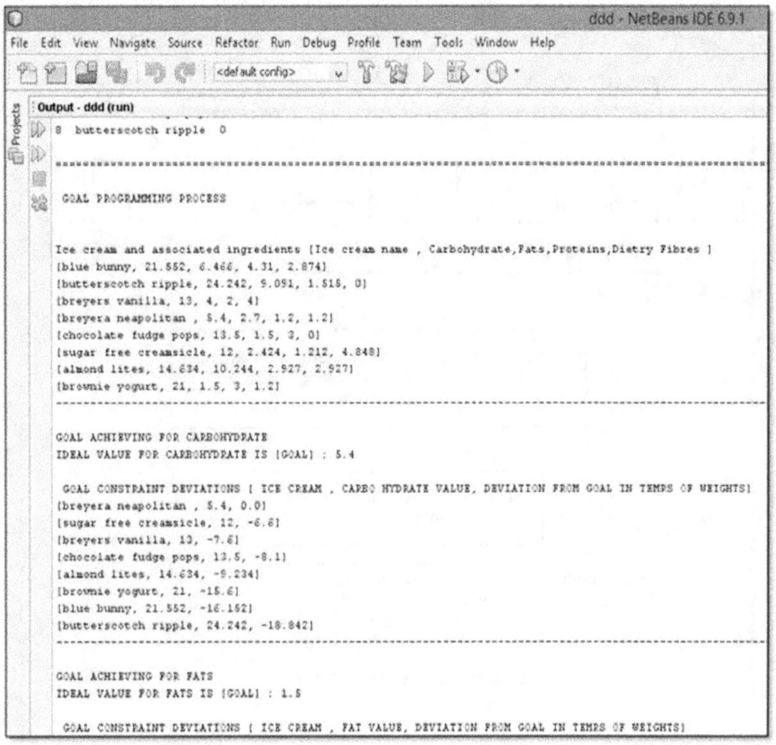

Figure 26. Ice cream recommendation through Goal Programming (Akash et al, 2016)

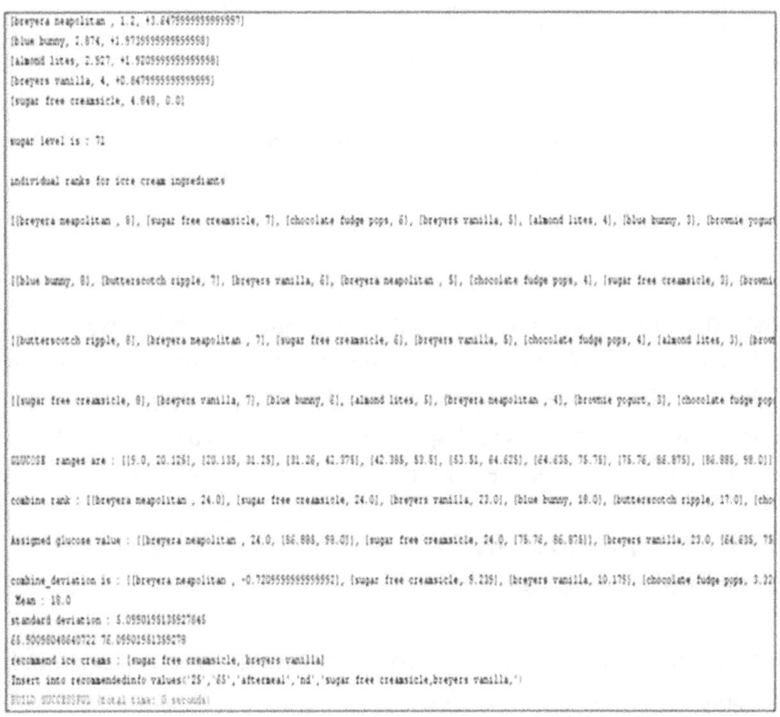

Figure 27. Research Outcome: Proposed Distributed Goal Programming

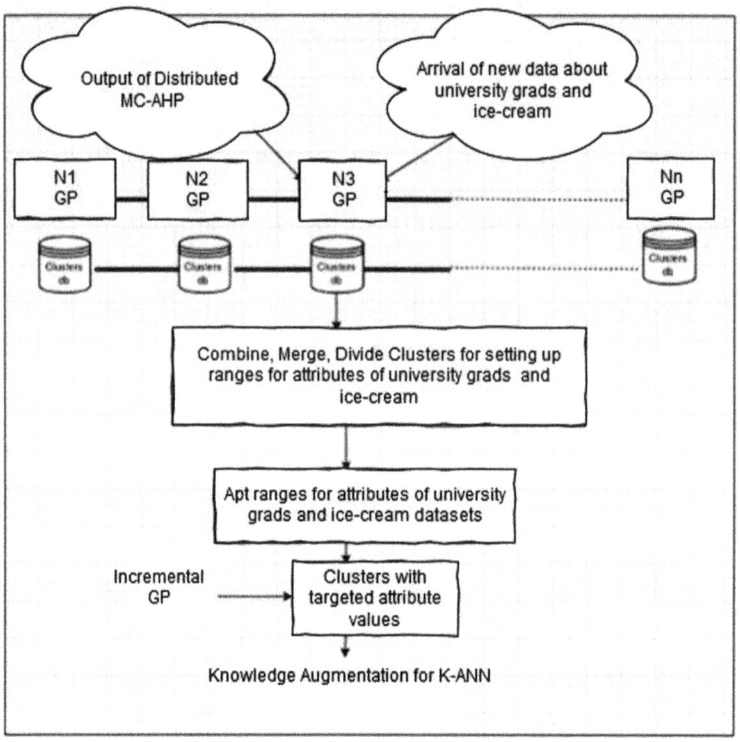

erudition method. Clustering does partitioning of fat datasets into dissimilar tiny subgroups. It is in a way provides ease to find out similarities among data.

Over the years different clustering methodologies get developed and are in use. The attractive property of clustering is that it desires less or no info for analysis of data. The underway study employs a novel tactics of K-Means coupled with ANN. The combination of K-Means and ANN generates background knowledge about recommending ice cream or ice creams to university grads.

K-Means

The K-Means does partitioning of data into "n" data points and into "K" clusters. The K -means was at first proposed by MacQueen in 1967 and later it was improved by Hartigan and Wong. Merging lands of K -means and algorithmic methodologies was demonstrated by Bottou and Bengio. It has been widely used for quantities of commonsensical chunks and applications of that type. The K-Means does an effective conversion of in-memory info to out-of-memory of resident datasets (Jin, Goswami, & Agrawal, 2006).

Significance of K-Means and ANN in This Ice Cream Recommendation Research

The problem with K-Means is that it investigates over entire dataset on each rotation. It needs many such rotations before focalizing to a valuable outcome. It makes costly to operate, especially for huge local diskette datasets. Researchers focused on attenuating passes needed for K - means. Thus, the performance of the algorithm gets enhanced. So, these methodologies give summarized results with deterministic limits of the results. A key soft spot of K-Means is that it merges to local minima (Kanungo, Mount, Netanyahu, Piatko, Silverman, & Wu, 2002). A fascinating question arises: can we have a method of calculation which obliges less number of passes on the entire dataset? Or can handle the same converging results as that of the basic K-Means? – that's the reason combo of "K-Means and ANN" used.

The combo K-Means and ANN is employed by using following three stages

1. In the first stage K-Means is used to generate dissimilar subsets for ice creams and health attributes of university students (Figure 28).
2. Based on these dissimilar sets, through ANN different neurons for ice creams recommendation get generated in the second stage (Figure 29).
3. In the last step, these neurons are used to develop apt ice cream recommendations.

Implementation of K-Means

By referencing Kanungo, Tapas (2002) work, this section represents K-Means implementation for underway problem. The input to K-Means is perceptions about ice creams, health attributes of university grads and outputs are ice creams and university grads data sets arranged into K clusters. The first step is to instate calculation by picking up centroids of K clusters. This is done by picking up K data objects from given input of university grads health attributes and ice cream composition. With these underlying K centroids, the K-Means algorithm works by using follows steps:

Figure 28. Research outcome: System diagram of this research focusing on cluster implementations

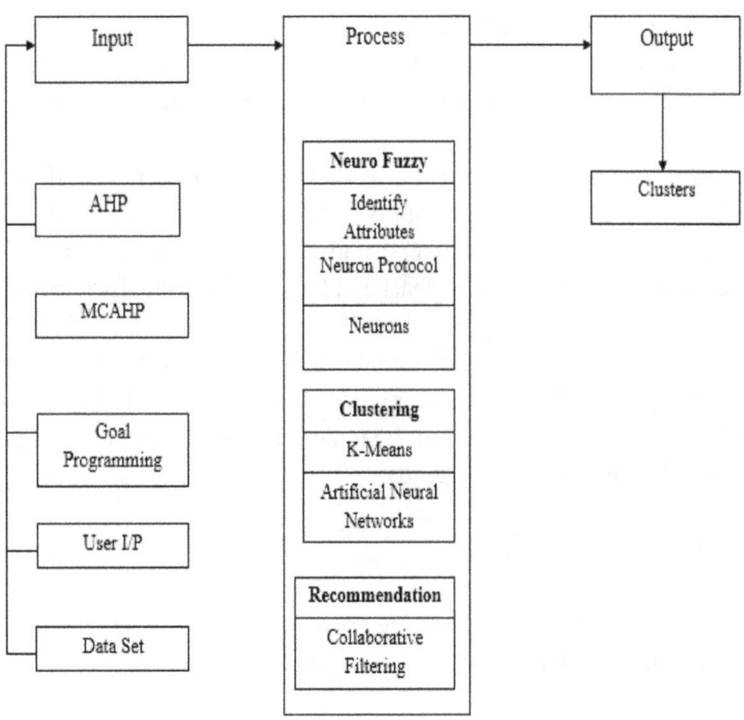

Figure 29. Cluster Formation for undertaken problem (Akash et al, 2016)

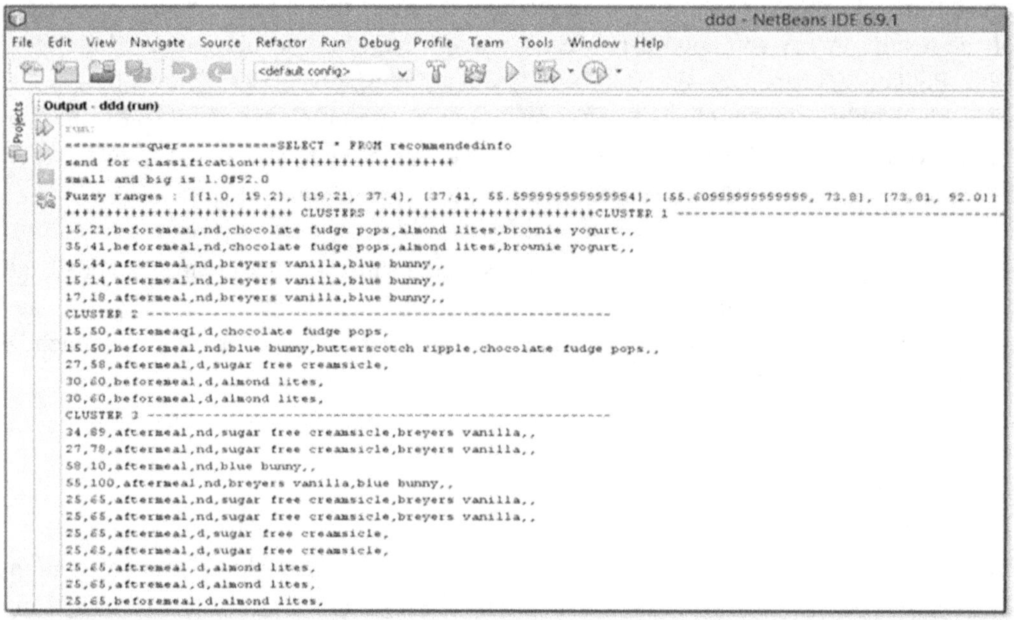

1. **Assignment:** Assignment is done for objects which are nearer to cluster centroids. After assignment re-computation of centroids takes place.
2. **Update Centroids:** Every cluster updates with a new centroid which is nothing but an average of its objects. For e.g., figuring out 'mean' of observations. It is to comprehend that K-Means is infamous for the situation of getting stuck in local minima. It implies that last result could not be the best one. To overcome this, K-Means run with various starting centroids. It selects centroid resulting in most errors. For each data object computation of error is done in terms of how close it is to its centroid. These errors summed up together to compute total error.

These progressions repeated until centroids quit moving. Inputs from the university grads, preferences to AHP, MCAHP and GP outputs are inputs to K-Means. Euclidian distances calculated using differences between ages and weights for university grads. These distances are arranged in ascending order of their values. The differences between least and largest Euclidian distances determined. The five ranges from zero to largest obtained. They are negative low, low, medium, high and positive high. Then age and weight pair of university grad matched with Euclidian distance having specific discrete range in generated clusters. In a way, plausible clusters for ice creams recommendation are generated. Figure 28 shows combo of K-Means and ANN applied in the undertaken study. Figure 29 shows clusters formed for ice cream recommendation to university grads.

Artificial Neural Networks (ANN)

ANNs are one of many models in machine learning used to polish raw data into useful decisions. ANNs are useful tools where data is collected without knowing their essential features. ANNs after getting unique initial data can find out abstractions about them. These abstractions can capture intricate dealings which are not palpable in the initial data. Capture of grave abstract numerical regularities leads to the prophecy in performance and simplification. The erudite features are often difficult to construe. ANNs have oodles of "ability" to confine intricate relationships. This ability comes at a cost. More ability means more responsive to input data patterns. ANNs are useful where observed data does not have too many "flukes" and models are not "fitting" to the flukes.

ANN in a simple form is nothing but the cluster of primitive artificial neurons. ANN provides enriched clusters by connecting distinct layers of underway implementation. This interconnection is a smart art to resolve real world complicated issues. Neurons take inputs to provide outputs as per accordance of users.

ANN Implementation

ANN accepts clusters formed though earlier implementation of K-Means as inputs and generates neurons as outputs. In this study, neurons consist of best ice creams recommendations. The 5 clusters from K-Means generate 10 different types of neurons. The knowledge developed through ANN can act as the catalysts to ice cream industry. It can also be useful for launching an appropriate variety of ice cream in university canteens.

Standalone Collaborative Filtering (S-CF)

The Impetus for CF is to get apt recommendations from someone who is having similar tastes as that of other. CF explores techniques that match alike interests of people and recommendations are build accordingly. CF cleanses data or information. This utilizes the strategy of collaboration among a variety of information sources and operators. The main drift of CF is to develop a product from created clusters. Collaborative filtering strategy makes predictions through historic data of user preferences. It is also through information from different collaborating clients. Labelling to the users' preferences is done during filtering process for matching the purpose or objective. Real-time collaborative filtering has applications on various types of data. For e.g. data from sensors (Inanloo, Ashouri, Gheibi, & Hemmatyar, 2012); administrative organizations coordinating many monetary sources (Linden, Smith, & York, 2003); electronic businesses and web applications focusing on client information and preferences (Schafer, Frankowski, Herlocker, & Sen, 2007), and so on.

Common pre-requisites for execution of S-CF algorithm are as follows:

1. Proper input for active data,
2. Representation of data based on interests of developed system,
3. Finally, the algorithm that matches similar interests from user viewpoints.

S-CF Workflow for underway problem is as given below:

1. Capture of university grads preferences in the developed system.
2. These preferences are further viewed as apt representation of considered ice creams.
3. Match of ratings about ice creams from university grads by considering common details.
4. For university grads with same set of health attributes, the system recommends ice cream with high rating.

A tricky issue in CF is how to combine and weigh preferences of university grads. The intermediate rating of ice creams leads to an accurate representation of university grads preferences about considered ice creams. The CF data space framework for undertaken problem is university grads preferences about ice creams. The rating is in the form of a triple viz., University grad, Ice cream, and Rating to ice cream.

This study considers different flavor, types of ice creams. The best recommendation has the least deviation from optimal solution of applied GP. If a particular ice cream recommendation is best for a university grad under considerable preferences. Then the same is best for the other university grads that have similar kind of preferences.

Proposed Distributed K-ANN and CF

Figure 31 shows proposed distributed version of K-ANN and it is augmented with distributed CF. Here also, K-ANN is to be run on each node. By transforming K-ANN into distributed version, dissimilar subsets for considered datasets are obtained. There are further utilized for generation of neurons for ice cream recommendation. These neurons are then further processed through CF along with user specific preferences to get sophisticated ice cream recommendations.

Proposed Research Is a Hybrid Mixed Recommendation System

Ramp-up problems are not part of Utility related KMS. Their recommendations are the accumulation of numerical proofs (Burke et al., 2002). In Utility KMS, the built system does utility functions across all shades of objects. One key benefit of this approach is ease addition of different factors to a product value. In the utility-based framework, the user articulates all considerations into a recommendation. Likewise this study is a utility related KMS as it articulated university grads health attributes into apt ice cream recommendations.

But, pure KM related recommender systems subjects to the negative aspect of all KMS. So, it does only knowledge acquisition. The study belongs to user-knowledge type of recommender system. The KM-based recommendation has some beneficial characteristics. It is appropriate for casual exploration. It demands less of the user than utility-based recommendation (Burke et al., 2002). So, it can make wide-range of recommendations as its knowledge base allows. The undertaken study suggests ice cream recommendations based on knowledge developed through usage of different DS techniques. Thus, this study is a "*Mix of Utility and KM related*" approach.

This study combines different DS techniques, university grads health attributes. CF combined with other earlier discussed DS technique is an attempt to avoid ramp-up problems. So, this study is also a "*Hybrid Mixed Recommendation System*". To make recommendations more realistic it considers recommendations from each of the employed DS techniques.

Ice Cream Recommendations Obtained Through S-CF

Following CF is obtained for user queries and accordingly apt ice cream recommendations are given

1. Age ='27', Weight='58', Food Status or Preference as "aftermeal", Health Status (Diabetic/Non-diabetic) as "d", the recommendation holds as 'sugar-free creamsicle' (neuron no. 4 in Figure 30).

2. Age ='34', Weight='89', Food Status or Preference as "aftermeal", Health Status (Diabetic/Non-diabetic) as "nd", the recommendation holds as ' sugar free creamsicle & breyers vanilla' (neuron no. 5 in Figure 30).
3. Age ='30', Weight='60', Food Status or Preference as "beforemeal", Health Status (Diabetic/Non-diabetic) as "d", the recommendation holds as 'almond lites' (neuron no. 3 in Figure 30).
4. Age ='25', Weight='65', Food Status or Preference as "aftermeal", Health Status (Diabetic/Non-diabetic) as "nd", the recommendation holds as ' sugar free creamsicle & breyers vanilla' (neuron no. 5 in Figure 30).

RESULTS

The Table 5 shows used DS methods and their results, other DS methods used to validate the earlier obtained results and figure or table to be referenced for the specified DS result.

CONCLUSION

Student's life style attributes considered in different phases of this study. AHP ranks different ice creams by considering their nutritional contents. AHP ranking shows students with high blood glucose level can consume sugar free ice cream(s). Also, non-diabetic can consume ice creams with high levels of carbohydrates and fats. Thus, best plausible ice cream's suggestions to both normal and diabetic students are possible.

Figure 30. Ice cream recommendation results received through implementation in this research based on neurons (Akash et al, 2016)

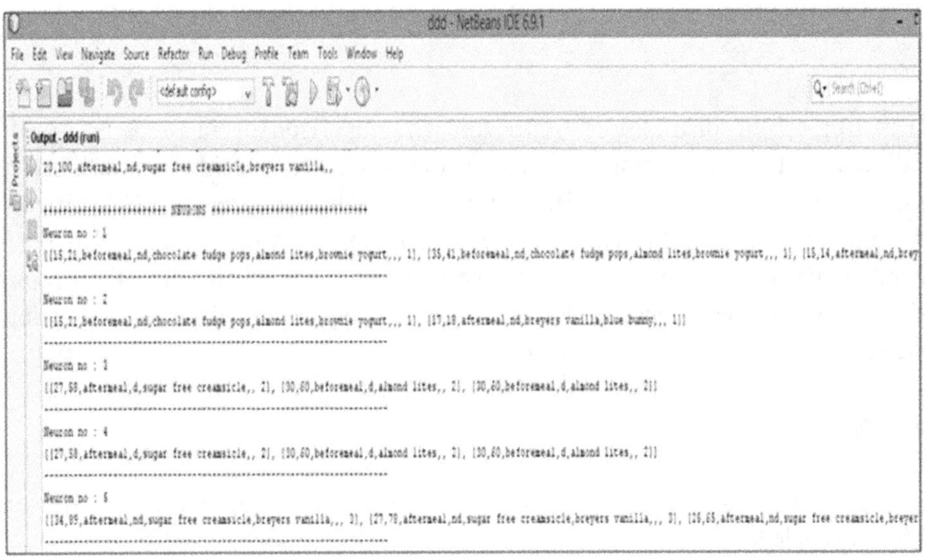

Figure 31. Research Outcome: Proposed Distributed K-ANN & CF

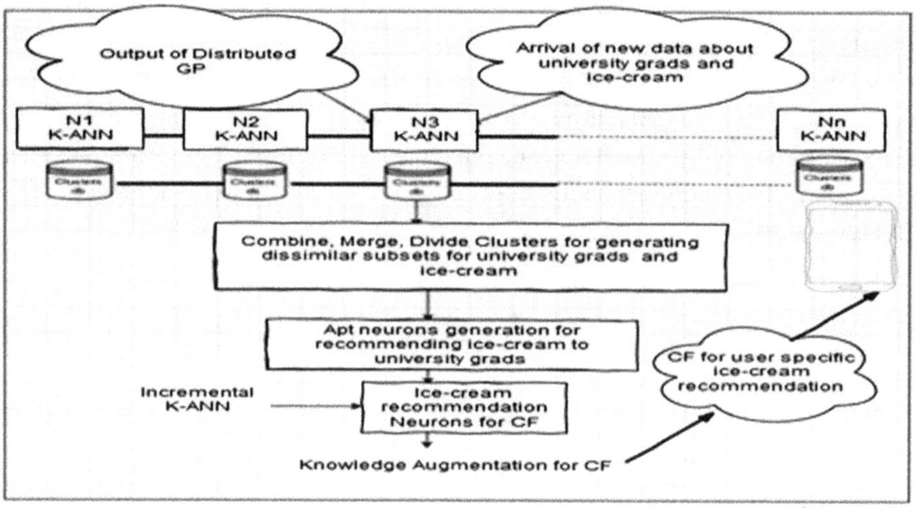

Table 5. Validations for used DS tactics

Sr. No.	Used DS Method	Results Obtained	DS Method Used for Further Validation	Figure or Table to Referenced
1	AHP	Breyers Vanilla, Blue Bunny, Butterscotch Ripple	MC-AHP	Figure 20
2	MC-AHP	Breyers Vanilla, Blue Bunny, Butterscotch Ripple	GP	Figure 20
3	GP	Combined ranking for Breyers Vanilla, Blue Bunny, Butterscotch Ripple in sequence	K-Means and ANN	Figure 26
4	K-Means and ANN	Cluster formation based upon user query for recommending Breyers Vanilla, Blue Bunny, Butterscotch Ripple	CF	Figure 26
5	CF	Filtered Recommendations about Breyers Vanilla, Blue Bunny, Butterscotch Ripple based upon preference distribution structure		Figure 30

MCAHP uses probability distribution to replicate each comparison several times. MC-AHP overcomes limits of traditional AHP by appending incremental concepts. It also considers uncertainty in judgments and proves that results are analogues to AHP. Later MC-AHP has powered by GP. Verified GP's results are inputs for cluster computing. In clustering, there is combo of K-Means and ANN. The results of this combo generate ten neurons from five clusters. These neurons give precise diabetic recommendations. The Table 5 shows validations about used DS tactics. In this way, through layered application of tact-tics successful ice cream recommendations can be achieved.

Future Scope

Knowledge generated through this research can develop healthy eating habits among students. This research can be extended

- For school students for developing healthy eating habits among them
- For Vegan, local and ice creams
- To channelize ice cream industry for new product planning.
- A tool for health care industries that are running their business on outcome based approach.
- By using fuzzy cluster computing or confusion matrix to get fuehrer classified data about ice cream recommendation.
- To implement full Knowledge Management Cycle for healthy eating behavior and to do Knowledge Augmentation.

REFERENCES

Alappanavar, P., Shewale, K., Markad, Y., & Patil, N. (2016). *Intrusion Detection System for Networks Using K-Means ANN Algorithm*. Academic Press.

Ataei, M., Shahsavany, H., & Mikaeil, R. (2013). Monte Carlo Analytic Hierarchy Process (MAHP) approach to selection of optimum mining method. *International Journal of Mining Science and Technology*, *23*(4), 573–578. doi:10.1016/j.ijmst.2013.07.017

Azadeh, A., Saberi, M., Anvari, M., & Moghaddam, M. (2010). An integrated ANN-K-Means algorithm for improved performance assessment of electricity distribution units. *Journal of Scientific and Industrial Research*, *69*, 672–679.

Balubaid, M. A., & Basheikh, M. A. (2016). Using the analytic hierarchy process to prioritize alternative medicine: Selecting the most suitable medicine for patients with diabetes. *International Journal of Basic and Applied Sciences*, *5*(1), 67. doi:10.14419/ijbas.v5i1.5607

Barlow, S. (2014). *Healthcare Data Warehouse Models Explained*. Retrieved June 20, 2016, https://www.healthcatalyst.com/best-healthcare-data-warehouse-model

Becker, P. (2010). *Improving Healthcare: A Data Mining Approach*. Academic Press.

Bijandi, M., Maddah, M. G., & Mogharabi, V. (2014). *Using a combined method of hierarchical analysis and Monte Carlo simulation in order to identify and prioritize the target market selection criteria (Case study: Food distribution companies of Mashhad, Iran)*. Academic Press.

Burke, R. (2002). Hybrid recommender systems: Survey and experiments. *User Modeling and User-Adapted Interaction*, *12*(4), 331–370. doi:10.1023/A:1021240730564

Chen, D., Wang, X., Liu, W., Zeng, Y., & Chen, Z. (2016). Ebd extended analytic hierarchy process (Ahp) approach to evaluating the effectiveness of engineering projects. *Journal of Integrated Design and Process Science*, *19*(2), 49–70. doi:10.3233/jid-2015-0012

Dadkhah, A., Bayati, N., & Khodadadi, A. (2016). *An investigation of the impact of size and location of dg on system reliability by employing sequential Monte Carlo simulation*. Academic Press.

Deliens, T., Clarys, P., De Bourdeaudhuij, I., & Deforche, B. (2014). Determinants of eating behaviour in university students: A qualitative study using focus group discussions. *BMC Public Health*, *14*(1), 1. doi:10.1186/1471-2458-14-53 PMID:24438555

Doust, D., & Walsh, Z. (2011). *Data mining clustering: A healthcare application*. Academic Press.

Gaikwad, S. M., Joshi, R., & Gaikwad, S. M. (2016, March). Modified analytical hierarchy process to recommend an ice cream to a diabetic patient. In *Proceedings of the Second International Conference on Information and Communication Technology for Competitive Strategies* (p. 138). ACM. doi:10.1145/2905055.2905198

Gaikwad, S. M., Joshi, R. R., & Kulkarni, A. J. (2015, December). Cohort Intelligence and Genetic Algorithm along with AHP to recommend an Ice cream to a Diabetic Patient. In *International Conference on Swarm, Evolutionary, and Memetic Computing* (pp. 40-49). Springer International Publishing.

Gaikwad, S. M., Joshi, R. R., & Kulkarni, A. J. (2017). Cohort Intelligence and Genetic Algorithm Along with Modified Analytical Hierarchy Process to Recommend an Ice cream to Diabetic Patient. In *Proceedings of the International Conference on Data Engineering and Communication Technology* (pp. 279-288). Springer Singapore. doi:10.1007/978-981-10-1675-2_29

Gaikwad, S. M., Joshi, R. R., & Mulay, P. (2015). Analytical Network Process (ANP) to Recommend an Ice cream to a Diabetic Patient. *International Journal of Computers and Applications*, *121*(12).

Gaikwad, S. M., Joshi, R. R., & Mulay, P. (2016). System Dynamics Modeling for Analyzing Recovery Rate of Diabetic Patients by Mapping Sugar Content in Ice cream and Sugar Intake for the Day. In *Proceedings of the Second International Conference on Computer and Communication Technologies* (pp. 743-749). Springer India. doi:10.1007/978-81-322-2517-1_71

Gaikwad, S. M., Mulay, P., & Joshi, R. R. (2015). Analytical Hierarchy Process to Recommend an Ice cream to a Diabetic Patient Based on Sugar Content in it. *Procedia Computer Science*, *50*, 64–72. doi:10.1016/j.procs.2015.04.062

Ganasegeran, K., Al-Dubai, S. A., Qureshi, A. M., Al-Abed, A. A. A., Rizal, A. M., & Aljunid, S. M. (2012). Social and psychological factors affecting eating habits among university students in a Malaysian medical school: A cross-sectional study. *Nutrition Journal*, *11*(1), 1. doi:10.1186/1475-2891-11-48 PMID:22809556

Granville, V. (2014). *16 analytic disciplines compared to data science*. Retrieved June 20, 2016, http://www.datasciencecentral.com/profiles/blogs/17-analytic-disciplines-compared

Gutierrez, D. (2013). *Data Science 101: Probability and Monte Carlo Methods*. Retrieved July 05, 2016, http://insidebigdata.com/2013/12/26/data-science-101-probability-monte-carlo-methods/

Health Care. (n.d.). Retrieved July 01, 2016, http://www.shimko1to1.com/health-care/

Hough, A. (2012). *Ice cream as 'addictive as drugs' says new study*. Retrieved June 22, 2016, http://www.telegraph.co.uk/news/science/science-news/9118768/Ice-cream-as-addictive-as-drugs-says-new-study.html

Hsu, P. F., Lin, E. P., & Tsai, C. W. (2016). Optimal Selection of Business Managers for Integrated Marketing Communications Companies Using AHP and GRA. *International Journal of Customer Relationship Marketing and Management*, 7(2), 16–29. doi:10.4018/IJCRMM.2016040102

Hsu, T. H., & Pan, F. F. (2009). Application of Monte Carlo AHP in ranking dental quality attributes. *Expert Systems with Applications*, *36*(2), 2310–2316. doi:10.1016/j.eswa.2007.12.023

Hunter, J. G., & Cason, K. L. (n.d.). *Healthy Eating Habits for Children*. Retrieved from http://www.clemson.edu/extension/hgic/food/pdf/hgic4109.pdf

Inanloo, M., Ashouri, M., Gheibi, S., & Hemmatyar, A. A. (2012, October). A new approach for multi-source data prediction in Wireless Sensor Networks: Collaborative filtering. In *Wireless Communications & Signal Processing (WCSP), 2012 International Conference on* (pp. 1-6). IEEE.

International Markets Bureau. (n.d.). *The Global Flavour Industry*. Retrieved from https://www.gov.mb.ca/agriculture/market-prices-and-statistics/food-and-value-added-agriculture-statistics/pubs/ma_global_flavours_industry_en.pdf

Jin, R., Goswami, A., & Agrawal, G. (2006). Fast and exact out-of-core and distributed K-Means clustering. *Knowledge and Information Systems*, *10*(1), 17–40. doi:10.1007/s10115-005-0210-0

Jing, L., Chen, B., Zhang, B., Li, P., & Zheng, J. (2012). Monte Carlo simulation–aided analytic hierarchy process approach: Case study of assessing preferred non-point-source pollution control best management practices. *Journal of Environmental Engineering*, *139*(5), 618–626. doi:10.1061/(ASCE)EE.1943-7870.0000673

Joanne, M., & Demand, M. (n.d.). *Advantages & Disadvantages of Ice cream to Human Health*. Retrieved from http://healthyeating.sfgate.com/advantages-disadvantages-ice-cream-human-health-2858.html

Joshi, R. R., Kadam, K. D., Shelke-Bembde, M., & Deshmukh-Joshi, V. (2015). PBR: Perspective Based Ranking of Selected State IT Policy Documents in India using AHP. *International Journal of Applied Engineering Research*, *10*(20), 41353–41356.

Kanungo, T., Mount, D. M., Netanyahu, N. S., Piatko, C. D., Silverman, R., & Wu, A. Y. (2002). An efficient K-Means clustering algorithm: Analysis and implementation. *IEEE Transactions on Pattern Analysis and Machine Intelligence*, *24*(7), 881–892. doi:10.1109/TPAMI.2002.1017616

Kou, G., Ergu, D., Peng, Y., & Shi, Y. (2012). *Data Processing for the AHP/ANP* (Vol. 1). Springer Science & Business Media.

Kulkarni, P. A., & Mulay, P. (2013). Evolve systems using incremental clustering approach. *Evolving Systems*, *4*(2), 71–85. doi:10.1007/s12530-012-9068-z

Laddha, A. R., Joshi, R. R., & Mulay, P. (2016). Enriching process of ice cream recommendation using combinatorial ranking of AHP and Monte Carlo AHP. *Journal of Theoretical & Applied Information Technology*, *85*(3), 298.

Linden, G., Smith, B., & York, J. (2003). Amazon. com recommendations: Item-to-item collaborative filtering. *IEEE Internet Computing*, *7*(1), 76–80. doi:10.1109/MIC.2003.1167344

Marie, J., & Media, D. *Advantages & Disadvantages of Ice cream to Human Health*. Retrieved June 28, 2016, http://healthyeating.sfgate.com/advantages-disadvantages-ice-cream-human-health-2858.html

Mingle, D. (n.d.). *4 big reasons why healthcare needs data science.* Retrieved July 10, 2016, http://www.cio.com/article/3001216/analytics/4-big-reasons-why-healthcare-needs-data-science.html

Momani, A. M., & Ahmed, A. A. (2011). Material handling equipment selection using hybrid Monte Carlo simulation and analytic hierarchy process. *World Academy of Science, Engineering and Technology*, *59*, 953–958.

Mudur, G. (2015). *App to pick right ice cream- Engineers propose tool to match tastes with health needs*, Retrieved June 29, 2016, http://www.telegraphindia.com/1150517/jsp/frontpage/story_20548.jsp#.V45o3qIzzIU

Mulay, P., & Kulkarni, P. A. (2013). Knowledge augmentation via incremental clustering: New technology for effective knowledge management. *International Journal of Business Information Systems*, *12*(1), 68–87. doi:10.1504/IJBIS.2013.050660

Nagaraj, R. (2016). Health care analysis for process deviation using alpha-fitness algorithm in process mining. *Journal of Theoretical & Applied Information Technology*, *88*(3).

O'Reilly, T., Loukides, M., Steele, J., & Hill, C. (2012). *How data science is transforming health care.* O'Reilly Media, Inc.

Papadaki, A., Hondros, G., Scott, J. A., & Kapsokefalou, M. (2007). Eating habits of university students living at, or away from home in Greece. *Appetite*, *49*(1), 169–176. doi:10.1016/j.appet.2007.01.008 PMID:17368642

Paul, R., & Hoque, A. S. M. L. (2010, July). Clustering medical data to predict the likelihood of diseases. In *Digital Information Management (ICDIM), 2010 Fifth International Conference on* (pp. 44-49). IEEE. doi:10.1109/ICDIM.2010.5664638

Preeti, M., Rahul, J., Aditya, A., Alisha, G., & Deepankar, G. (2017). *Threshold based clustering algorithm analyzes diabetic mellitus.* Academic Press.

Raychaudhuri, S. (2008, December). *Introduction to monte carlo simulation. In 2008 Winter Simulation Conference* (pp. 91–100). IEEE. doi:10.1109/WSC.2008.4736059

Revelant, J. (2014). *4 shocking ways sugar affects your kid's health.* Retrieved from http://www.foxnews.com/health/2014/08/17/4-shocking-ways-sugar-affects-your-kids-health.html

Rosen, J. A. (n.d.). *Data science solutions for healthcare.* Retrieved from https://www.leidos.com/sites/default/files/Leidos%20WP%20-%20Data%20Science%20Solutions%20for%20Health%201.15.pdf

Saaty, T. L. (2008). Decision making with the analytic hierarchy process. *International Journal of Services Sciences, 1*(1), 83-98.

Salleh, S. (2013). *When Multiattribute Decision Analysis Needs Monte Carlo.* Retrieved from http://www.lumina.com/blog/when-multiattribute-decision-analysis-needs-monte-carlo

Schafer, J. B., Frankowski, D., Herlocker, J., & Sen, S. (2007). Collaborative filtering recommender systems. In *The adaptive web* (pp. 291–324). Springer Berlin Heidelberg.

Siddique, H. (n.d.). *Sugar should be no more than 5% of daily calories, say nutrition experts*. Retrieved from https://www.theguardian.com/society/2015/jul/17/cut-recommended-daily-allowance-sugar-5-percent-daily-calories-report

StatCrunch. (2012). *Ice cream Survey Report*. Retrieved June 10, 2016, http://www.statcrunch.com/5.0/viewreport.php?reportid=25427

Subramaniam, S., Dhillon, J. S., Ahmad, M. S., Teoh, C., Hassan, N. H., Ismail, Z., & Ranjan, K. S. (2016). Integrating health behavioural change theories in the design of prediabetes self-care applications: A systematic literature review. *Journal of Theoretical and Applied Information Technology*, *88*(2).

Suhas, G., Rahul, J., & Preeti, M. (2015). Cluster mapping with the help of new proposed algorithm and MCF algorithm to recommend an ice cream to the diabetic patient. *International Journal of Applied Engineering Research, 10*(8), 21259-21266.

Tweets by @regionalvoice. (2014). *Open data in health+care- a blueprint*. Retrieved June23, 2016, http://www.regionalvoices.org/node/230

Van Der Aalst, W. (2012, July 1). Process mining: Overview and opportunities. *ACM Transactions on Management Information Systems*, *3*(2), 7. doi:10.1145/2229156.2229157

VanderMey, A. (2014). *Do we still scream for ice cream?* Retrieved June 10, 2016,http://fortune.com/2014/07/24/ice-cream-sales/

Yaraghi, N., Tabesh, P., Guan, P., & Zhuang, J. (2015). Comparison of AHP and monte carlo AHP under different levels of uncertainty. *IEEE Transactions on Engineering Management*, *62*(1), 122–132. doi:10.1109/TEM.2014.2360082

Zhang, S., Huang, Z., Sun, Y., & Guo, K. (2016). A Fuzzy Integrated Multi-Criteria Decision Approach to Select Green Logistics Provider for Sustainable Supply Chain. *Transylvanian Review, 24*(4).

Zhang, Y., & Li, W. (2012, March). AHP Construct Mining Component strategy applied for data mining process. In *2012 IEEE International Conference on Information Science and Technology* (pp. 591-595). IEEE. doi:10.1109/ICIST.2012.6221714

Chapter 12
Improved Health Monitoring Informatics by New Similarity Measures

Vijayalakshmi Kakulapati
Sreenidhi Institute of Science and Technology, India

V.V.S.S.S. Balaram
Sreenidhi Institute of Science and Technology, India

P. Vijay Krishna
Mahindra École Centrale (MEC), India

ABSTRACT

This research will identify different patient's online behaviours and similarities that can help patient-clinician communications to improve to discover the future or additional threats to raise awareness of causes and consequences. To scale the model, the prototype will rely on the High Performance Computing (HPC) platform running Hadoop file system for storing patient data at distributed locations and Map-reduce paradigm with machine learning algorithms will be deployed to detect the symptoms. In this approach the authors protect online data of patients from privacy issues. In this, the author's effort this difficulty by means of a new advance utilising new similarity measures between patients. The authors are also providing a research investigation on grouping behavior which is affecting by diverse series demonstration, diverse distance similarity measures, the number of genuine patients, and the number of online doctors obtainable, similarity among patient symptoms, minimizing the feasibility, the number of patients for sittings, and the number of clusters to form.

1. INTRODUCTION

Now- a-day healthcare moving towards huge health issues and maintain records. These records are providing for analysis and providing personalized recommendations to patients. The author's research belongs to multiple health symptoms of diabetic and thyroid from patients using online profiles based, using their online interaction on healthcare applications specially belongs for patients to actively developed

DOI: 10.4018/978-1-5225-5222-2.ch012

Copyright © 2018, IGI Global. Copying or distributing in print or electronic forms without written permission of IGI Global is prohibited.

different patterns. Many organizations and researchers are working on different predictive analytics on healthcare systems. The authors approach an efficient method for finding similarity between Patients of diabetic and thyroid and find it comfortable to communicate directly with other patients via social networks. This research will identify different patient's online behaviors and similarities that can help patient-clinician communications to improve to discover the future or additional threats to raise awareness of causes and consequences. To scale the model, the prototype will rely on the High Performance Computing (HPC) platform running Hadoop file system for storing patient data at distributed locations and Map-reduce paradigm with machine learning algorithms will be deployed to detect the symptoms. In this approach the authors protect online data of patients from privacy issues. In this, the author's effort this difficulty by means of a new advance utilizing new similarity measures between patients. The proposing function utilizes online records by considering the similarity between patients and provides recommendation for medicines to the patient. For a large number of patients, the new measure assists the minimization of risk and realistic. The authors have established the framework comparison of performance on the assimilation of bunch utilizing algorithm. The authors are also providing a research investigation on grouping behavior which is affecting by diverse series demonstration, diverse distance similarity measures, the number of genuine patients, and the number of online doctors obtainable, similarity among patient symptoms, minimizing the feasibility, the number of patients for sittings, and the number of clusters to form.

Healthcare systems is a promising area which apprehensions itself with experimental, data processing, intelligence tasks of therapeutic observation, learning and investigate in medical domain inclusive of the technologies to sustain these undertakings. Healthcare systems can be defined as "Integration of the theory and practice of information and data management and use in all characteristics of health-care deliverance and public health". A number of health informatics disciplines is allows exploring the implementation, advance applications, techniques and instruments.

Healthcare systems create electronic health record (EHR) (C.Sunil kumar et al 2012) to progressing the processes of:

1. Health and patient-care data storage, retrieval and communication of data for medical research.
2. Medical knowledge is learning and transmission.

In the last decade healthcare applications have developed quickly. Primary health centres moved towards a consecutive healthcare process support from inaccessible systems. Various systems include health practitioners, societies; utilize the technological advances in computing healthcare environments. There is a need for information sharing amongst healthcare systems in interactive systems. The relevant patient medical information is required to available easily for healthcare professionals whenever they need to analyze the information which improves the health care quality. The specific situation is characterized by:

1. Healthcare applications can be support by hardware and software solutions in heterogeneous systems also.
2. Consumption of EHR is suitable for various healthcare applications in the Heterogeneities structure.

The typical problem in healthcare applications is heterogeneities. Every EHR is unique, which means that the framework of EHR and the processes utilized for interchanging their content may diverge significantly. This interchanging becomes a complication for distribution health information between hospitals.

Improvement of health in health care systems is the analysis, therapeutics, and avoidance of sickness, ill health, sprain, and other natural and psychological ruination in public. Health practitioners are conveyed about medical care associated with medical practitioners, doctors, associate doctors, dental care, maternology, attending, drug etc. Health care systems providing primary care, secondary care, and tertiary care for the health for public.

The initiation of online medical records and huge corpora of health information produces an increasing demand for recommendation methods adapted to retrieving health related information [W. Hersh et al., 2009]. An insightful health file provides challenges which are terminology mismatch are ubiquitous as the same perceptions can be communicated utilizing diverse words. The most challenging situations are where significance must be contingent. To overcome these requires capable retrieval systems of accurately determining the similarity between health conceptions. Health informatics utilized similarity measures including: medicinal discovery [P. Agarwal, 2009], gene clustering (P. Glenisson, 2003), and ontology erection (S. Cederberg, 2003).

Big data have datasets that are huge and difficult to the transaction with these data sets, and observes various challenges; those are including attaining, accumulating, analyzing, investigating, distributing, relocating, inquiring, revising, data confidentiality and visualizing. A collection of related sets of information is known as a data set which can be expressed by a single or multidimensional attributes. These datasets contain large volumes of data such that conventional database systems cannot hold such amounts of data. Today, many organizations are using big data due to its popularity in need of advanced data intensive technologies. Due to the increasing size of datasets leads to the vast demand for efficient clustering techniques which persuades the limitations of memory utilized, the number of files progression and implementation time. The most demanding issues in big data are to the collection of data that the data in the similar group is similar to each other in the identical cluster than new groups. Telecommunications, health care, bioinformatics, banking, ecommerce, online libraries, policies, constructions, geographical and spatial studies are examples of big data applications.

2. CLUSTERING IN HEALTH INFORMATICS

To reveal unknown structures and "clusters" originate in huge data sets by using statistical techniques which is frequently using Cluster analysis (Minlei Liao et. al, 2016). However, this classification has not been utilized in huge healthcare databases; the expenditure of data distribution is strictly twisted. by grouping attribute values, Cluster analysis is a technique that helps entities, devices, positions with similar type into homogenous clusters while expanding heterogeneity across clusters [Dilts D, 1995 and McLachlan GJ, 1992). Attribute values of concern are clustered as one based on attributes that formulate similar, discriminate these attributes by grouping into comparable and dissimilar attributes into different clusters. Each cluster within homogeneous systems aim to relatively identical solution which leads to these clusters has high intra-class similarity whereas clusters heterogeneity maximization leads to low inter-class similarity. The cluster attributes are close together, at the same time as their distance with cluster is not together. Cluster analysis is helps to entities in which group these entities belongs to; consequently, it assists to recognize a underlying structure within a dataset [Romesburg HC, 1984].

Distance based clustering is a extremely popular technique to grouping the attributes. The clusters attributes with in a cluster have a minimum distance value and attribute from different clusters have a maximum distance value.

3. HEALTH INFORMATICS SIMILARITY MEASURES

Here, briefly discussed about a general overview of similarity measures used in health informatics for health research. Firstly, an extensive definition of similarity measures, the chapter illustrates the utilization of similarity measures in patient symptoms of health informatics which leads to investigation of the information created by the online platforms. This information provides promising potential to predict public attitude on diverse concerns and it is also used for improved analysis and avoidance of ailments. Comparing health informatics research methods with traditional research methods and emphasize their strengths and weaknesses.

3.1. Mathematics in Patient Similarity Analytics

Now a day's Thyroid and diabetic are common diseases currently addressed in public health. Most of the people suffer these diseases. For the demonstration of the effectiveness of similarity symptoms in patients, suggestions provided based on their similarities and providing useful suggestions in medicine. In some research work, a patient can be characterized by a Euclidean vector for determining patient similarity metric (Lee, J., et al, 2015 and Li, L et al., 2015). Lab results taken as predictor variables or fundamental symptoms can be describing as a multi-dimensional attribute values. Cosine angle can be calculated among two patients and dot product can utilize for calculation. The cosine patient similarity metric is defined as:

$$\textit{Patient similarity measures}\left(P_1, P_2\right) = \frac{P_1 \; P_2}{\left\|P_1\right\| \left\|P_2\right\|}$$

In this, $P_1 i$ and $P_2 i$ *correspond to* a single predictor variable vector for two patients, · and Euclidean vector magnitude is ||||. Cosine similarity is normalizes between minimum possible similarity -1 and maximum possible similarity 1. These two predictor variable vectors are in the exact opposite direction and angle between them is 180o and then compute a patient similarity metric of −1. If the angle between these two variables is 0o then these vectors are overlapping and then compute a patient similarity metric of 1. Similarly, before the entire similarity can be computed that predictor variable vector normalized between the range of -1 and 1 (Lee, J., et al, 2015). Cosine similarity is computed for every attribute in the dataset and comparative to an index *P*1. N index is utilized as a training set and testing for confirmation, with prediction of diagnosis. Subsequent to validation this representation can be utilized for epidemiologic or medical research. Cosine similarity recognized three sub groups of patients (Li, L et al., 2015).

Patients with diabetic heart disease and diabetic cancer are belongs to first subgroup.

Diabetic People be inclined to extend heart disease at a younger age than non diabetic people. Heart disease and heart stroke are more common in adult diabetic patient causes of death. Diabetic Adults are dying due to heart disease or heart stroke when compared with non diabetic patient. The main symptom of heart disease is Chest pain.

Diabetic patient have these symptoms to attain a heart stroke

- Chest tenderness that preceding more than a few minutes
- Uneasiness in one or both of arms or shoulders or back, neck, or jaw

- Breathing problems
- Panic
- Upset stomach
- Annoying

Physicians diagnose heart attack in diabetic people

- Observing symptoms of patient
- Medical and family history
- Patient heart attack frequency
- A bodily assessment
- Tests and methods results

3.1.1. Heart Disease Caused by Thyroid

Normal function of heart can alter by the thyroid gland, causing symptoms and resulting in significant complications. For analysis of heart affected by thyroid is essential to understand the working condition of heart beat.

Blood is circulated around the body due to muscular chambers which exits in heart. Due to valves in the heart, blood circulates in one direction. Heart channels blood everywhere throughout the body through the circulatory structure, giving oxygen and supplements to the tissues and killing carbon dioxide and different scatters.

Thyroid patient can understand two principles.

1. Heart requires oxygen to working and gets oxygen from coronary courses. In the event that there is a blockage in inside the lumen and lessening of blood stream causes the heart works with poor oxygen provide and chest agony or "angina" can be produced.
2. Heats beat in a intended manner and remove blood easily and productively, the heart is animated to agreement in a coordinated manner by particular tissues inside the heart which lead electrical driving forces. The motivation typically begins at the highest point of the correct chamber and spreads down through the heart.

3.1.2. Patient of Hyperthyroidism Symptoms and Signs

In hyperthyroidism, the thyroid gland produces huge amounts of thyroxin hormone that will stimulate the heart to beat more rapidly. This rapid heart rate felt initially is termed as tachycardia. The physician can examine this but cannot be perceived by the patient. When this tachycardia becomes severe they can be perceived by the long-suffering as palpitations. This is caution of the sensitivity against the chest barrier. These are sometimes physiological i.e can be felt in normal individuals due to extreme work out or overwhelming a large amount of caffeine. However, if this occurs at rest, then it is considered abnormal. These palpitations can likewise be seen in different sorts of coronary illness, yet in the event that caused because of hyperthyroidism overactive thyroid organ, they don't really demonstrate a genuine basic coronary illness. In a few patients, this drawn out incitement of the heart because of thyroxin may prompt an in coordination of the conduction of electrical driving forces inside the heart and atria fibrillation may result. This is the place the impulses arising emerging in the correct chamber, as opposed to be led typically into the ventricles, frame a short out inside atria and quickly go round in hovers causing in composed atrial constriction and loss of general incitement of the ventricle with a sporadic pulse.

Increase in blood pressure caused by extended stimulation of heart called as systolic hypertension. The diastolic circulatory strain is not ordinarily expanded. The expanded compression of the heart with expanded cardiovascular yield causes a quick heartbeat that is effortlessly felt at the wrist and adds to warm damp with sweat hands.

3.1.3. Symptoms and Signs of Hypothyroidism

This is opposite of hyperthyroidism as the production of thyroxin hormone is decreased which causes slow heart beat and low blood pressure. The patient neither of these symptoms usually have. Delayed hypothyroidism causes metabolic changes in the body and may deliver increased levels of cholesterol. People know that a few sorts of increased cholesterol may obtain gathered in the arterial wall causing narrowing of the coronary corridors. Be that as it may, as heart rate and circulatory strain are additionally brought down, the intricacies of angina or heart assault are moderately unprecedented.

Diabetic patients has cancer and cardiovascular diseases belongs to second subgroup

Diabetes is commonly partitioned into two noteworthy subtypes, type 1 and type 2 diabetes, and furthermore certain different types of diabetes are available, while tumor is ordinarily grouped by its anatomic starting point (of which there are more than 50, e.g., lymphoma, leukemia, lung, and bosom disease) and inside which there might be various subtypes (e.g., leukemia).

Diabetic type 2, insulin resistance usually makes the body create more insulin than ordinary because of expanded glucose levels in the blood. Another motivation behind why a connection might be available is that an unsafe way of life may prompt heftiness and along these lines higher dangers of both type 2 diabetes and growth.

The following cancers may be cause by type 2 diabetes:

- Pancreatic tumor
- Liver tumor
- Uterine tumor

A littler expanded risk, of 20% to 50% is seen for the accompanying types of tumor

- Colorectal tumor
- Bladder tumor
- Breast tumor
- Blood tumor

Type 2 diabetes has positive effect that frequency of prostate tumor is lower

The International Diabetes Foundation highlights the following symptoms that signal the need for diabetes testing:

- Polyuria- increased urine excretion
- Weight loss

- Lack of energy
- Polydypsia- excessive thirst

3.1.4. Caner Affected by Thyroid Patients

Thyroid tumor is an illness that patient get when unusual cells start to develop and increase in patient thyroid organ. The thyroid organ is formed like a butterfly and is situated before your neck. It produces hormones that direct the digestion systems in the body.

This type of tumor is not a general category. The majority of patients have superior prediction as the tumor is typically discovered early and the medications function admirably.

Thyroid tumor causing symptoms are:

- Neck swelling
- Soreness in neck and ears
- Trouble in swallowing
- Trouble in breathing
- Throaty tone
- Recurrent cough without cold.

Few patients don't have any symptoms but physicians finding a swelling in the neck for the duration of a routine checkup

3.2. Patient Similarity Measures

This measures can possibly change Systems Medicine, which is Systems Biology connected to health-care frameworks. The characteristics of natural science are cells, tissues, organisms, or other thorough organic units as entire frameworks. This determines, how changes in single part of the human body can influence the conduct of the entire body and frequently concentrates on prescient demonstrating of the framework in gap bed state. Patient characteristics could be created similarity analytics of the patient in human body, and compare these to a multitude of similar patients.

The assessment of similarity metrics of Patient (Jimeng Sun et al) is necessary in the context of patient contingent recognition for analysis of clinical applications; this leads to distinguish the appropriate and helpful to derived utilization of electronic health record information for enhancing persistent result without bringing about extra exertion from doctors. These are principle objective of the significant reuse of electronic health records. The main goal of this patient symptoms similarity is to determine a similarity measure between symptoms of patients in view of their EHR.

3.3. Patient Similarity Analytics

In healthcare prescription in commercial genomics, transcriptomics, proteomics, microbiomics, are diverse components. Besides, reproduction of physiology at the level of the particle, cell, tissue, organ, and life form ought to be solidified as a complete comparability highlight to give a more extensive perspective of communications among organ systems. Predictive models of a patient's illness irritations or analysis appropriate to the patient are provided by patient similarity analytics. These predictive models would consent to assessment of how new diagnoses or treatments could affect the performance of the entire patient. Integrating the larger part of these healthcare medicine tools into patient similarity analytics is latent the next border line in healthcare informatics for at least a few reasons.

Investigation of patient similarity analytics by perspective of patient's characteristic by reviewing number of patients to deliver a significant and helpful outcome. One may compete that patient comparability not exactly closely resembles genomics, since a person's genome is believed to be consistent all through their lifetime. This is not any more fundamentally the case, because of the present advance of genome editing tools. In fact, these analytics is analogous from these different omics with the possibility to change patient lifetime. In cell genome is the supplement of DNA; a similarome is the supplement of patients observed. It can recognize subgroups of patients that are an index patient within similarome based on comorbidities or prescriptions relevance to the patient. In diagnosis of diabetes, the presence or absence of a particular gene feature, genotyping would allocate the presence or absence of genotyping feature. The presence and absence of a specific feature is determined by genotype, simotyping is assign the presence or absence of a specific feature. Similarity wide association study has the objective of finding clusters of patient's persistent and distinguishing features that associate with precise outcomes for instance, intricacies, methods, hospitalizations, or demise. Diabetic patient are more likely associate with non-healing leg ulcers, critical limb ischemia, or gangrene leading to limb amputation.

Variety of omics and systems medicine tools are to bring together by Patient similarity analytics that is effective, accurate, consistent, and computationally efficient. Many researchers proposed various methods of aggregating omics and monitoring these for each patient. Coordinating these techniques with patient similarity can launch drug promote into a future. patient similarity will probably progress towards in systems Medicine.

3.4. Statistical Measures

Diverse statistical measures (Schatten M and V. Kakulati et al, 2010] for replicating the removal of two random variables (X,Y) from autonomy. One of such measure is Pearson Correlation Coefficient (PCC is derived by Galton). The formula is

$$PCC = \frac{1}{N-1}\sum_{i=1}^{N}\left(\frac{x_i - \mu_x}{\sigma_x}\right)\left(\frac{y_i - \mu_y}{\sigma_y}\right)$$

3.4.1. JDM (Jaro Distance Metric)

Two patients *s* and *t*, let *s'* be the symptoms of *s* which is common with *t*, and let *t'* be the symptoms of *t* which is "common with" *s*; a symptom *a* in *s* is in common with *t* if *a* appears in *t*. Let the number of transpositions of symptoms in *s'* relative to *t' is Ts,t.* The formula for *s* and *t* is

$$J(s,t) = \frac{1}{3}\times\left(\frac{|s'|}{|s|} + \frac{|t'|}{|t|} + \frac{|s'| - T_{s',t'}}{2|s'|}\right)$$

3.4.2. Jaro Winkler

"Jaro winkler" is a similarity measure between two patients. The Jaro measure is the weighted summation of the percentage of matched symptoms from each file and transposed symptoms. Winkler adds to this measure by pairing initial symptoms, and then recycled it by a chunk wise function, whose intervals and weights depend on the type of patient (first name, last name, disease, etc.).

$$JW\left(s,t\right) = J\left(s,t\right) + \left(l * p * \left(1.0 - J\left(s,t\right)\right)\right)$$

3.4.3. Hamming Distance

This is defined only for patients of the same symptoms. Two patients' s and t, H(s, t) is the number of symptoms explains about patients have different symptoms.

3.4.4. LD (Levenshtein Distances)

LD is to examine the similarity between patient's s and t where s refereed as the source and t referred as the target. The number of removals, additions or exchanges required to convert the distance form s into t. LD(s,t) = 0, means no alterations are required. Patient symptoms are the same. If LD(s,t) = 1, one substitution is adequate to alter s into t. Levenshtein distance greater, the further diverse the keys are.

3.4.5. Needleman-Wunsch Distance

The primary assumption of algorithm LD is "all insertions or conversions costs same". Sometimes these causes to hide considerable distances and this behavior may not be desirable. The existing Levenshtein distance algorithm got updated to overcome this limit. This updated model is called as NWD (Needleman-Wunsch distance) algorithm that takes individual costs as the matrix along with the other input parameters. Individual costs will be submitted as the matrix that includes two matricies those includes costs for every duo of symptoms to translate from and to.

Due to the different gap cost and distance methods this NWD gives a diverse consequential assessment for the same group but dissimilar categorization is alternated. These methods can be adapted to the information implicated in the similarity measure.

3.4.6. Latent Semantic Analysis (LDA)

This is a statistical model that allocates sets of studies to be clarified by unobserved clusters that is why a number of patient symptoms are similar. Every patient may be observed as a combination of various symptoms where every patient is considered to have a set of symptoms that are allocated to it via LDA. In fact, results are added practical grouping of symptoms in a patient.

Latent Dirichlet Allocation, underlying set of treatment behavioral symptoms from the patient storage area. Patient similarities between symptoms can be measured efficiently by using consequential treatment performance. Text document corpus utilized LDA to model the procedure for summarizing topics. In this chapter, a patient symptom is a combination of underlying treatment performances. Here, the authors are identifing treatment performances as a group of medical events,

LDA explains the behavioral similarity of patient Symptoms by cluster medical measures into the ignored group. For every patient symptom s, a combination of symptom percentage $\Theta_s \sim$ Dir (α) is tested from a Dirichlet parameterized distribution by α.

Determine the treatment performance of patients, latent Dirichlet allocation (LDA) which is based on a probabilistic graphical model used (Zhengxing Huang).

4. DISTANCE METRICS USED FOR CLUSTERING

To measure the similarity between the attribute values distance metrics are more efficiently gives the result. Distance metric calculation is required in a precise problem is to attain a suitable distance similarity measure. Similarity distance function is a distance between attribute values of a set (Joaquin Perez Ortega et al). Metric space is defined by a set with metric (Archana Singh, 2013). Clustering techniques mainly utilized the distance similarity metrics. K-means clustering algorithm utilized Euclidean distance similarity metric for comparing similarity between patient symptoms. In general, the work is to describe a Similarity (P, S) function, where P and S are two entities (patient, symptoms) of a patient class, and the function significance describes the extent of "similarity" among the entities (Archana Singh, 2013).

Here the authors discussed different similarity measures commonly utilized for clustering techniques

4.1. Euclidean Distance

It is most popular distance metric for similarity measures. It is defined as the general distance between two entities. It is most popularly utilized in clustering problems. This is default distance metrics in K-means algorithm. It is defined as

$$Dist_{PS} = Max_K \ |P_{iK -} P_{jK}|$$

4.2. Cosine Distance

This distance measure is defined as similarity among two non-zero vectors of an inner product space that establish the angle between two vector measures.

$$\Theta = \arccos \frac{P_1 . P_2}{\|P_1\| \, \|P_2\|}$$

4.3. MD (Manhattan Distance)

It is defined as the addition of the unconditional value of the differences of the coordinates.

$$Dist_{PS} = Max_K \ |P_{iK -} P_{jK}|$$

4.4. CD (Chebyshev Distance)

This distance is defined on a vector space where the distance among two vectors and computes the unconditional degree of the dissimilarity among brings together a couple of attribute values and also known maximum value distance.

$$\text{Dist}_{PS} = \text{Max}_K \,|P_{iK} - P_{jK}|$$

4.5. MinD (Minkowski Distance)

A normed vector which can be considered as the generalization of Euclidean distance and Manhattan distance is referred as Minkowski distance metric which can be utilized for ordinal variables and quantitative performance.

$$Disp, s = \left(\sum_{i=1}^{n} \left| P_{i,k}, P_{j,K} \right|^{1/v} \right)^{v}$$

4.6. Distance Metrics in Clustering Limitations

Capturing correlations between attribute values by using distance metrics are not always efficient. Survival of related data patterns between the set of attribute values even if they are distant from one another as calculated by similarity metrics is an elevated probability (Kulkarni et al.,2015]. Distance metrics calculate the physical distance among data point to find similarity and are not enough by capturing the performance of the information sequence. Association and disassociation between patterns of attribute values can be captured by information sequence, that carry the proximity among attribute values [Haixun Wang et al, 2002]. For measuring similarities between patient symptoms, utilize the performance analysis approach. One of such measure is Latent Dirichlet Allocation, which is a probabilistic graphical model utilized to determine patient treatment performances [Zhengxing Huang et al].

5. METHODOLOGY

5.1 Hadoop

Hadoop is a huge information storage engine. The main advantage of Hadoop is combining information storage and information processing. MapReduce is the main processing engine which is the most popular big-data processing framework. It makes possible seamlessly integrate accessible data storage in processing MapReduce soles various problems like analysis of a log, information sorting, processing text, search patterns, processing graphs, methods of machine learning, and many more.

Data set in MapReduce data set the job splits into break parts of data such that the map tasks processes in an equivalent manner. The output of maps sort by the framework, then the output is input to reduce tasks. File-system stored both the input and output jobs. The mapReduce framework will do scheduling tasks, observing jobs and re-performs the unsuccessful tasks. HDFS is a distributed file system which has master/slave structural design and proficient of accumulating large volumes of data.

Two principles are utilizing by Hadoop those are one is MapReduce and another one is HDFS (hadoop distributed File system).

5.1.1 MapReduce

In this the computations are performed on a cluster of nodes in parallel to carry out large scale data operations in a reasonable amount of time that are scalable and feasible with increased complexity or data size to perform such computations. The capability of MapReduce to work in parallel on several clusters of computers makes it easy to scale to very large datasets.

Information parallelization programming the representation in map reduce, the dataset is divided into free splits and communicated, every split in the dataset following similar guidelines simultaneously to progression and generating massive measures of datasets (Sharmila K et al., 2015).

MapReduce programs are tailored to manage unlimited measures of data in parallel.

It includes of two principles:

Map is the individual tasks takes a set of the data and transform set of data to intermediate records. The output records of Map task is taken as input of the Reduce task and combines these intermediate records into a smaller set of tuples.

5.1.2. HDFS

HDFS associated with circulated record structure and Java-based distributed system which is adaptable and consistent information storage, and intended to extent huge bunches of product servers. The hadoop file system is elevated error understanding and intended utilizing low-cost hardware than the general distributed file system; it is reveals fabrication adaptability of capable of two hundred Petabytes of storage space and a particular bunch of 4500 servers, sustaining secure billions of files and blocks.

5.2. K–Mean Clustering

This algorithm sort attribute values into clusters in accordance of similar attributes (Can A et al., 2013). The most popular and broadly utilized algorithm for bunch is K-means. The categorizations of data points are easy to understandable and utilized grouping strategy (Zhao W et al, 2009). Various characterization applications are utilized this clustering. By taking k as parameter, and parts a collection of n items into k clusters in order that the successive intra-cluster similarity is elevated though the inter cluster similarity is low. By calculating the significance assessment of attribute values is called as “center of gravity”.

6. THE RESULT EVALUATION

In this chapter, implement a distance measure algorithm such as, *k-means or k-medoids* for the datasets of thyroid, diabetic given.

Clustering for Diabetic Dataset to - *Non-Diabetic (0) and Diabetic (1)*

Clustering for Heart Attack Datasets to - *Healthy (0) and Sick (1, 2, 3, 4)*

Clustering for Thyroid Datasets to - *Compensated hypothyroid, Primary hypothyroid, Secondary Hypothyroid and Negative*

Results will be clustered data records.

Accuracy Analysis will be computed between clustered and existing record class.

The clustering evaluation has performed over 3 datasets accumulated from the UCI repository related to "Diabetes", "Heart" and "Thyroid". The Diabetes dataset consists of 8 attributes which are Preg, plas, pres, skin, insu, mass, pedi, age, related to observation and a class attributes, similarly, Heart Dataset has 76 raw attributes out of these attributes use only 14 attributes which are Age, sex, chest, resting_blood_pressure, serum_cholestoral, fasting_blood_sugar, resting_electrocardiographic_results, maximum_heart_rate_achieved, exercise_induced_angina, oldpeak, slope, number_of_major_vessels. thal . However, for the experiments evaluation 14 attributes are referred which are highly impacting, and the Thyroid dataset consists of 29 attributes those are lass_hyperthyroid, class_hypothyroid, class_binding_protein, class_general_health. class_replacement_theory, class_antithyroid_treatment, class_discordant_results. age, sex, on_thyroxine, query_on_thyroxine, on_antithyroid_medication, sick, pregnant, thyroid_surgery, I131_treatment, query_hypothyroid, query_hyperthyroid, lithium, goitre, tumor, hypopituitary, psych, TSH_measured, TSH, T3_measured, T3, TT4_measured, TT4, T4U_measured, T4U, FTI_measured, FTI, TBG_measured TBG and a class attributes.

The experiment executed the popular *k*-mean algorithm. The grouping method comprises a deterministic efficient method for the minimization of the grouping inaccuracy so as to make use of the method as a confined exploration procedure and progress in an additional technique to explain the grouping problem.

The following are the steps of algorithm.

1. The Health dataset which contains both +ve and –ve values then go to step otherwise go to step 4.
2. In the given Health dataset find the min attribute value.
3. Reduction of min values from data values.
4. Calculate the distance of every attribute value from Centroid.
5. The out of step 4 is sorted with respect to the distance of every attribute value.
6. Divided the sorted attribute values into k identical sets.
7. For every set, capture the center as the initial Centroid.
8. calculate the distance between every attribute value.
9. xi (1 <= I <= n) to all the initial centroids oj (1 <= j <= k). (x is distance and o is origin)
10. do again
11. For every attribute value xi, find the nearest Centroid oj and allocate xi to bunch j.
12. Set bunchId[i]=j. // j:Id of the nearest bunch.
13. Set NearestDist[i]= x(xi, oj).
14. For every bunch j (1 <= j <= k), recalculate the centroids.
15. For every attribute value xi,
    a. Calculate its remoteness from the Centroid of the present closest bunch.
    b. If xi ≤ the present nearest distance, the attribute values exists in the same bunch.
16. Else
    a. For every Centroid oj (1<=j<=k) compute the distance x(xi, oj).
17. End for;
    a. Until the appropriate criteria is reached.

Output is K number of clusters.

A repetitive experiment has performed varying the *k* value from 2 to 6, and the output values are used to measure the error rate and accuracy of the cluster as discussed below.

The generated cluster's accuracy rate percentage is measured for the 3 datasets in comparison with the number of cluster classes given in the datasets as shown in Figure 1, 2 and 3. All the 3 dataset results demonstrate that increasing the number of *k* value decreasing the clustering accuracy and increasing incorrectly clustered instances i.e., error rate.

Even it was observed that the clustering accuracy depends on the number of attributes being utilized. Here, the dataset of Diabetes has 8 attributes, Heart has 14 attributes and Thyroid has 29 attributes, so according to this when $k=2$, the rate of accuracy is diabetes datasets shows an average of 6% higher in comparing with other 2 datasets, but in case of higher $k=6$ it shows the 9% higher error rate in compared with others. It concludes that less number of attributes can be efficient for the minimum number of clustering, but in case of large number clustering more attributes is effective and will be accurate shows in Table 1, 2 and 3.

Table 1. Diabetes error and accuracy rate

Diabetes		
Cluster - K	**Error Rate**	**Acc. Rate**
2	33.2	66.8
3	48.3	51.7
4	48.04	51.96
5	54.29	45.71
6	65.75	34.25

Figure 1. k cluster Accuracy for Diabetes Datasets
Time taken for clustering 0.06 seconds

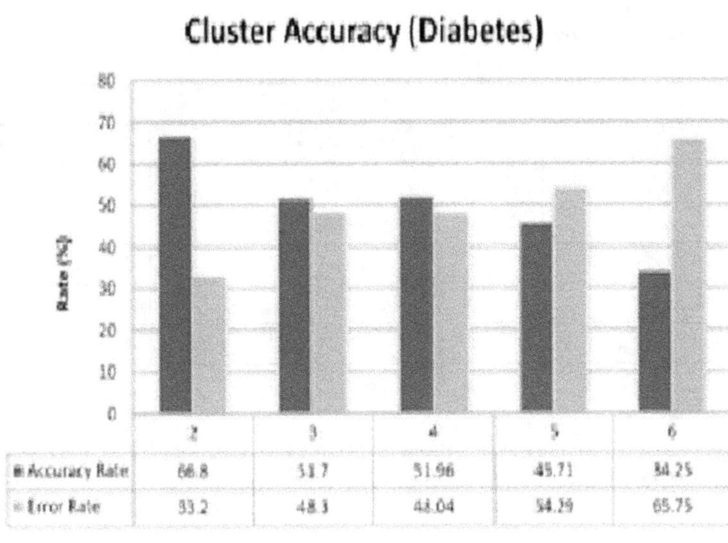

Table 2. Heart disase error and accuracy rate

Heart Attack		
Cluster - K	**Error Rate**	**Acc. Rate**
2	40.74	59.26
3	43.33	56.67
4	43.7	56.3
5	56.66	43.34
6	56.66	43.34

Figure 2. k cluster Accuracy for Heart Datasets
Time taken for clustering 0.02 seconds

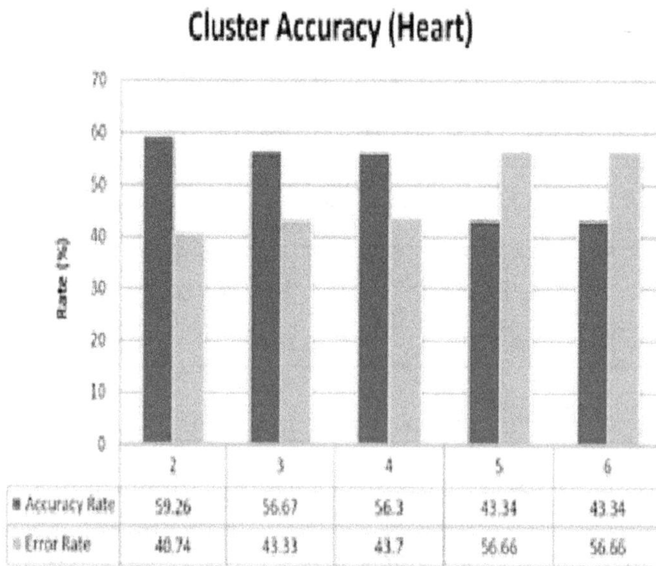

Table 3. Diabetes error and accuracy rate

Thyroid		
Cluster - K	**Error Rate**	**Acc. Rate**
2	51.41	48.59
3	59.88	40.12
4	67.15	32.85
5	67.44	32.56
6	64.47	35.53

Figure 3. k cluster Accuracy for Thyroid Datasets
Time taken for clustering 09 seconds

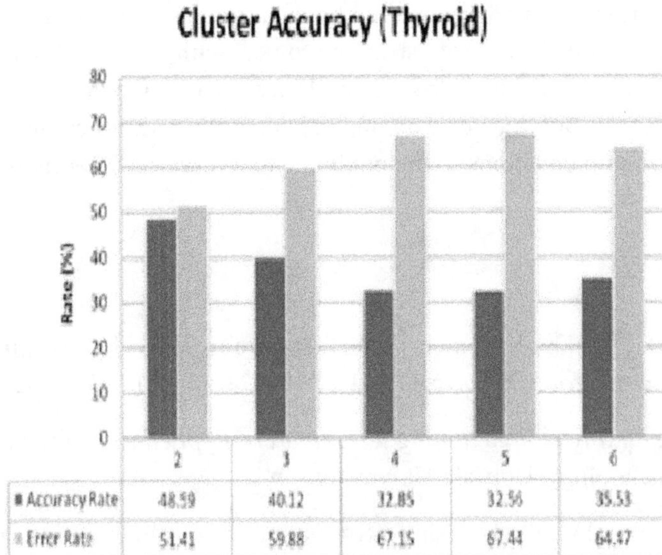

Figure 4. Accuracy and error rate

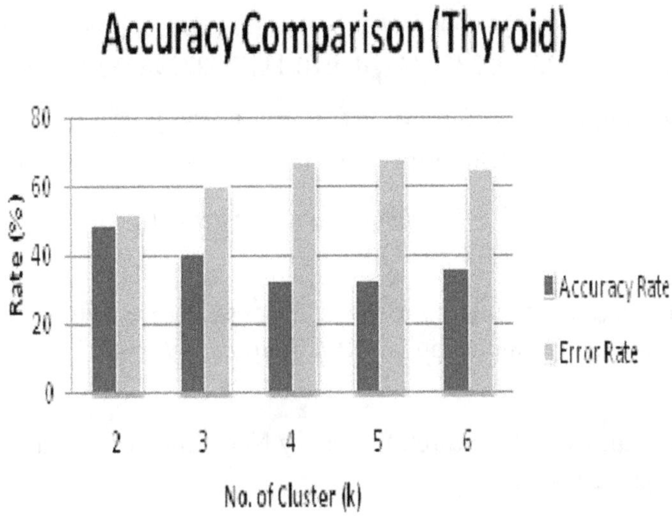

7. CONCLUSION

Clustering techniques are applied to patient symptoms. Different similarity measures are discussed in this work. Clustering based on distance operations are facilitated with similarity measures. Different types of similarity measures on the huge datasets utilize under diverse assessment metrics by comparing with other clustering methods. The proposed method significantly improved clustering performance. The experiment results demonstrates that the Apache Hadoop cluster shows potential model for flexible implementation when the dataset size is large.

8. FUTURE ENHANCEMENT

The system can also improve to support clustering on data streams. In the future, the authors would like to develop the patient symptoms' similarity structure to deal with other healthcare applications such as relative treatment assessment and pattern based similarity clustering method. Various clustering algorithms implemented on huge volumes of data and calculate their accuracy and based on comparative analysis give the best recommendations to the public, which serves efficiently for the problem.

REFERENCES

Agarwal, P., & Searls, D. B. (2009, November). Can literature analysis identify innovation drivers in drug discovery? *Nature Reviews. Drug Discovery*, *8*(11), 865–878. doi:10.1038/nrd2973 PMID:19876041

Can, A. (2013). *Benchmarking of data mining techniques as applied to power system analysis*. Department of Information Technology, Uppsala University.

Cederberg, S., & Widdows, D. (2003). Using LSA and noun coordination information to improve the precision and recall of automatic hyponymy extraction. *Proc of CoNLL'03*. doi:10.3115/1119176.1119191

Cohen, T., & Widdows, D. (2009). Empirical distributional semantics: Methods and biomedical applications. *Journal of Biomedical Informatics*, *42*(2), 390–405. doi:10.1016/j.jbi.2009.02.002 PMID:19232399

Dilts, D., Khamalah, J., & Plotkin, A. (1995). Using cluster analysis for medical resource decision making. *Medical Decision Making*, *15*(4), 333–347. doi:10.1177/0272989X9501500404 PMID:8544677

Glenisson, P., Antal, P., Mathys, J., Moreau, Y., & Moor, B. D. (2003). Evaluation Of The Vector Space Representation In Text-Based Gene Clustering. *Proc Pacific Symposium of Biocomputing*, 391–402.

Hersh, W. (2009). *Information retrieval: a health and biomedical perspective* (3rd ed.). New York: Springer Verlag. doi:10.1007/978-0-387-78703-9

Huang, Dong, Duan, & Li. (n.d.). Similarity Measure Between Patient Symptoms for Clinical Pathway Analysis: Problem, Method, and Applications. *IEEE Journal of Biomedical and Health Informatics, 18*(1), 4-14.

Kakulapati, V. (2011). Improved Web Search Engine by New Similarity Measures. *Proc of TREC'11*. doi:10.1007/978-3-642-22726-4_30

Kulkarni, A., Tokekar, V., & Kulkarni, P. (2015). Discovering context of labeled text documents using context similarity coefficient. Procedia Computer Science, 49C(9), 118-127.

Kumar. (2012). A Framework for Integration and Standardization of Data from Heterogeneous Sources. *American Journal of Database Theory and Application*. DOI: 10.5923/j.database.20120101.01

Lee, J., Maslove, D. M., & Dubin, J. A. (2015). Personalized mortality prediction driven by electronic medical data and a patient similarity metric. *PLoS ONE*, *10*(5), e0127428. doi:10.1371/journal.pone.0127428 PMID:25978419

Li, L., Cheng, W.-Y., Glicksberg, B. S., Gottesman, O., Tamler, R., Chen, R., & Dudley, J. T. et al. (2015). Identification of type2 diabetes sub groups through topological analysis of patient similarity. *Science Translational Medicine*, *7*(311), 311ra174. doi:10.1126/scitranslmed.aaa9364 PMID:26511511

Liao, M., Li, Y., Kianifard, F., Obi, E., & Arcona, S. (2016). Cluster analysis and its application to healthcare claims data: A study of end-stage renal disease patients who initiated hemodialysis. *BMC Nephrology*, *17*(1), 25. doi:10.1186/s12882-016-0238-2 PMID:26936756

McLachlan, G. J. (1992). Cluster analysis and related techniques in medical research. *Statistical Methods in Medical Research*, *1*(1), 27–48. doi:10.1177/096228029200100103 PMID:1341650

Romesburg, H. C. (1984). *Cluster analysis for researchers*. Belmont: Lifetime Learning Publications.

Romesburg, H. C. (1984). *Cluster analysis for researchers*. Belmont: Lifetime Learning Publications.

Schatten, M., & Kakulapati, V. (2010). Reasoning about Social Semantic Web Applications using String Similarity and Frame Logic. *Proceedings of Central European Conference on Information and Intelligent System.* Doi:10.13140/2.1.4489.2163

Sharmila, K., & Vethamanickam, S. A. (2015). Application of mapreduce in diabetic dataset using hadoop platform. *International Journal of Applied Engineering Research.*, *10*(60), 15–20.

Singh, A., Yadav, A., & Rana, A. (2013, April). K-means with Three different Distance Metrics. *International Journal of Computers and Applications*, *67*(10).

Sun, J. (n.d.). Supervised Patient Similarity Measure of Heterogeneous Patient Records. *SIGKDD Explorations*, *14*(1). doi:10.1186/s12882-016-0238-2

Wang, H., Wang, W., Yang, J., & Yu, P. S. (2002). Clustering by Pattern Similarity in Large Data Sets. *Proceeding SIGMOD '02,* 394-405. doi:10.1145/564691.564737

Zhang, P. (2014). Towards personalized medicine: Leveraging patient similarity and drug similarity analytics. *AMIAJt. Summits Transl. Sci. Proc.*, *2014*, 132–136. PMID:25717413

Zhao, W., Ma, H., & He, Q. (2009). Parallel K-means clustering based on mapreduce. *Springer-Verlag Berlin Heidelberg.*, *5931*, 674–679.

Chapter 13
Usage and Analysis of Big Data in E-Health Domain

Sushruta Mishra
C. V. Raman College of Engineering, India

Hrudaya Kumar Tripathy
KIIT University, India

Brojo Kishore Mishra
C. V. Raman College of Engineering, India

Soumya Sahoo
C. V. Raman College of Engineering, India

ABSTRACT

Big data analytics is a growth area with the potential to provide useful insight in healthcare. Big Data can unify all patient related data to get a 360-degree view of the patient to analyze and predict outcomes. It can improve clinical practices, new drug development and health care financing process. It offers a lot of benefits such as early disease detection, fraud detection and better healthcare quality and efficiency. This chapter introduces the Big Data concept and characteristics, health care data and some major issues of Big Data. These issues include Big Data benefits, its applications and opportunities in medical areas and health care. Methods and technology progress about Big Data are presented in this study. Big Data challenges in medical applications and health care are also discussed. While many dimensions of big data still present issues in its use and adoption, such as managing the volume, variety, velocity, veracity, and value, the accuracy, integrity, and semantic interpretation are of greater concern in clinical application.

INTRODUCTION

Over the past 20 years, data has increased in a large scale in various fields. According to a report from International Data Corporation (IDC), in 2011, the overall created and copied data volume in the world was 1.8ZB ($\approx$ 1021B), which increased by nearly nine times within five years (Gantz, J. & Reinsel, D. 2011). This figure will double at least every two years in the near future. Under the explosive increase

DOI: 10.4018/978-1-5225-5222-2.ch013

Copyright © 2018, IGI Global. Copying or distributing in print or electronic forms without written permission of IGI Global is prohibited.

of global data, the term of big data is mainly used to describe enormous datasets. Compared with traditional datasets, big data typically includes masses of unstructured data that need more real-time analysis. Recently, industries become interested in the high potential of big data, and many government agencies announced major plans to accelerate big data research and applications (Fact sheet 2012). In addition, issues on big data are often covered in public media, such as The Economist (Cukier, K. 2010, Drowning in numbers 2011), New York Times (Lohr, S. 2012) and National Public Radio (Yuki, N. 2011). Two premier scientific journals, Nature and Science, also opened special columns to discuss the challenges and impacts of big data (Big data 2008,Special online collection 2011). The era of big data has come beyond all doubt (Manyika, J. et al. 2011)The current international population exceeds 7.2 billion (Worldometers 2014), and over 2 billion of these people are connected to the Internet. Furthermore, 5 billion individuals are using various mobile devices, according to McKinsey (2013). As a result of this technological revolution, these millions of people are generating tremendous amounts of data through the increased use of such devices. In particular, remote sensors continuously produce much heterogeneous data that are either structured or unstructured. This data is known as Big Data (Che, D.,et al. 2013). Figure 1. groups the critical issues in Big Data into three categories based on the commonality of the challenge.

Big data is a largest buzz phrases in domain of IT, new technologies of personal communication driving the big data new trend and internet population grew day by day but it never reach by 100%. The need of big data generated from the large companies like face book, yahoo, Google, YouTube etc for the purpose of analysis of enormous amount of data which is in unstructured form or even in structured form. Google contains the large amount of information. So; there is the need of Big Data Analytics that is the processing of the complex and massive datasets this data is different from structured data in terms of five parameters –variety, volume, value, veracity and velocity (5V's). The five V's (volume, variety, velocity, value, veracity) are the challenges of big data management shown in Figure 2 which are:

Figure 1. Challenges in Big Data

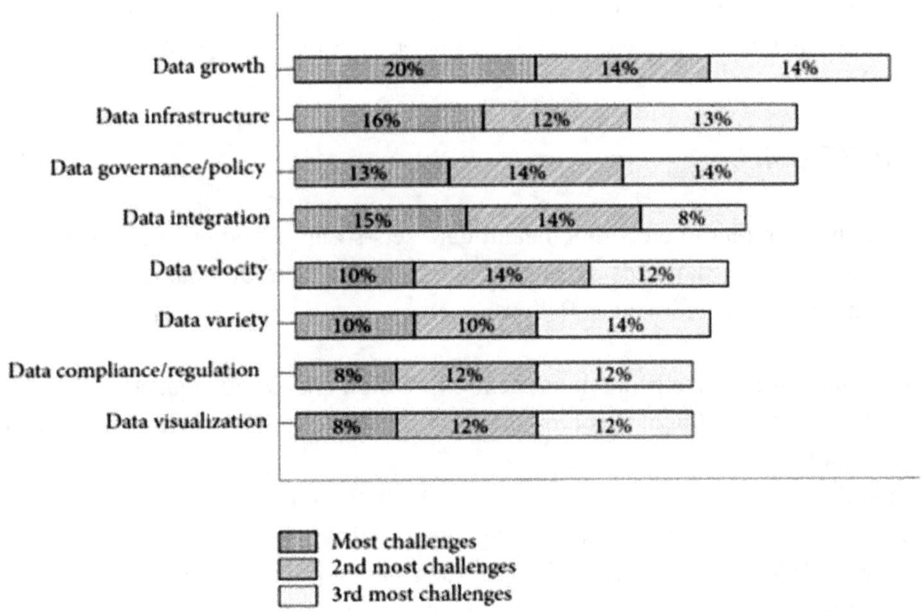

Figure 2. The five dimensions of big data

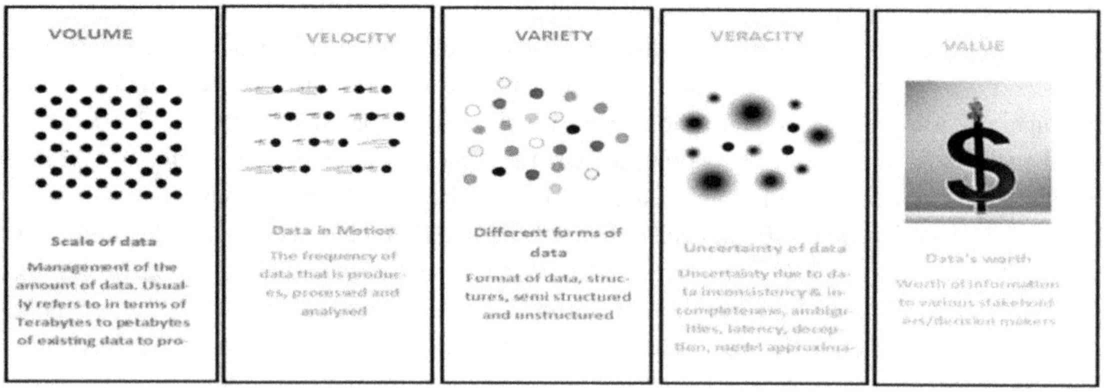

- **Volume:** Data is ever-growing day by day of alltypes ever MB, PB, YB, ZB, KB, TB of information. The data results into large files. Excessive volume of data is main issue of storage. This main issue is resolved by reducing storage cost. Data volumes are expected to grow 50 times by 2020.
- **Variety:** Data sources are extremely heterogeneous. The files comes in various formats and of any type, it may be structured or unstructured such as text, audio, videos, log files and more. The varieties are endless, and the data enters the network without having been quantified or qualified in any way.
- **Velocity:** The data comes at high speed.Sometimes 1 minute is too late so big data is time sensitive. Some organisations data velocity is main challenge. The social media messages and credit card transactions done in millisecond and data generated by this putting in to databases.
- **Value:** It is a most important v in big data. Value is main buzz for big data because it is important for businesses, IT infrastructure system to store large amount of values in database.
- **Veracity:** The increase in the range of values typical of a large data set. When we dealing with high volume, velocity and variety of data, the all of data are not going 100% correct, there will be dirty data. Big data and analytics technologies work with these types of data.

HEALTH CARE DATA

Big data in healthcare refers to electronic health data sets so large and complex that it is difficult to manage with traditional or common data management methods and traditional software and/or hardware Data in healthcare can be categorized as follows:

- **Genomic Data:** It refers to genotyping, gene expression and DNA sequence.
- **Clinical Data:** About 80% of this type data are unstructured documents, images and clinical or transcribed notes.
- Structured data (e.g., laboratory data, structured EMR/HER).
- Unstructured data (e.g., post-op notes, diagnostic testing reports, patient discharge summaries, unstructured EMR/HER and medical images such as radiological images and X-ray images).
- Semi-structured data (e.g., copy-paste from other structure source).

- **Behaviour Data and Patient Sentiment Data:** Web and social media data (Search engines, Internet consumer use and networking sites (Facebook, Twitter, Linkedin, blog, health plan websites and smartphone, etc.).
- Mobility sensor data or streamed data (data in motion, e.g., electroencephalography data). They are from regular medical monitoring and home monitoring, tele-health, sensor-based wireless and smart devices.
- **Health Publication and Clinical Reference Data:** Text-based publications (journals articles, clinical research and medical reference material) and clinical text-based reference practice guidelines and health product (e.g., drug information) data.
- **Administrative, Business and External Data:** Insurance claims and related financial data, billing and scheduling.
- **Biometric Data:** Fingerprints, handwriting and iris scans, etc.
- **Other Miscellaneous Data:** Device data, adverse events and patient feedback, etc.
- The content from portal or Personal Health Records (PHR) messaging (such as e-mails) between the patient and the provider team; the data generated in the PHR.

BENEFITS OF BIG DATA IN MEDICAL APPLICATIONS

Big data is recognized as a multidisciplinary information processing system. Areas of business, government, media, and in particular healthcare, are increasingly incorporating big data into information processing systems. To make effective use of the potential of big data in healthcare, an understanding of what the 2.5 quintillion bytes of data consists of, where they reside, are they raw, processed or derived artifacts, and what the delineation between public and private access is required. Effective large-scale analysis often requires the collection of heterogeneous data from multiple sources. For example, obtaining the 360-degrees health view of a patient(or a population) benefits from integrating and analyzing the medical health record along with Internet available environmental data and then even with readings from multiple types of meters (for example, glucose meters, heart meters, accelerometers, among others).Applying advanced analytics to patient profiles, characteristics and the cost and outcomes of care can help identify the most clinically and cost effective treatments, proactively identify individuals who would benefit from preventative care or lifestyle changes. Big Data could help reduce waste and inefficiency in the following three areas:

1. **Clinical Operations:** Determine more clinically relevant and cost-effective ways to diagnose and treat patients.
2. **Research & Development:** (1) lower attrition and produce a leaner, faster, moretargeted R&D pipeline in drugs and devices with the help of predictive modeling; (2) improve clinicaltrial design, thus reducing trial failures and speeding new treatments to market; and (3) identify follow-on indications and discover adverse effects before products reach the market.
3. **Public Health:** (1) analyze disease patterns and track disease outbreaks and transmission to improve public health surveillance and speed response; (2) faster develop more accurately targeted vaccines and (3) turn large amounts of data into actionable information.

Big Data benefits in medical applications and health care can be summarized as follows:

1. Improvement of health outcomes through more accurate and precise diagnoses; identification of patients who are at risk of adverse outcomes; and customization of care at the level of the individual patient (personalized medicine).
2. Reduction of costs through earlier detection of disease; elimination of unnecessary and duplicate care; reduction in variations in care; and elimination of erroneous and improper claims submissions.
3. Predicting and managing obesity and health risks; detecting health care fraud more quickly and efficiently (Certain developments or outcomes may be predicted and/or estimated based on vast amounts of historical data).
4. Decreasing inappropriate Emergency Department (ED) utilization by using statistical models to identify the best ED services or care alternatives that are more appropriate, more convenient and lower in cost according to health conditions, prior use of health care.

OPPORTUNITIES OF BIG DATA IN HEALTH CARE

Big Data can provide support across all aspects of health care. Big Data analytics has gained traction in genomics; epidemic spread prediction, clinical outcome, fraud detection, pharmaceutical development and personalized patient care, etc. There are potential applications in these areas. The specific applications of Big Data in the areas are as follows.

- **Genomics Analytics:** Genomic data is becoming critical to the complete patient record. Combining patient genomic data with clinical data helps cancer treatment.
- **Flu Outbreak Prediction and Control:** In public and population health, continuously aggregating and analyzing public health data helps detect and manage potential disease out breaks. Big Data analytics can mine web-based and social media data topredict flu outbreaks based on consumer search, social content and query activity.
- **Clinical Outcome Analytics:** Clinical analytics can be performed through unifying clinical, financial and operation data for efficient clinical decisions. Blue Cross and Blue Shield of North Carolina, USA has provided several promising examples of how Big Data can be used to reduce the cost of care, predict and manage health risks and improve clinical outcomes.
- **Fraud Detection and Prevention:** Identifying, predicting and minimizing fraud can be implemented by using advanced analytic systems for fraud detection and checking the accuracy and consistency of claims. Big Data predictive modeling can be used by health care payers for fraud prevention. Fraud waste and abuse analytics can be performed in analyzing claims and benefits of Veterans benefits and education fraud.
- **Medical Device Design and Manufacturing:** Big Data tools enable a broader set of anatomical configurations, device materials, delivery methods and tissue interactions to be evaluated. Computational methods and Big Data can play an important role in medical device design and manufacturing.
- **Personalized Patient Care:** Healthcare is moving from a disease-centered model towards a patient-centered model. In a disease-centered model, physicians' decision making is centered on the clinical expertise and data from medical evidence and various tests. In a patient-centered model, patients actively participate in their own care and receive services focused on individual needs and preferences. The patient-centric model creates a personalized disease risk profile, as well

as a disease management plan and wellness plan for an individual. Personalized healthcare is a data-driven approach. With the increase in the use of electronic medical records, Big Data will facilitate to bring proactive and personalized patient care. In the near future, new big data-derived linkages will prompt timely updates of patient triage, diagnostic assistance and clinical guidelines to allow more precise and personalized treatment to improve clinical outcome for patients.

- **E-Consultation and Tele-Diagnosis:** In the future, the aggregated ECG and images from hospitals worldwide will become big data, which should be used to develop an e-consultation program helping on-site practitioners deliver appropriate treatment. Real-time tele-consultation and tele-diagnosis of ECG and images can be practiced via an e-platform for clinical, research and educational purposes. Big Data analytics can predict over 50% deaths with fewer false positives as compared with the traditional ECG analysis, conducted based on a smaller segment of ECG signals.
- **Pharmaceuticals and Medicine:** The ability of pharmaceutical companies to continue bringing new life-saving/life enhancing medicines to patients in a timely, yet cost-effective manner will dependent on their ability to manage big data generated during all phases of pharmaceutical development. Integration of clinical, healthcare, patents, safety and public research data will provide key insights into decision making for target selection and lead optimization through Big Data analytics for drug discovery.
- **Medical Education:** Visual analytics was explored as a tool for finding ways of representing big data from the medical curriculum of an undergraduate medical program. A possible use of Big Data in the medical education context is to: (1) identify data connections and the relations between them; (2) determine data's roles in the lowest level of a course and in the overall picture of the medical program; (3) perceive and analyze the curriculum in terms of identifying whether knowledge, skills and attitude are constructed through the alignment of teaching methods and assessment towards learning outcomes and (4) perform gap analysis by comparing different states in which data can be found to identify possible discrepancies.
- **Smart Health and Wellbeing:** Business Intelligence and Analytics (BI&A) and the related field of Big Data analytics have become increasingly important in the business communities. Big Data has brought great opportunities in medical applications and health care. Big Data applications will expand to more areas (such as telemedicine and digital hospitals), further improve medical service and deliver extensive value-based care. Big Data applications and opportunities need technology support.

APPLICATION OF BIG DATA IN RURAL HEALTHCARE

Problem Statement

Health care is one of the greatest concerns in India. While, those living in cities and big towns have access to high end health services, the millions of people living in rural India, particularly in the remote parts of the country face problems of inadequate facilities and poor access to healthcare. Many experts, including researchers, policy makers and practitioners identified that, there is a big gap in the knowledge about innovations in public and private health financing and delivery. The inefficiencies and inequities in the public health care access in India have pushed forward the need for creative thinking and innovative solutions to strengthen the same. The problems existing in the health care scenario provides apparent calls for the need to change the existing structure of the present health care services by applying big data analytics. This section identifies the massive shortage of proper health care facilities and addresses how to provide greater access to primary health care services in rural India. The objective is to present the reforms in the health care sector and boosts the discussions on how government can harness innovations in the big data analytics to improve the rural health care system. Now, the digital health care solutions has transformed the health care system to become much more efficient, less expensive and achieve better quality than before with the introduction of Big data analytics in health care. To offer better services to the people, the health care system needs to evolve and innovate continuously. The following are the key points that make the performance of health center better and people live healthier.

- Measure, store and analyze the data to improve treatment quality.
- Manage revenue costs by reducing un-necessary tests.
- Improve preventive care and increase patient & physician's satisfaction.

Adoption of big data in healthcare (Liu,W. & Park, E.K. 2014)significantly increases security and patients primary concerns and recommends the patient information to be stored in data center's with varying levels of security. As per the health insurance acts, EHR security must be taken as a high priority to ensure patient safety. As per the above discussions, the e-Health service data can be considered as a Big Data because of its variety of data with huge volumes flowing with high velocity. Some of the solutions to the e-Health service big data include the predominant current technologies (Harsh,K.P. &Ravi Seshadri.R) like HDFS, Map Reduce, Hadoop, STORM etc. At present, with the increase in number of hospitals and rural health care centers, the health care system seems to have improved. Also, it is observed that e- Health care doctors, technicians, nurses and other administration staff are not in good pace with the kind of growth that the health care is exhibiting, the report says that, US spends 18% of its GDP on health care, where as India spends only 4% of GDP. D. Peter Augustine (Peter A.D.,Leveraging 2014) has noticed the need for big data analytics in India's health care system and concludes how to overcome the realistic challenges involving the government and its policies. The doctors, medical professionals and others using this technology suggest how to achieve better outcomes at lower costs.This section describes the existing health care in India while focusing on the problems in the existing healthcare system. It provides the big ideas to provide better health care to the rural population of India, presenting the big data analytics in health care system

Existing Healthcare in Rural India

Rural India contains over 68% of India's total population, and half of all residents of rural areas live below the poverty line, struggling for better and easy access to health care and services. Accessing primary health care to the population residing in rural India is still a challenge. Health issues being experienced by rural people are many and diverse – from severe malaria to uncontrolled diabetes, from a badly infected wound to cancer.

Mr. Arnab Mukherji (Mukherji, A) has pointed out that, the main issue in the Indian health care system is inequity in Healthcare. To overcome the inequity in healthcare system, the Government of India has launched the National Rural Health Mission (NHRM) in 2005. The aim of this mission is to provide effective healthcare to India's rural population. The thrust of this mission is on establishing a fully functional, community owned, decentralized health delivery system with inter-sectoral convergence at all levels, to ensure simultaneous action on a wide range of determinants of health such as water, sanitation, education, nutrition, social and gender equality. Institutional integration within the fragmented health sector was expected to provide a focus on outcomes, measured against Indian Public Health Standards for all health facilities. Though it is hard to believe, the fact is, compared to government health sector the private health sector has highly skilled doctors and the facilities are world-class using the latest laboratory equipment's and innovative technology. Though, the aim of National Rural Health Mission (NRHM) is to provide effective health care to rural population, the hospitals located in remote villages are not equipped with well qualified doctors and sophisticated equipment due to several unknown reasons like the doctors may not be interested to reside in village to serve the rural population, lack of funds to procure and supply required infrastructure to all the remote hospitals. To access the high-end private sector facilities, people are spending large amounts of money on treatment which in-turn affects their livelihoods and slowly poor people are becoming poorer. In such cases, the concept of Telemedicine along with big data analytics is the better alternative to treat the patients in rural areas.

The Rural public health care system in India as depicted in Figure 3 has three different levels of health care access. At the lowest level, we have Sub Centre (SC) and on top of that there will be a Primary Health Centre (PHC). This PHC is the referral unit for 6 sub centers and PHC contains 4 to 6 beds and Medical officer in-charge along with 14 subordinate paramedical staff. After the Primary health center, a 30 bedded hospital called Community Health Centre (CHC) which will be a referral unit for 4 PHC's. To access primary health care services, the rural patient's visits the Sub center. The Health workers at the sub center first take note of the vitals and symptoms of the patient, record them using the proposed system and if possible, they will try to resolve the issues themselves. If the case is too complex to handle,

Figure 3. Structural Outline of Rural Public Health Care System in India

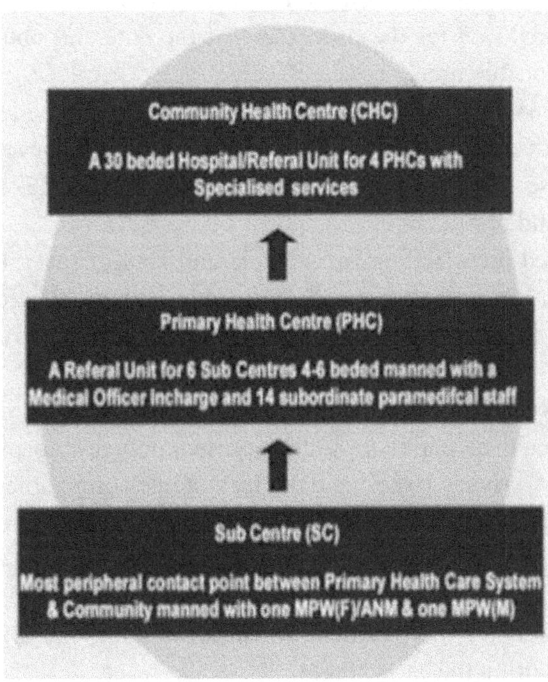

they send the corresponding criticality level and escalate it to the next level i.e. primary health center, this level consists of a pool of medical officers connected to the network via our proposed method. Any medical officer available online at this level will try to resolve this issue by requesting for more information or by providing suitable recommendations. But, if a medical officer feels that the case cannot be resolved at this level, He / She suggests an immediate short time remedy, modifies criticality level if necessary and escalates it to the next level. i.e., the community health center. At this level, a similar pool of specialist doctors available online will try to resolve the case with their medical expertise. If, however the case is too critical for them as well, they provide their immediate suggestions and escalate the case to the city hospital level. Who, being the final point of contact will resolve the issue of the patient. At any point in this process, if a doctor feels that a physical consultation is necessary, he/she can suggest the same through our system to the patients and diagnose the patient physically. Electronic Health Records (EHR's) in the proposed system are sorted first by criticality and then by timestamp and also the proposed system should not allow two doctors at the same level to handle the case simultaneously.

Big Ideas to Fix Rural Healthcare in India

Seven big ideas are presented here to fix rural health care in India and bridge the gap between quality and affordability in government hospitals. These ideas will enable us to access the services on par with the private super specialty hospitals. Further, the implementation of these ideas will provide cheaper, better and easier health care facilities to the citizens of India.

- **E-Health File:** The creation of a e-Health care file for each patient, where all health care providers and patients themselves were able to submit information (with the consent of the patient). Both subjective data, symptom diaries, lab data, image diagnostics, pathology reports etc., could be filed. To overcome the information overload from the massive amounts of data, Big Data Analytics could be employed for the processing of the data and obtain the desired results with great accuracy in reasonable time.
- **Creating Awareness With Chronic Diseases:** The system must identify and create awareness among the people with the common chronic diseases at particular areas, through which we can prevent diseases. These chronic diseases are responsible for the 75% of health care spending due to lack of awareness and prior care.
- **Prescribe:** Paper based prescriptions are archaic and lead to several miseries each year due to errors in prescription. But if every doctor is provided with an electronic prescription system, it would improve safety by making prescriptions easier to read and providing instant checks on drug interactions, dosages, and a patient's medication history.
- **Electronic Medical Records:** Medical Experts agree that electronic medical records (EMRs) are a must for the better health care in India. But, at present only few hospital are maintaining EMR's, mainly because of cost, privacy issues, and the lack of one compatible, easy-to-use infrastructure.
- **Stop Unnecessary Treatments:** Doctors should avoid trial and error type of medication. The problem must be examined thoroughly by performing the required diagnostic tests during the preliminary days of disease. The right treatment should be suggested at the first visit only which avoids the disease to become more critical. Most of the issues are arising with the misdiagnosis and wrong treatment during the early stages.

- **Reduce Infant Mortality:** The Infant Mortality rate in our country is substantially large compared to other countries. Though, the government has several schemes for the pregnant women, those were not yielding better results due to the lack of proper medical care. If the proper care is taken towards the pregnant women, definitely the new-born baby will be healthy in all aspects to make India healthy.
- **Tele Medicine:** Doctors can often diagnose or prescribe without seeing the patient. The patient has to physically appear before the nearby health centre, where the nurses or health workers will diagnose at first level, note the symptoms and informs the high level specialist doctors about the case. After examining the reports, the specialist doctor suggests the treatment through health worker which reduces costs and creates satisfaction by virtual communication of patients and doctors to discuss medication changes and test results through an online system.

Applying Big Data Analytics in Health Care

We live in the age of big data. The amount of data created in the world up to and including 2005 is now created every two days. Big data is a platform for importing, storing and analyzing data to uncover information not previously known. This explosion of the data changing the way people think about everything. From the cutting edge scientific research to the monetization of social media and exchanging the way people think about healthcare analytics too. However, the health care has not kept pace with big data. Big Data Healthcare is the drive to capitalize on growing patient and health system data availability to generate healthcare innovation. By making smart use of the ever-increasing amount of data available, we find new insights by re-examining the data or combining it with other information. In healthcare this means not just mining patient records, medical images, diagnostic reports etc., for insights, diagnoses and decision support device, but also continuous analysis of the data streams produced for and by every patient in a hospital, at home and even while on the move via mobile devices (Mohanty, S . et al. 2013)Even today the majority of health care analytics is performed by doing monthly data refreshes in relational databases that produce pre-processed reports. A fair gap is often missing lab test is often 45 days old, as the data flow move from batched data fields to real time fields from transactional systems and streaming data from analytical modeling devices. This old model of analytics will fail. Analysis will need to be done on that spot moment not in the pre-processed form. Data refreshes need to be done in real-time not once in a month. The data analysis tools of today are likely yellow pages phone book in the era of Internet Search Engine. They are becoming more obsolete with each passing day. The traditional health care analytic tools are built on tools developed by IBM in 1970, more than 40 years ago.If all the three parties (payer, provider, pharmaceutical company) (Edwin M.F) work collaboratively and share data/insight, disease management programs will become cost-effective and deliver improved patient outcomes at a scale that will further optimize overall health-care cost structure.The term "E-health" (Zwicker,M. et al.2012)defined by WHO: "a new term used to describe the combined use of electronic communication and information technology in the health sector". E-health is the main driver for three significant changes within the health care environment(Zwicker,M. et al.2012)

- Patients to become better informed.
- Patients to become more active and empowered in their health care.
- Healthcare to become more efficient.

It is referred in the Cognizant 20-20 insights by Cognizant, (. Hamilton,B 2012)Big data solutions attempt to cost-effectively solve the challenges of large and fast-growing data volumes realize its potential analytical value. For instance, trend analytics allow you to figure out what happened, while root cause and predictive analytics enable understanding of why it happened and what it is likely to happen in future. All healthcare constituents – patients, payers, providers, groups, researchers, governments etc. – will be impacted by big data, which can predict how these players are likely to behave, encourage desirable behavior. These applications of big data can be tested, refined and optimized quickly and inexpensively and will radically change healthcare delivery and research. The healthcare domain has been an easy target for people who seek easy money by using fraud methods (Konasan,V. et al. 2012) Healthcare fraud is expected to continue to rise as people live longer. The white paper by trend analytics (Konasan,V. et al. 2012) reveals that healthcare fraud prevention has resulted savings of nearly $4.1 billion in 2011. A big data platform has ability to sift through a huge amount of historical data in relatively shorter amount of time, so that the business transactions can use fraud detection on real time. Though, the big data analytics in healthcare plays a crucial role to provide better health care services, provide analysis on the historical data to uncover hidden information, the big data analytics has the challenges like Heterogeneity and Incompleteness of data, scale, timeliness, privacy and Human Collaboration(Konasan, V. et al. 2012) The future research is all about to overcome the challenges and use big data analytics in healthcare to uncover the knowledge from the raw unstructured data.

Concluding Remarks

Big data analytics in healthcare is evolving into a promising field for providing insight from very large data sets and improving outcomes while reducing costs. In this section, an overview of the issues faced by the rural population residing in remote parts of the country in accessing the primary health care is addressed in detail. Also, discussed how the big data analytics are beneficial to transform rural healthcare by gaining insight from their clinical and other data repositories and make informed decisions. It discusses about the big data and its characteristics, methods and challenges and suggests how to overcome the underlying problems being faced by the health care industry. Also presents the big ideas to fix the healthcare system in India. Achieving better outcomes at lower costs has become very important for health care which can be achieved through the implementation of this section using Hadoop HDFS and MapReduce to uncover the information lying in big health data sets.

CONCLUSION

Big Data is going to continue growing during the next years, and each data scientist will have to manage much more amount of data every year. This data is going to be more diverse, larger, and faster. Big Data is becoming the new Final Frontier for scientific data research and for business applications. Big Data is based on data obtained from the whole process of diagnosis and treatment of each case. Big Data analytics can perform predictive modeling to determine which patients are most likely to benefit from a care management plan. It is moving forward quickly in population health and quality measurement. Big Data offers a lot of benefits such as disease prevention, reduced medical errors and the right care at the right time and better medical outcomes. In addition, Big Data can improve the Research and Development (R&D) and translation of new therapies. Big data has great potential to improve medicine, guide clinicians in delivering value-based care. Big Data has challenges in medical applications and healthcare. These challenges include consolidating and processing segmented data, aggregating and analyzing unstructured data, indexing and processing continuously streaming data, privacy, data leakage, information security and lack of infrastructure and unified standards, etc. Our study discusses about the big data and its characteristics, methods and challenges and suggests how to overcome the underlying problems being faced by the health care industry. It also presents the big ideas to fix the healthcare system in India. The implementation part can be done using HDFS (Hadoop File System) for the huge data storage and Hadoop Map Reduce with Amazon Web Services. The use of big data analytics across the healthcare organization and healthcare industry will mine the doctor's lab transcript's using text mining and co-relation to patient outcomes and location aware application analytics for enhancing customer experience. Achieving better outcomes at lower costs has become very important for health care which can be achieved through the implementation of this chapter using Hadoop HDFS and Map Reduce to uncover the information lying in big health data sets.

REFERENCES

Big data. (2008). Retrieved from http://www.nature.com/news/specials/bigdata/ index.html

Che, D., Safran, M., & Peng, Z. (2013). From Big Data to Big Data Mining: challenges, issues, and opportunities. In *Database Systems for Advanced Applications* (pp. 1–15). Berlin, Germany: Springer. doi:10.1007/978-3-642-40270-8_1

Cukier, K. (2010). *Data, data everywhere: a special report on managing information. Economist Newspaper*.

Drowning in numbers - digital data will flood the planet - and help us understand it better. (n.d.). Retrieved from http://www.economist.com/blogs/daily chart/2011/11/bigdata-0

Edwin, M. F. (n.d.). *Big Data Healthcare, An overview of the challenges in data intensive health care*. Discussion Paper. Academic Press.

Fact sheet. (2012). *Big data across the federal government*. Retrieved from http:// www.whitehouse.gov/sites/default/files/microsites/ostp/big data fact sheet 3 29 2012.pdf

Gantz, J., & Reinsel, D. (2011). Extracting value from chaos. *IDC iView*, 1–12.

Hamilton, B. (2012). *Big Data is the Future of Healthcare*. Cognizant 20-20 Insights.

Harsh, K.P., & Seshadri, R. (n.d.). *Big data security and privacy issues in healthcare*. Academic Press.

Konasani, V., Biswas, M., & Koleth, P.K. (2012). *Healthcare Fraud Management using Big Data Analytics*. A Whitepaper by Trendwise Analytics.

Liu, W., & Park, E. K. (2014). Big Data as an e-Health Service. *International Conference on Computing, Networking and Communications*, 982-988.

Lohr, S. (2012). The age of big data. *New York Times*, p. 11.

Manyika, J., Chui, M., Brown, B., Bughin, J., Dobbs, R., Roxburgh, C., & Byers, A.H. (2011). *Big data: The next frontier for innovation, competition, and productivity*. Report McKinsey Global Institute.

Mohanty, S., Jagadeesh, M., & Srivatsa, H. (2013). *Big Data Imperatives*. Apress Publications. doi:10.1007/978-1-4302-4873-6

Mukherji, A. (n.d.). *Indian Healthcare system: Challenges and Opportunities*. Retrieved from http://tejas.iimb.ac.in/interviews/41.php

National Rural Health Mission (NRHM). (n.d.). Retrieved from http://nrhm.gov.in/

Peter, A. D. (2014). Big Data Analytics and Hadoop in Developing Indias Healthcare Services. *International Journal of Computers and Applications*, *89*(16), 44–50. doi:10.5120/15719-4622

Special online collection: dealing with big data. (2011). Retrieved from http:// www.sciencemag.org/site/special/data/

Worldometers. (2014). *Real time world statistics*. Retrieved from http://www.worldometers.info/world-population/

Yuki, N. (2011). *Following digital breadcrumbs to big data gold*. Retrieved from http://www.npr.org/2011/11/29/142521910/thedigitalbreadcrumbsthat-lead-to-big-data

Yuki, N. (2011). *The search for analysts to make sense of big data*. Retrieved from http://www.npr.org/2011/11/30/142893065/the-searchforanalyststo-make-sense-of-big-data

Zwicker, M., Seitz, J., & Wickramasinghe, N. (2012). Identifying Critical Issues for Developing Successful E-Health Solutions. *Proceedings of the Pacific Asia Conference on Information Systems (PACIS)*. Retrieved from http://aisel.aisnet.org/pacis2012/33

Chapter 14
Exploration of Healthcare Using Data Mining Techniques

Anindita Desarkar
Birla Institute of Technology Mesra – Kolkata, India

Ajanta Das
Birla Institute of Technology Mesra – Lalpur, India

ABSTRACT

Huge amount of data is generated from Healthcare transactions where data are complex, voluminous and heterogeneous in nature. This large dataset can be used as an ideal store which can be analyzed for knowledge discovery as well as various future predictions. So, Data mining is becoming increasingly popular as it offers set of innovative tools and techniques to handle this kind of data set whereas traditional methods have limitations for that. In summary, providing the better patient care and reduction in healthcare cost are two major goals of application of data mining in healthcare. Initially, this chapter explores on the various types of eHealth data and its characteristics. Subsequently it explores various domains in healthcare sector and shows how data mining plays a major role in those domains. Finally, it describes few common data mining techniques and their applications in eHealth domain.

INTRODUCTION

eHealth is an emerging field which uses the combination of medical informatics, public health and business to satisfy the needs of common people including patients, healthcare professionals, healthcare service providers and policy makers as well (Sartipi et al., 2008). Nowadays huge amount of complex and heterogeneous data is generated from healthcare industry rapidly. It includes data from various medical devices, electronic patient record, hospital resource details, diagnosis results etc. This large amount of dataset is a major source of resources which can be processed and analyzed for knowledge discovery. It can be used for future prediction, appropriate decision making and cost savings as well. But processing and analyzing become a challenge here as data volume is large and it's diverse in nature. These challenges include technical difficulty of matching patients' records, data exchange among various EHR systems and geographies and properly extract relevant information from the huge dataset so that it can be used effectively and efficiently by healthcare providers.

DOI: 10.4018/978-1-5225-5222-2.ch014

Copyright © 2018, IGI Global. Copying or distributing in print or electronic forms without written permission of IGI Global is prohibited.

Data mining is a methodology of finding relevant, innovative and useful patterns in data. This includes various numbers of techniques like clustering, classification, data summarization, change analysis etc. It comes into the picture here as it offers a set of innovative tools and techniques which can be used to process and analyze this large amount of data to discover the hidden patterns. These tools have the ability to work with such complex dataset though the files are huge in volume and heterogeneously structured. Healthcare professionals are benefited to a large extend in the decision making by using this knowledge source. For instance, data mining can be the solution to find the most effective treatment for a specific condition, patterns can be identified which are due to medicine side effect or readmission in the hospital. It also helps the patient to identify the most cost effective treatment for a specific disease (Koh & Tan, 2011). There are good number of data mining tools already available in the market which includes ODND, NCC2 which is used in the area of heart disease, WEKA – used for the betterment of cancer patients, K-means clustering for brain cancer, WEKA 3.6 for HIV/AIDS, SNP for Hepatitis C, RST for kidney related problems.

The organization of the chapter is as follows. Background section talks about the related work. The next section describes various features and sources of big data and analyses the eHealth data in the light of big data. Section 2 explores eHealth data with the help of various well known data mining techniques. It includes brief overview of data mining, motivations behind exploration of e-Health data, major dimensions of healthcare industry where data mining applications are used, few well known data mining techniques along with their detailed application in the healthcare domain. Next section concludes the chapter.

BACKGROUND

Data mining which is a newer technology, came into picture predominantly only in 1994. After that it was used in almost every domains including healthcare management. Various data mining applications can be created to measure the efficiency of current medical treatments. It can generate a report regarding the most appropriate and effective action on that condition by analyzing the causes, symptoms and course of treatments. As example, the patient's condition can be compared after applying different drugs for a specific disease to find the most appropriate and cost effective treatment. United Healthcare has implemented it by mining its treatment record data to provide better treatment to its patients in reduced cost (Durairaj & Ranjani, 2013).

Jayanthi Ranjan already presented the discovery and extraction of useful data patterns to find observable patterns from huge volume. It proves the advantages of data mining in pharma industry in decision making process along with other issues like adverse reactions to the drugs (Ranjan, 2007).

K. Srinivas, B. Kavitha Rani and Dr. A. Goverdhan had used classification based data mining techniques on huge data set to predict the likelihood of having heart diseases for a patient. It takes age, sex, blood pressure, blood pressure as inputs from the patient profile (Srinivas, 2010).

Shweta Kharya had discussed the application of various data mining techniques in breast cancer diagnosis and prognosis decision tree was found to be the best predictor having 93.26% accuracy on benchmark data as well as SEER data set. Elias Lemuye discussed the application of Apriori algorithm and WEKA 3.6 tool in predicting the HIV virus (Kharya, 2012).

IDENTIFICATION OF E-HEALTH DATA AS BIG DATA

e-Health data majorly includes clinical data, claims and cost related data, pharmaceutical R&D data, patient behavior and sentiment data. Clinical data means electronic medical records and medical images whereas claims and cost related data describes the provided services and the process of their reimbursement. Pharmaceutical R&D data indicates drugs' therapeutic mechanism of action, their target behavior on the body, side effects etc and patient behavior and sentiment data includes patient activities and their preferences (Groves, 2016). All these kind of data are growing rapidly as number of patients are increasing day by day across the globe. They also have various structures as they are stored in various places with various formats. So all these dataset have the basic features of big data - volume, variety and velocity. The following sections describe various features of eHealth data in a more detailed manner.

Big Data and Its Characteristics

Big data refers enormous data set which can have the characteristics of structured as well as unstructured and coming from different regions of the world. Majorly three 'V's – Volume, Variety and Velocity exist which defines Big Data. Data is large in volume as produced across the globe. Variety defines its diverse sources and various data formats whereas Velocity describes the arrival of data at an unprecedented speed. Another major area of concern is the difficulty of capturing, processing and managing it through traditional software tools in a cost-effective manner. So a new set of tools, applications and frameworks are required for managing all the processes (Abinaya, 2015).

Big data is well described by primarily three 'V's – Volume, Variety and Velocity. Though, an additional 'V'–Veracity should also be considered to describe big data characteristics. Other two 'V's which are discussed in the summit are - Validity and Volatility. Explanation of all 'V's are as follows.

- **Volume:** Data is large in volume which is getting generated from multiple sources like machines, human interactions etc.
- **Variety:** Variety is associated with thedata source variationas well as data types. Data can be available in both the forms like structured and unstructured. Structured data includes spreadsheets and relational databases whereas unstructured data includes emails, phones, videos, audios, monitoring device data etc.
- **Velocity:** Velocity refers the pace at which data is generated from different sources. The following data talks about this feature clearly.
    - 40 Zeta bytes of data will be available by 2020
    - 18.9 billion network connections will exist by 2016
    - More than 1 TB of data generated during each trading session at NSE (National Stock Exchange of India Ltd.).
- **Veracity:** Veracity describes the biases, noise and irregularity in data. These incorrect data causes lots of problems for consumer as well as organizations.
- **Validity:** Validity means the accuracy of data for intended use. So valid data is the key of taking right decision.
- **Volatility:** Volatility refers the time span for data validity which means how long the data is valid. Depending on that, data will be archived or stored.

Various Sources of Big Data

In today's world, data size is increasing tremendously because it's coming from almost every possible domain. Few such domains are described briefly in the following.

- **Manufacturing & Sales Sector:** The enormous data volume generated from this industry can be used to identify machinery and process variations which can be the pointers of quality problems. The effective analysis helps to increase sales as well as optimizing assignment of sales resources and accounts, product mix and other operations.
- **Banking Sector:** Huge amount of transactional data is generated from this industry where Big data analytics can be used to suggest better investment proposals to customers and as a result, business growth comes automatically.
- **Telecom Industry:** Various studies indicates that the implementation of analytics tools will see a substantial growth in this industry also.
- **Retail Sector:** Retailers analyses Big Data so that they can offer personalized shopping experiences to the consumers. According to a study, around 66% of retailers have made financial gains in customer relationship management by analyzing existing big data.
- **Healthcare Domain:** Healthcare industry mainly comprises data regarding electronic medical record (EMR) system where appropriate tools and techniques can be used for overall cost reduction and patient care improvement.
- **Media and Entertainment:** The Media and Entertainment industry is also witnessing a change as it provides users and viewers a much more personalized and enriched experience through proper analysis of big data. It's also used for revenue increase, customer sentiment analysis, increasing marketing effectiveness and ratings and viewership.
- **Tourism Industry:** People can enjoy much more detailed itineraries with the help of big data.

Analyzing E-Health Data

e-Health data primarily includes huge amount of data generated from Electronic Health Record (HER) system which is always expanding. It's because the massive increase of patients in regular basis. This is considered as big data as it possesses all the major characteristics like volume, variety and velocity. It's large in volume as patient number is extremely large, increasing rapidly and heterogeneous in nature as coming from various sources and stored differently.

EXPLORING E-HEALTH DATA USING DATA MINING ALGORITHMS

Data mining algorithms have a great impact in the healthcare domain as it's capable of identifying hidden patterns from the huge dataset. Few application areas where data mining algorithms can be applied are fraud detection in healthcare insurance, availability of medicines in a cheaper rate to the patients, detection of appropriate causes of diseases in more effective and efficient way along with its remedy. A big challenge in health domain data is its vastness and complexity. So regular tools and technologies are not very suitable to complete the task whereas an innovative tools and techniques are required to deal with the problem. Data mining comes here into picture as it's able to provide meaningful insights from these complex and heterogeneous datasets. Hence healthcare system is improved as the performance of patient management task is also increased. One such analysis may be grouping the patients with similar diseases so that they can receive appropriate treatments from healthcare organizations. Data mining techniques are used successfully to identify the reasons behind any disease like food habit, work environment, education level, living style, condition of drinking water, availability of nearby health care services.

Brief Overview of Data Mining

Data mining came into the real world in the middle of 1990s and became one of the most essential technologies in the domain of big data. It's empowered to detect hidden information or pattern from the huge, complex and heterogeneous dataset. Decision making has been improved to a great extend as a result of this discovery of unknown things in advance.

Motivations of Exploring E-Health Data

Pharmaceutical companies are increasing rapidly across the globe and swamped with data but finding timely actionable insights from this huge data set is missing. The primary reason is the inability to effectively manage the evolving needs with the traditional tools and techniques. Following are few problem areas which works as the motivators of exploring this huge e-health data so that appropriate actions can be taken on the same.

- Patient classification based on similar health pattern.
- Evidence based suggestion – Information is extracted from the dataset to find similar cases so that best medical treatment can be suggested to the patients. Here the system is acted as a support system for the healthcare professionals and provides appropriate advices.
- Predict treatment cost and patient's approximate stay in hospital.
- Identifying the most profitable customers.
- Choosing appropriate hospital based on need from patient's perspective.
- Planning for effective information system management.
- Future planning of resources based on patient load.

Few other major challenges faced by pharmaceutical industry include declining research and development productivity, globalization of supply chain, regulatory compliance requirement specific to country and rising commercial demand. These challenges can be addressed effectively by mining e-health data and taking actions accordingly

Key Dimensions of Data Mining in Healthcare

Huge amount of data is produced in the healthcare industry today which deals with patients, hospitals, electronic patient record, medical devices etc. Appropriate analysis of this kind of data make life hazard free as decision making becomes much easier. Following are the various domains of healthcare industry where data mining plays a major role.

Diagnosis and Treatment Effectiveness

Different data mining applications have been developed which are used to a large extent to find the effectiveness of medical treatments across the globe. The analysis can guide the medical practitioners about the appropriate course of treatments by comparing and contracting various similar cases from the past incidents.

Healthcare Management

Chronis healthcare related issues can be dealt more effectively by identifying the high risk patients in advance by analyzing their existing health reports, lifestyle etc. As a result, hospitalization admission rate is reduced.

Customer Relationship Management

Customer relationship management indicates interaction between commercial organizations and their customers. In healthcare domain, it deals with call centers, hospital billing departments, physician's offices etc. This can be managed in more efficiently and effectively by implementing various data mining techniques.

Fraud and Anomaly Detection

Fraud detection is a very significant aspect of any domain. Healthcare is not an exception. It faces various issues like forged prescriptions or referrals, inappropriate insurance and medical claims etc. Appropriate implementation of data mining tools and techniques can identify these kind of fraudulent cases and abuses by analyzing the huge dataset.

Medical Device and Pharmaceutical Industry

Pharmaceutical industry includes various stuffs, out of which medical devices definitely demands the priority. Mobile communications and low-cost of wireless bio-sensors are two major aspects which shows a great avenue in the way of developing the mobile healthcare applications. It supplies a safe and secured way of constant monitoring of patients effortlessly.

Data Mining Techniques

Various well-known data mining techniques are described in the following section which are widely used in the eHealth domain for doing different analysis and prediction accordingly (Patel & Patel, 2016) (Rogers & Joyner, 1997).

Descriptive Models

Descriptive modelling refers to a mathematical process which includes mainly four aspects: customer segmentation, value based segmentation, behavior based segmentation and needs based segmentation.

Clustering, association, summarization, sequence discovery are some well-known data mining techniques which come under this category.

Clustering Techniques

Clustering technique refers the creation of clusters on the given dataset based on the similarities present within it. It divides the dataset in such a way that objects having similar properties come under same cluster. It comes under unsupervised learning which basically finds natural grouping of instances within the unlabeled dataset. There are different types of clustering algorithms, out of which few well known are partitioning algorithms, hierarchical algorithms, density-based algorithms, grid based algorithms and model based algorithms. k-means and k-medoids are two widely used partitioning algorithms. In k-means technique, center of the cluster represents every cluster whereas one of the objects in the cluster represents each cluster in the k-medoid technique.

k-means technique consists the following steps.

1. A number (K)of cluster centers - centroids (at random) should be picked
2. Every item should be assigned to its nearest cluster center (e.g. using Euclidean distance)
3. Movement needs to be done for each cluster center to the mean of its assigned items
4. Step 2 and Step 3 need to be repeated until convergence

k-means has the advantages like simplicity, understandability, automatic assignment of items to the clusters along with some disadvantages like number of clusters need to be chosen in advance, often termination at a local optimum, too much sensitivity to outliers.

k-medoid is the similar kind of technique of k-means where the only difference is medians are used instead of means. Here median value of the object in a cluster is considered as a reference point.

Hierarchical clustering produces a tree based hierarchical taxonomy from a bunch of unlabeled examples. Recursive application of a standard clustering algorithm can create a hierarchical clustering.

Density based clustering produces clusters based on density. Here each cluster consists considerable higher density of points than outside of the cluster. DBSCAN is the widely used density based clustering technique.

Association Techniques

Predictive Models

Predictive modelling is a widely used technique for predicting future behaviors It analyses historical and current dataset to generate a model which helps to predict future outcomes. As a first step of predictive modelling, it collects data from various sources. The next part is data cleansing and transformation in the required format so that analysis can be done easily. Once the dataset is ready, various models and business understanding are used to identify the useful business insights from the data.

Classification Techniques

Classification is a well-known technique which basically finds the group in which a particular data instance is associated with in a given dataset. It classifies data into various classes based on some constraints. Few common classification techniques include ID3, decision tree, genetic algorithm, k-nearest neighbor, naïve Bayesian, SVM, k-means, apriori algorithm etc.

ID3

ID3 was originally introduced by J. Ross Quinlan, the classification algorithm at the Sydney University. ID3 builds a decision tree from the fixed set of dataset based on the theory of information gain. The resulting tree is used to predict the future dataset. Information gain is the measurement of the goodness of a given attribute for separating training dataset into targeted classes. The attribute having the highest information gain is selected for the deciding node as the attribute contains most useful information for classification. Information gain is again measured against entropy, an important concept of information theory. Entropy measures the amount of information in an attribute (Han et al., 2011).

The following Figure 1 summarizes ID3 algorithm.

Entropy H(S) which is a measure of uncertainty present in dataset S, can be defined in the following Equation 1.

$$H\left(S\right) = -\sum_{x \in X} p\left(x\right) \log_2 p\left(x\right)$$

where

S: The current dataset for which Entropy is being calculated
X: Set of classes present in S
p(x): The proportion of the number of elements in class x to the number of elements in set S

Information gain is again calculated based on this Entropy. It is the measure of Entropy difference from before to after the set S is split on an attribute A. It is presented in the following Equation 2.

$$IG\left(A, S\right) = H\left(S\right) - \sum_{t \in T} p\left(t\right) H\left(t\right)$$

Figure 1. Outline of ID3 algorithm

1. **Calculate the entropy of every attribute using the data set**
2. **Split the set into subsets using the attribute for which the resulting entropy (after splitting) is minimum (or, equivalently, information gain is maximum)**
3. **Make a decision tree node containing that attribute**
4. **Recurse on subsets using remaining attributes.**

where

H(S): Entropy of set S
T: The subsets created from splitting set S by attribute A such that $S = \mathrm{U}t \ \& t \in T$
p(t): The proportion of the number of elements in t to the number of elements in set S
H(t): Entropy of subset t

Decision Tree

Decision tree classifier is one of the most common and straightforward classification techniques across various domains. It organizes a bunch of questions and conditionsin a tree structure. In this classifier, the root node as well as the internal nodes consist attribute test conditions to differentiate among the records having different characteristics. All the leaf nodes are assigned a class label Yes or No. After construction of a decision tree, a test record classification is a straightforward job. Beginning from the root node, test condition is applied to the record and appropriate branch is followed depending on the result of the test. After that, it suggests to take another internal node where a new test condition can be applied or to a leaf node. After reaching to the leaf node, the class label is assigned to the record which is basically associated with the leaf node. The outline of the algorithm is summarized in the following Figure 2.

Genetic Algorithm

Genetic algorithm is another one widely used classification algorithm which works on the policy of selecting the best and discarding the rest. It's a search technique which is used in computation for finding approximate solutions to optimize and search related problems. It's basically inspired by Darwin's theory of evaluation. The basic principle of the algorithm is presented below.

Figure 2. Outline of Decision Tree algorithm

buildtree (*examples, questions, default*)
/* examples: a list of training examples
questions: a set of candidate questions, e.g., "what's the value of feature *xi*?"
default: default label prediction, e.g., over-all majority vote */
IF empty(*examples*) THEN return (*default*)
IF (*examples* have same label y) THEN return(y)
IF empty(*questions*) THEN return(majority vote in *examples*)
q = best_question(*examples, questions*)
Let there be n answers to q
- Create and return an internal node with n children
- The ith child is built by calling
    Buildtree ({*example*|q=ith answer}, *questions*\{q}, *default*)

- The algorithm is started with a bunch of solutions which is called as population. These solutions are represented by chromosomes.
- Solutions created by the population are taken and again a new population is formed. Basically the objective is to create more effective solution set.
- The selection of solution from the population is done depending on the value of the fitness function. Basically the offspring population will be better if the parent is selected appropriately.
- This is repeated until some specific condition is satisfied. The condition may be reaching to the specific value or within the value range.

The basic version of the algorithm is as follows.

```
Calculate initial population;
WHILE stop condition not satisfied DO
BEGIN
Choose individuals for reproduction;
Generate offspring's by crossing individuals;
Eventually mutate some individuals;
Calculate new generation
END
```

k-Nearest Neighbor

k- Nearest Neighbor(KNN) is one of the easiest classification algorithms though able to provide highly competitive results (Tomar & Agarwal, 2013). In general, three aspects are looked into while computing the effectiveness of any algorithm, which includes easiness in interpreting output, computation time and prediction power. KNN scores well in all these three domains. Itis also used in regression problems along with classification domain. The main objective of this algorithm is to predict appropriately the classification of a new sample point in a database where existing data points are separated into various distinct classes. The basic algorithm can be depicted in the following way.

1. A positive integer k needs to be mentioned which is accompanied with the new sample
2. k entries are selected in the database which are nearest to the new sample
3. The most common classification of these entries are found
4. The classification is given to the new sample

Naive Bayesian

Naive Bayesian is a supervised as well as a statistical method in the classification domain. It's one of the fastest classification algorithm also. This technique is named after Thomas Bayes who introduced the Bayes theorem and it works based on this principle. The initial guess of this classifier is that no relation should exist between the occurrences of specific feature in a class with the occurrence of any other feature. The approach is quire suitable for the large data sets (Tomar & Agarwal, 2013).

Posterior probability P(c|x) can be computed based on Bayes theorem with the help of P(c), P(x) and P(x|c). The following Figure 3 describes the theorems.

Figure 3. Bayes Theorem

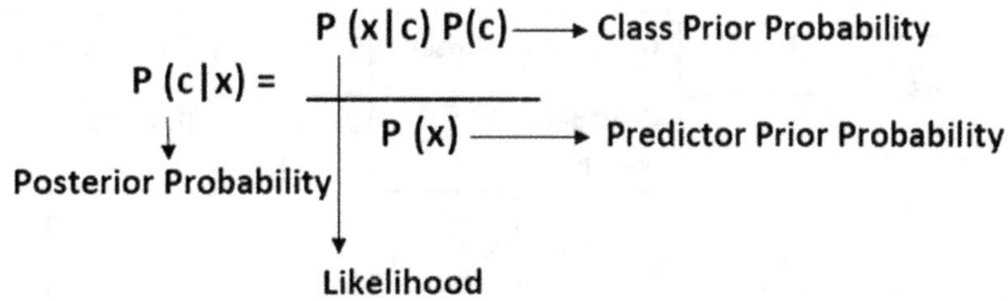

$$P(c|x) = P(x_1|c) * P(x_2|c) * \ldots\ldots * P(x_n|c) * P(c)$$

It's most commonly used in the cases like real time prediction, multi class prediction, analysis of sentiment etc.

Support Vector Machine

Support vector machine is a classification approach applicable both for linear and non-linear data (Seetha Lakshmi & Isakki, 2017). It uses a nonlinear mapping for transforming the original data set to the higher dimension. Then it searches the linear optimal separating hyperplane (also called as decision boundary) with the help of new dimension. This hyperplane can be used for classification, regression or other tasks. SVMs can be applied in various real life problems like text and hypertext categorization, image classification etc.

Apriori Algorithm

Apriori algorithm is a well-known data mining algorithm which is used for frequent itemset mining and appropriate association rules. It is mainly suitable for the e-commerce related applications where the database contains loads of transactions. It's very effective tool in market based analysis where customers can buy their items more easily as well as sales are increased.

The basic algorithm is divided into two steps as mentioned in the following.

Step 1: Minimum support should be applied to search all the frequent sets with k items in a database.
Step 2: A self-join rule should be used to search the frequent sets with k+1 items with the association of frequent k-itemset. The complete process should be repeated from k=1 to the point where applying the self-join rule in not possible.

The approach here is called "bottom up" approach as it works to extend a frequent item set one at a time. The outline of the flow is given in the following Figure. The major advantages of this algorithm include its easy implementation process as well as its simplicity. Though it has few limitations like sometimes it may require to find a large number of candidate rules which may be computationally expensive. Traversal of entire database is another reason of its expensiveness. The following Figure 4 describes the algorithm steps.

Figure 4. Outline of Apriori Algorithm

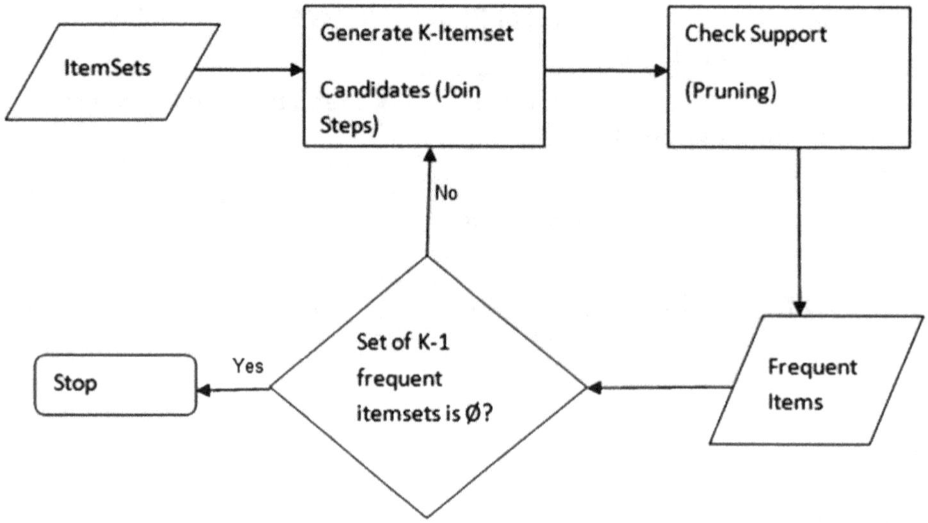

Regression Techniques

Regression refers a data mining function by which a number can be predicted. This methodology is very useful for predicting profit, sales, mortgage rates, house values, square footage, temperature or distance.A dataset is the starting point of a regression task where target values are defined. In the training process, a regression algorithm evaluates the target value as a function of the predictors for each case in the build data. Subsequently, a model summarizes the relationships between predictors and target. This model can be used further on a separate data set where target values are not known to us.

Testing of Regression models are done through the computation of various statistics which measures the variation between the predicted values and the expected values. There are majorly two categories of data sets for the historical data for a regression project. The data sets include building the model and testing it.Few well known real life applications of regression modelling includes trend analysis, business planning, marketing, financial forecasting, time series prediction, biomedical and drug response modeling, and environmental modeling.

Time Series Analysis

A time series represents a set of data points which are ordered sequentially. Typically, it's measured at successive times spaced at uniform time intervals. Daily value of stock market index is an example of time series data. Time series analysis refers the methodology of evaluating time series data for extracting meaningful statistics, rules and patterns. In the future, forecasting models can be built based on these rules and patterns for predicting future developments. The major applications areas include stock market analysis, forecasting in sales, health care domain.

Prediction

Prediction is a well-known technique in data mining which creates pattern to predict forthcoming events based on the available input data. The major objectives include anticipating inhabitant actions, finding anomalies, predicting the appropriate actions, providing information for decision making. Common prediction techniques include classification based approaches and sequential behavior modelling. Classification based approaches include Nearest Neighbor, Neural Network, Bayesian Classifiers, Decision Trees whereas Sequential Behavior Modeling includes Hidden Markov Models, Temporal Belief Networks.

Application of Data Mining Techniques in Healthcaredomain

Classification Technique for the of Heart, Cancer, HIV/AIDS, IVF Diseases

HIV, AIDS, cancer, various types of heart diseases are one of the major threats in the healthcare domain across the globe, especially in all developing countries. Various types of classification techniques like Decision trees, Naïve Bayes classification model, support vector machine (SVM) are applied in this area for various predictions as earlier prediction is the key of success.It reduces the human effort and increases the diagnostic accuracy. Here data is collected from different places and then it's divided into two classes, one as a training set and another is test set. The classifier model has been developed by using the training dataset. And after that the model tests its accuracy by using the test dataset. If the accuracy reaches to the expected level, the generated model can be used for future reference. It will predict the outcome of the new cases successfully. Few data preprocessing techniques are used before applying the classification model on the new data set. The techniques include data cleansing, feature selection and data discretization. Following are few tools and techniques which has been successfully implemented in this area (Priyavadana et al., 2015).

- ODND, NCC2 are the data mining tools which are used for treating various heart diseases by applying the Naïve Bayes algorithm.
- WEKA is a widely used tool for treating cancer patients by using rules and decision tables. Also, the blood blank sector is dependent on this tool. Tuberculosis is also treated with the help of this tool.
- HIV/AIDS are treated with the help of a data mining tool, WEKA 3.6. It uses J48 as the basic algorithm.
- k-means clustering is a very common approach in the treatment of brain cancer.

Clustering Technique for Brain Tumor Detection

Various segmentation and edge detection techniques are used as the first step of brain tumor grading. Here patient's stage is determined for taking various decisions like medicine is sufficient or C-section is required (Mandwel & Anjum, 2013). Clustering techniques are also used for segmentation of the brain MRI images for tumor detection. A cluster is formed with the group of pixels which are satisfying a specific relationship. Here k-means clustering algorithm is used for image segmentation which is followed by morphological filtering. It detects the presence of tumor from the brain MRI images. The process has the following major steps.

- As a first step, the input MRI image is collected.
- Pre-processing is done on the input data.
- k-means clustering algorithm is applied for image segmentation.
- Morphological filtering is used as the next step for tumor detection.
- The output is shared with medical professional for taking final decisions.

Naïve Bayes Classifier for Tuberculosis

Tuberculosis is one of the most widely spread disease in India. As a first step, data has been collected from various TB centers (Priyavadana et al., 2015). These huge data set are used to analyze and finding hidden patterns which can be used to diagnose and predict the disease. Naïve Bayes classification and KNN are two most effective techniques which are used to categorize tuberculosis affected patients into two categories: least probable and most probable. Though pathological tests (sputum test, x-ray and skin test) are required to detect TB completely, these are not required for the least probable cases. Following is the outline of the above mentioned methodology (Maniya & Hasan, 2011).

- Here a set of cases are taken as the input and the model is trained with this dataset in such a way that the probabilities of all the classes along with all conditions are computed.
- The result is stored in a database.
- Probabilities for various classes are generated as output based on the given symptom values present in the test data.
- Based on this probability, decision can be taken regarding the patient's condition like patient should belong to the class with the highest probability.

Information Gain for Hepatitis C

Bioinformatics research largely depends on the mining of appropriate information from huge experimental dataset. One major obstruction is to select the genomic markers in Hepatitis B Virus (HBV) which are related with liver cancer. This can be done with the comparison of complete genomic sequences of HBV among patients with having liver cancer and those without this. An innovative data mining framework has been introduced which works as a solution of the above problem. It has the features like molecular evolution analysis, clustering, feature selection, classifier learning, and classification. As a first step, data has been collected for HBV DNA sequences, either genotype B or C. Then in the molecular evolution analysis and clustering, three subgroups have been recognized in genotype C and a clustering method has been created to create the subgroups separately. Potential markers are chosen based on Information Gain for further classifier learning in the feature selection process, In the next step, meaningful rules are learnt with the help of Evolutionary algorithms.

Decision Tree in Various Predictions

Dengue is reoccurring throughout the tropical world, also leads to death for multiple cases. The initial symptoms appear to be similar with other febrile illness, especially in the early stage of the disease. As a result, diagnosis is often delayed with other diseases which takes a toll on patient care (Tanner et al, 2008). A decision algorithm has been introduced to address the above limitation. It's able to discriminate patients with dengue illness from the rest having other causes of fever with an accuracy of 84.7% by using body temperature and laboratory test results on blood samples of these patients. Another decision algorithm can predict successfully whether a dengue patient can go to the critical stage as indicated by an eventual drop in the platelet count to 50,000/mm^3 blood or below.

Genetic Algorithm(GA) in Diabetes and Cancer Treatment

Genetic algorithm is widely used to receive the chromosome accuracy and for evaluating the diabetes in diabetic patient. A bidirectional connection exists in fuzzy system and genetic algorithm. In one way, genetic algorithms are used to deal with different optimization problems through fuzzy systems (Sapna et al, 2012). Challenge in optimizing fuzzy inference rules in fuzzy controllers is the area for which genetic algorithm has been proved as very appropriate. In another way, fuzzification is possible for classical genetic algorithms. The resulting fuzzy genetic algorithms has been proved as more efficient for few applications.

Diabetes is a disease where human body is unable to produce insulin or use properly. As a result, low blood sugar and other various problems can arise which can lead to severe complications. Here, by using GA, chromosome optimization can be obtained and depending on the rate of old population, diabetes can be restricted within new population to receive chromosomal accuracy.

Two major methods, the fuzzy-based systems and the evolutionary genetic algorithms were used to find a computer aided diagnosis system that will help medical professional for diagnosing bread cancer in earlier stages. The result shows that the fuzzy-genetics approach creates systems which produces high classification performance, with simple and well interpretive rules and a greater confidence level.

Knowledge Discovery and Future Prediction

Data mining has great impact in the healthcare domain and it refers comprehensive process which needs detailed information of the necessity of healthcare organizations. Data mining tools and techniques are used to obtain successful decisions which improves the success of healthcare organizations as well as the patients. Another advantage of datamining is the continuous knowledge discovery once it's implemented. Its primary potential lies within the huge dataset in healthcare domain. Various clinical diagnosis and predictions can be done based on analysis of this hidden pattern. Healthcare organizations can be benefited by using these tools and techniques which can predict future requests, requirements and patient conditions and able to decide the appropriate route required for their treatments.

CONCLUSION

The data mining applications and techniques have a huge impact on healthcare industry in terms of its incredible potential and usefulness. Though the real success of this field lies in the presence of noise free healthcare data. So it's very crucial for healthcare industry to give adequate effort on data capture, storage, preparation and mining to get clean data. Few possible directions include the standardization of clinical vocabulary and exchanging data among organizations to improve the advantages received from data mining applications.

REFERENCES

Abinaya, K. (2015). Data Mining with Big Data e-Health Service Using Map Reduce. *International Journal of Advanced Research in Computer and Communication Engineering, 4*(2).

Durairaj, M., & Ranjani, V. (2013). Data mining applications in healthcare sector: a study. *Int. J. Sci. Technol. Res., 2*(10).

Groves, P., Kayyali, B., Knott, D., & Kuiken, S. V. (2016). *The big data revolution in healthcare: Accelerating value and innovation.* Academic Press.

Kharya, S. (2012). Using data mining techniques for diagnosis and prognosis of cancer disease. *International Journal of Computer Science, Engineering and Information Technology, 2*(2).

Koh, H. C., & Tan, G. (2011). Data mining applications in healthcare. *Journal of Healthcare Information Management, 19*(2), 65. PMID:15869215

Lemuye, E. (2011). *HIV Status Predictive Modeling Using Data Mining Technology* (Doctoral dissertation). AAU.

Mandwel, A. A., & Anjum, A. (2013). Detection of Brain Tumor Using K-Means Clustering. *International Journal of Science and Research, 5*(6).

Maniya, H., Hasan, M. I., & Patel, K. P. (2011). Comparative study of Naïve Bayes Classifier and KNN for Tuberculosis. *International Conference on Web Services Computing (ICWSC).*

Patel, S., & Patel, H. (2016). Survey of data mining techniques used in healthcare domain. *International Journal of Information, 6*(1/2).

Priyavadana, V., Sivashankari, A., & Senthil Kumar, R. (2015). A comparative study of data mining applications in diagnosing diseases. *International Research Journal of Engineering and Technology, 2*(7).

Ranjan, J. (2007). Applications of data mining techniques in pharmaceutical industry. *Journal of Theoretical and Applied Information Technology, 3*(4), 61–67.

Rogers, G., & Joyner, E. (1997, March). Mining your data for health care quality improvement. *SAS User Group International Conference*, 641-647.

Sapna, S., Tamilarasi, A., & Pravin Kumar, M. (2012). Implementation of Genetic Algorithm in Predicting Diabetes. *International Journal of Computer Science Issues, 9*(1).

Sartipi, K., Najafi, M., & Kazemzadeh, R. S. (2008). *Data and mined-knowledge interoperability in eHealth systems.* INTECH Open Access Publisher. doi:10.5772/6413

Seetha Lakshmi, G., & Isakki, P. (2017). A Comparative Study of Data Mining Classification Technique Using HIV/AIDS and STD data. *International Journal of Innovative Research in Computer and Communication Engineering, 5*(1).

Sharma, A., & Gupta, P. C. (2012). Predicting the number of blood donors through their age and blood group by using data mining tool. *International Journal of Communication and Computer Technologies, 1*(6), 6-10.

Srinivas, K., Rani, B. K., & Govrdhan, A. (2010). Applications of data mining techniques in healthcare and prediction of heart attacks. *International Journal on Computer Science and Engineering*, *2*(02), 250–255.

Tanner, , Schreiber, M., Low, J. G. H., Ong, A., Tolfvenstam, T., Lai, Y. L., & Ooi, E. E. et al. (2008, March). Decision Tree Algorithms Predict the Diagnosis and Outcome of Dengue Fever in the Early Phase of Illness. *PLoS Neglected Tropical Diseases*, *2*(3), e196. doi:10.1371/journal.pntd.0000196 PMID:18335069

Tomar, D., & Agarwal, S. (2013). A survey on Data Mining approaches for Healthcare. *International Journal of Bio-Science and Bio-Technology*, *5*(5), 241–266. doi:10.14257/ijbsbt.2013.5.5.25

Chapter 15
Kernel-Based Machine Learning Techniques:
An Innovative Way of Designing Healthcare Systems and Services

Kumar Vijay
Manav Rachna International University, India

Saxena Arti
Manav Rachna International University, India

Kumar Suresh
Manav Rachna International University, India

ABSTRACT

Health care is considered as the fundamental right of every citizen and it is principle duty of every country to provide good health care facilities. Many developed countries spend substantial amount of gross domestic product (GDP) on healthcare. In this chapter, we discuss kernel based machine learning techniques, i.e., k-PCA (Kernel principal component analysis) and its related properties with a aim to prescribe cost effective treatments and easy diagnosis of diseases. This objective could be met only by the serious collaboration between physician and data scientist. We discussed that how we could construct a kernel and exact features based on the given dataset. Also, we compared the proposed method with the other methods. For the sake of easy understanding, applications of the proposed method are included in the text.

1. INTRODUCTION

A robust health care system is the foremost factor and the need that can contribute to the personal health of everyone in the changing environment. Unfortunately, health care is a costly affair. [WHO, 2015], world health organization (WHO) revealed that United States alone spent 17.0% of gross domestic product (GDP) on health care in 2012, which is the highest among the globe and the expenditure in terms of

DOI: 10.4018/978-1-5225-5222-2.ch015

Copyright © 2018, IGI Global. Copying or distributing in print or electronic forms without written permission of IGI Global is prohibited.

percentage of GDP is also growing, which is up from 13.1% in 1990. Every developed country spends substantial amount of their GDP on providing health care facilities to their citizens. The estimated details of some developed countries are as:

1. France spent 11.6% of GDP on health in 2012, which is up from 10.1% in 1990.
2. Germany spent 11.3% of GDP, which is up from 10.4% in 1990.
3. Canada increased spending from 10.9% of GDP in 2012 to 8.7% in 1990.
4. United Kingdom spent 9.3% of GDP in 2012, which is up from 6.9% in 1990.

Overall, the trend represents that one should increase the budget of health care, which is not feasible for the countries with low GDP. Therefore, certain reforms in health care solutions need to be incorporated. Globally, health care systems should be efficient enough at treating patients as well as reducing costs of the treatments.

[Blumenthal, 2010], to keep this in mind, the United States established the Health Information Technology for Economic and Clinical Health (HITECH) Act in 2009. The purpose of the act is to establish programs to improve the quality of health care, safety and efficiency by using information technology in health care to make meaningful use of electronic health records (EHR) and secure electronic sharing of information. The ultimate aim of the act is to create more information-based, higher-quality based health care system. Also, the act provide incentives to eligible professionals and health care centers, who adopt, implement, upgrade or demonstrate meaningful use of e- health records (EHR) technology. Therefore, health care providers have collected huge amount of structured and unstructured data, which this data helps in the improvement of the existing health care systems with a goal to reduce the cost of the treatments.

World Health Organization (WHO) estimates that the expenditure on health care reveals a trend of increasing costs, the existing health care systems are not efficient enough to treat the patients at reasonable cost. Various incentives and programs were proposed by the authorities to develop information based e-health care systems by using machine learning tools in medicine. These tools will definitely enhance the level of existing system of health care.

In this chapter, we propose new methods for the modeling of individual response to the treatment. It also improves the collaboration between machine learning experts and clinicians.

2. BACKGROUND

No doubt, machine learning is a tool to deal with the large datasets with the outcome to produce meaningful information but the real challenge is that what to do with all the available data. These larger datasets includes more relational, temporal, unstructured data in complex form collected through multiple sources. These heterogeneous datasets urges the technology to develop new tools for practical purposes. [Page, 2015], machine learning offers variety of new tools for the analysis of data that can be used to improve health care among patients. [Mitchell, 1997], machine learning is the generalized area of artificial intelligence which focuses on algorithms, learns from the concerned datasets and construct models used for the purpose of decision making. We encountered with many applications of machine learning without even thinking of it.

For example, Google uses the tools of machine learning in search engine to forecast which pages are most relevant to the searched keywords. Amazon uses machine learning to suggest products to the users, based on which they are likely to buy it.

Machine learning has already being implemented in business for the purpose of analytics with companies like Google, Amazon etc. Also, it has shown similar impact in healthcare analytics and demonstrated many innovative healthcare techniques for the purpose of medical diagnosis of diseases and treatments.

3. MACHINE LEARNING IN MEDICINE

This chapter focuses on demonstrating new methods in machine learning to improve health care and investigates the following statement:

Machine learning algorithms provide various tailor made clinically-relevant approaches to meet the objectives of medical decision making. These models should be incorporated in clinical practices so as to improve the existing model and refine it to meet the expectations. Many machine learning techniques are already in application to optimize their performance measures. To apply machine learning models into useful clinical applications, we need to re visit and modify standard measures of performance to meet the clinical objectives of decision making.

In our work, we demonstrated kernel method, which improves the scope of collaboration between the mathematicians and clinicians. This helps in the development of models that will more effectively address the real clinical objectives. [Radcliffe and Surry, 1999], modeling individual's response to the treatment, building machine learning techniques originally developed in the marketing domain.

In the next section, we will discuss some insights that how some clinical practice works and how it could be improved.

4. PROPOSED INNOVATIVE HEALTH CARE SUPPORT SYSTEM

Health care practitioners may have to deal with many different patients with different diseases and may also have a great amount of information about the status of the patients. It is the job of the practitioner to use this information to correctly diagnose the diseases and treat them. To use this information, they shall prepare a knowledge base containing the relevant information about the diseases, treatments, expected outcomes etc.

It is very uneasy and ridiculous at the end of the practitioner to manage e-health records and do the necessary proliferation of the health records. Although these records are critically important for providing support to the health care systems. This additional burden of maintaining the data needs some another skill set that must be learned by the practitioner. [Roshanov, 2013], medical care is a variable and often suboptimal across health care systems. Therefore, decision support systems assist practitioners in diagnosing processes and help them in approximately treating patients. [Roshanov, 2013, Kawamoto, 2005, Chaudhry, 2006, Ash, 2012], there are many such systems already available to increase adherence and improve health care in total. These tools may come in any form, but in our work we will focus only on those techniques which deal with machine learning. In this chapter, we will discuss kernel method, which has advantage over Support Vector Machine methods and have the potential to develop other algorithms for non-linear modeling of data and reduce the complexity of the kernel expansion. In the next section, we will discuss the basics of kernels.

5. BASICS OF KERNELS

In machine learning problems, kernel is introduced as a similarity measure that can be found as a dot product in feature space.

[Schurmann, 1996], let us consider that χ is a subset of vector space $\mathbb{R}^N, \left(N \in \mathbb{N}\right)$ presented with the canonical dot product. Suppose that $x \in \chi$ be the pattern where most information is contained in the dth order products (called monomials) of entries $\left[x\right]_j$ of x,

$$\left[x\right]_{j_1} \cdot \left[x\right]_{j_2} \cdots\cdots\cdots \left[x\right]_{j_d} \tag{5.1}$$

where $j_1, j_2, \ldots\ldots, j_d \in \left\{1, 2, \ldots\ldots, N\right\}$

These monomials are called as product features and these features form the basis of many algorithms. This can be done by extracting product features and then applying learning algorithms to these features. In other words, patterns are preprocessed by mapping into the product space H of all products of d entries. This approach works only for small dimension problems but happens for N - dimensional patterns, there exist $N_H = C_d^{d+N-1}$ different monomials of degree d of dimension N_H in product space H.

Using non linear kernels in the input space $\mathbb{R}^N$, one can compute dot products in high dimensional feature spaces without explicitly mapping into the spaces, and the subsequent processing can be carried out by using dot products(rotationally invariant) exclusively.

To compute dot products of the form $\left\langle \Phi\left(x\right), \Phi\left(x'\right) \right\rangle$, we use kernel of the form

$$k\left(x, x'\right) = \left\langle \Phi\left(x\right), \Phi\left(x'\right) \right\rangle \tag{5.2}$$

This allows us to compute the value of the dot product in feature space H without explicitly computing the function Φ.

In the context of polynomial approximation, the polynomial kernel is defined as:

Let us consider the map $f_d : x \rightarrow f_d\left(x\right); \quad \forall x \in \mathbb{R}^N$

$\exists$corresponding kernel, where dot product of vectors mapped by f_d is

$$k\left(x, x'\right) = \left\langle f_d\left(x\right), f_d\left(x'\right) \right\rangle = \left\langle x, x' \right\rangle^d \tag{5.3}$$

Kernel learning algorithms are applicable to large number of situations where the representation of the data in vector form is not available and one can directly work with pair wise distances or similarities between the non-vector objects.

Some basic terminologies of the kernels are as:

5.1. Positive Definite Kernel

[Parthasarathy, 1972], let $\mathbb{N}$, $\mathbb{C}$ and $\mathbb{R}$ be the set of natural, complex and real numbers. $\forall \ i, j = 1, 2, ..., m$

5.2. Gram Matrix

Let $x_1, x_2, ..., x_m \in \chi$ be the set of patterns. Given a function $k : \chi^2 \rightarrow K$, where, $K = \mathbb{C} \ or \ \mathbb{R}$, then the matrix $\left[K\right]_{m \times m}$ with elements

$$K_{ij} = k\left(x_i, x_j\right) \tag{5.1.1}$$

is called the Gram Matrix or kernel matrix of k with respect to $x_1, x_2, ..., x_m$.

5.3. Positive Definite Matrix

A matrix $[K]_{m \times m}$ satisfying $\sum_{i,j} c_i . \bar{c_j} K_{ij} \geq 0$ is called positive definite matrix.

$\forall C_i \in \mathbb{C} \ or \ \mathbb{R}$ and $\bar{c_j}$ denotes complex conjugate.

5.4. Positive Definite Kernel

Let χ be a non empty set. A function K on $\chi \times \chi$ be a positive definite Gram matrix of order $m \times m$ is called a positive definite kernel or simply a kernel.

$\forall m \in \mathbb{N}$

and

$x_1, x_2, ..., x_m \in \chi$.

5.5. Cauchy- Schwarz Inequality for Kernels

If k is a positive definite kernel and $x_1, x_2 \in \chi$, then

$$\left|k\left(x_1, x_2\right)\right|^2 \leq k\left(x_1, x_1\right).k\left(x_2, x_2\right) \tag{5.1.2}$$

5.6. Feature Space

Let χ be a non empty set and k be a real-valued positive definite kernel.

Define a map, $\mathbb{R}^{\chi} = \left\{ f : \chi \to \mathbb{R} \right\}$, $\Phi : \chi \to \mathbb{R}^{\chi}$ and $x \to k\left(.,x\right)$ (5.1.3)where, $\Phi\left(x\right)$ denotes the function that assigns the value $k\left(x',x\right) \to x'$ i.e. $\Phi\left(x\right)\left(.\right) = k\left(.,x\right)$

Here, we turned each pattern into a function, with a view that a pattern represents similarity to all the points in the input domain χ as shown in Figure 1.

There are many ways to construct feature spaces for any given kernel, they can even differ in terms of dimensionality.

In the Figure 1, kernel is assumed to be bell shaped, i.e. $k\left(x,x'\right) = \exp\left(-\left\|x - x'\right\|^2 / \left(2\sigma^2\right)\right)$.

There are certain postulates by virtue of which we can construct feature space associated with Φ and are defined below as:

1. Turn the image of Φ into vector space.
2. Define the positive definite bilinear form of a dot product.
3. Show that dot product satisfies $k\left(x,x'\right) = \left\langle \Phi\left(x\right), \Phi\left(x'\right) \right\rangle$

Note

1. To get the vector space, taking the linear combination of the form

$$f\left(.\right) = \sum_{i=1}^{m} \alpha_i . k\left(., x_i\right) \tag{5.1.4}$$

where

$m \in \mathbb{N}$, $x_i \in \chi$

and

$\alpha_i \in \mathbb{R}$

Figure 1. Feature map associated with a kernel representing each pattern by a kernel (5.1.3) shaped function

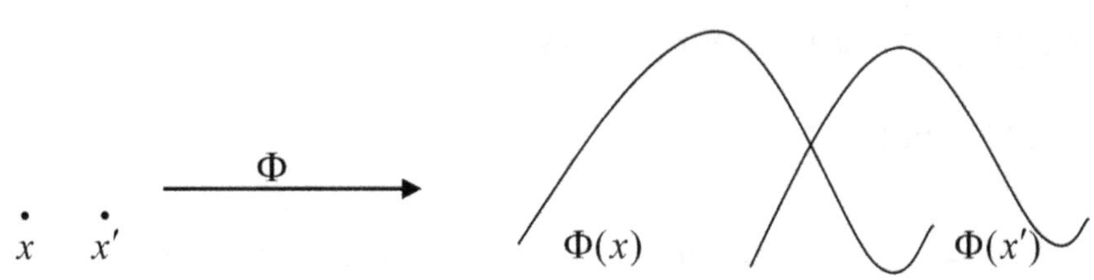

2. Establish dot product between f and another function,

$$g(.)=\sum_{j=1}^{m'}\beta_j k(.,x_j') \tag{5.1.5}$$

$\forall\ m' \in \mathbb{N}, \beta_j \in \mathbb{R}$

and

$x_1', x_2', ----, x_j' \in \chi$

$$\langle f,g\rangle=\sum_{i=1}^{m}\alpha_i g(x_i) \tag{5.1.6}$$

Equation (5.1.6) is the bilinear form.

3. Since positive definiteness of k for any function f, re-write equation (5.1.4) we have

$$\langle f,f\rangle=\sum_{i,j=1}^{m}\alpha_i\ \alpha_j\ k(x_i,x_j)\geq 0 \tag{5.1.7}$$

Please note that any algorithm formulated in terms of a positive definite kernel k, one can construct an alternative algorithm by replacing k by another positive definite kernel $\tilde{k}$.

5.7. Proposition

Let $x_1, x_2, \ldots., x_m$ be the data values and k be the kernel such that kernel gram matrix $K_{ij}=k(x_i,x_j)$ is positive definite, then the necessary and sufficient condition for a function Φ on m-dimensional feature space H is that the matrix K_{ij} is positive definite.

It is commonly known as Data-Dependent kernel map. By virtue of these properties, positive definite kernels k are also called as reproducing kernels as given by [Aronszajn, 1950, Berg, 1984, Saitoh, 1988, Wahba, 1990, Scholkopf, 1997, Girosi, 1998].

5.8. Examples and Properties of Kernels

5.8.1 Polynomial Kernel

Let $x \in \mathbb{R}^N$, $k(x,x')=\langle x,x'\rangle^d$, commonly known as homogeneous polynomial kernel.

5.8.2. Gaussian Kernel

[Boser, 1992, Guyon, 1993, Vapnik, 1965] suggests Gaussian radial basis function kernels and applied it in pattern recognition problems [Bashkirov, 1964]

$$k\left(x, x'\right) = \exp\left(-\left\|x - x'\right\|^2 / \left(2\sigma^2\right)\right), \sigma > 0$$

5.8.3. Sigmoid Kernel

$$k\left(x, x'\right) = \tanh\left(k\left\langle x, x'\right\rangle + \theta\right), k > 0, \theta < 0$$

Sigmoid kernel is not actually positive definite, therefore not much in practice.

5.8.4. Inhomogeneous Polynomial Kernel

$$k\left(x, x'\right) = \left(\left\langle x, x'\right\rangle^d + C\right)^d, d \in \mathbb{N}, C \geq 0$$

5.8.5. Invariance of Kernel

$$k\left(x, x'\right) = k\left(U_x, U_{x'}\right)$$

if

$$U^T = U^{-1}$$

For complex numbers, $U^* = \overline{U}^T$

5.8.6. Radial Basis Function (RBF) Kernels

$$k\left(x, x'\right) = f\left(d\left(x, x'\right)\right)$$

where, $d\left(x, x'\right) = \left\|x - x'\right\| = \sqrt{\left\langle x - x', x - x'\right\rangle}$ is a metric on χ and f is a function in $\mathbb{R}_0^+$

In this chapter, we confined only to positive definite kernel.

6. DESIGNING OF KERNELS

In order to write algorithms to get promising results, designing of kernels is the foremost requirement. The choice of a kernel depends on the selection of certain factors as: similarity measure for the data, linear representation of the data, a function space for learning, a regularization term, a covariance function for correlated observation and apriori over the set of functions.

In other words, the choice of kernel indicates the prior knowledge of the problem at hand and there is no free lunch in choosing kernel.

7. CONSTRUCTION OF KERNELS

[Berg, 1984, Cressie, 1993, Abrahamsen, 1992, Burges, 1998, MacKay, 1998, Scholkopf, 1999, Cristianini, 2000], discussed certain results, which are used to construct positive definite kernels and are explained below as:

1. **Sum of Kernels:** Let us consider that k_1 and k_2 are kernels and $\alpha_1, \alpha_2 \geq 0$ are scalars, then $\alpha_1 k_1 + \alpha_2 k_2$ is also a kernel.
2. **Limits of Kernels:** If $k_1, k_2, ...$ are kernels, then k is a kernel if $k(x, x') = \lim_{n\to\infty} k_n(x, x')$ exists for all x, x'.

From (7.1) and (7.2), it is concluded that the set of kernels form a convex cone, closed under point wise convergence.

3. **Product of Kernels:** If k_1 and k_2 are kernels, then $k_1.k_2$ is also a kernel

i.e. $(k_1.k_2)(x, x') = k_1(x, x').k_2(x, x')$

4. **Conformal Transformation of Kernels**

$$k_f(x, x') = f(x)k(x, x')f(x'); \quad f(x) > 0$$

RHS is obtained by multiplying kernel k with a rank one kernel,i.e. $k'(x, x') = f(x)f(x')$

5. [Burges, 1999], the necessary condition for the dot product $k(x, x') = k(\langle x, x' \rangle)$ is that it has to satisfy $k(t) \geq 0, k'(t) \geq 0$ and $k'(t) + tk''(t) \geq 0, \forall t \geq 0$.
6. [Schoenberg, 1942], the power series of the dot product kernels $k(x, x') = k(\langle x, x' \rangle)$ defined with a power series expansion $k(t) = \sum_{n=0}^{\infty} a_n t^n$ is a positive definite kernel if $a_n \geq 0, \forall n$.
7. **Fourier Criterion Kernel:** A translation invariant kernel,

i.e. $k(x,x') = k(x-x')$ is a positive definite kernel if $F[k](w) = (2\pi)^{-\frac{N}{2}} \int_x e^{-i\langle w,x\rangle} k(x)\,dx > 0$ where, $F[k](w)$ is called Fourier Transform.

Note: In the process of the constructing kernels, it is useful to compute the kernels from mapping into some dot product space. i.e. $k(x,x') = \langle f_x, f_{x'}\rangle^d$ where, $\langle f_x, f_{x'}\rangle = \int f_x(x).f_{x'}(x)\,dx$

8. **Tensor Product:** If k_1 and k_2 are kernels defined on $\chi_1 \times \chi_1$ and $\chi_2 \times \chi_2$ respectively, then tensor product,

$$(k_1 \otimes k_2)(x_1, x_2, x_1', x_2') = k_1(x_1, x_1').k_2(x_2, x_2')$$

is a kernel on $(\chi_1 \times \chi_2) \times (\chi_1 \times \chi_2)$, where $x_1, x_1' \in \chi_1$ and $x_2, x_2' \in \chi_2$

9. **Direct Sums:** [Haussler, 1999, Scholkopf, 1999], if k_1 and k_2 are kernels defined on $\chi_1 \times \chi_1$ and $\chi_2 \times \chi_2$ respectively, then direct sum $(k_1 \oplus k_2)(x_1, x_2, x_1', x_2') = k_1(x_1, x_1') + k_2(x_2, x_2')$ is a kernel on $(\chi_1 \times \chi_2) \times (\chi_1 \times \chi_2)$ Where $x_1, x_1' \in \chi_1$ and $x_2, x_2' \in \chi_2$
10. R **-Convolution of Kernels:** [Haussler, 1999]

$$(k_1 * k_2 * --- * k_D)(x, x') = \sum_R \prod_{d=1}^{D} k_d(x_d, x_d')$$

where, the summation of RHS of the term runs over all possible ways in which we can decompose x into $x_1, x_2, ..., x_D$ and x' into $x_1', x_2', ..., x_D'$, $\forall (x_1, x_2, ..., x_D, x_1', x_2', ..., x_D')$ such that $R(x_1, x_2, ..., x_D, x)$ and $R(x_1', x_2', ..., x_D', x')$.

It is commonly known as R -convolution of $k_1, k_2, ..., k_D$.

11. **ANOVA Kernel:** [Wahba, 1990, Burges, 1995, Vapnik, 1998, Stitson, 1999], for some set S and kernels $k^{(i)}$ on $S \times S$, $\chi = S^N$, the ANOVA kernel of order D is defined as:

$$k_D(x, x') = \sum_{1 \le i_1 < --- < i_D} \prod_{d=1}^{N} k^{(id)}(x_{id}, x_{id}'), i = 1, 2, ----N$$

Note

1. If $D = N$, then $k = k^{(1)} \otimes .... \otimes k^{(N)}$ for which $(i_1, i_2, ..., i_D) = (1, 2, ..., N)$.
2. If $D = 1$, then $k = k^{(1)} \oplus .... \oplus k^{(N)}$ and the products collapse to one factor each.

3. For intermediate values of D, we get kernels that lie in between tensor products and direct sums. Also, it is possible to use ANOVA kernels to interpolate between ordinary products and sum of kernels.

Here, we are more interested in some moderated values of D, which explain the order of the interaction between attributes χ_{id}.

8. NATURAL KERNELS

[Jaakkola, 1999], for a strictly positive definite natural matrix M, the corresponding natural kernel is given by

$$k_{m}^{nat}\left(x,x'\right) = V_{\theta}\left(x\right)^{T} M^{-1} V_{\theta}\left(x'\right)$$

$$= \nabla_{\theta} \ln\left[p\left(x|\theta\right)\right]^{T} M^{-1} \nabla_{\theta} \ln\left[p\left(x'|\theta\right)\right]$$

where, $l\left(x|\theta\right) = \ln p\left(x|\theta\right)$ is log likelihood, $p\left(x|\theta\right)$ is called density function and the derivative of $l\left(x|\theta\right)$ is called score.

$$V_{\theta}\left(x\right) = \left(\partial_{\theta^{l}} l\left(x,\theta\right),\ldots\ldots,\partial_{\theta^{r}} l\left(x,\theta\right)\right) = \nabla_{\theta} l\left(x,\theta\right) = \nabla_{\theta} \ln p\left(x|\theta\right)$$

For $p\left(x|\theta\right)$ to be a normal distribution, then $\theta = \left(\mu,\sigma\right)$, where μ is the mean vector and σ is the covariance matrix of Gaussian. The magnitude of components of $V_{\theta}\left(x\right)$ specifies the extent to which a change in a particular component of θ changes with the probability of generating the object x.

Since $\ln\left[p\left(x|\theta\right)\right]$ is Riemannian and the metric defined on the spaces of the scores, with metric tensor given by the inverse of the Fisher information matrix.

$$I = E_{p}\left[V_{\theta}\left(x\right)V_{\theta}\left(x\right)^{T}\right]$$

i.e. $I_{if} = E_{p}\left[\partial_{\theta^{i}} \ln\left[p\left(x|\theta\right)\right] . \partial_{\theta^{r}} \ln\left[p\left(x|\theta\right)\right]\right]$

where, E_{p} = expectation with respect to the density p.

Note

1. For $M = I$, we will get Fisher kernel and for $M = 1$, we obtain a plain kernel i.e. $k_m^{mt}\left(x, x'\right) = \exp\left(-\left\|V_\theta\left(x\right) - V_\theta\left(x'\right)\right\|^2 / C\right)$

9. KERNEL FEATURE EXTRACTION

Using Support Vector Machines (SVMs), we will get valuable results and mapped the data implicitly into a high-dimensional feature space. In this chapter, we are discussing kernel based method for performing non-linear form of principal components analysis (PCA), commonly known as kernel PCA (k-PCA). Through positive definite kernels, we can compute principal components in high dimensional feature spaces related to some non-linear maps. PCA is a powerful technique for extracting structure from high dimensional data sets and is performed by means of iterative algorithm, which estimates principal components. It is an orthogonal transformation of the coordinate system in which we describe our data and the new coordinate system is obtained by projecting onto the principal axis of the data and is called principal components or features and sometimes called factors of the data. The standard PCA algorithm is follows as:

1. Given a set of observations $x_i \in \mathbb{R}^N, i = 1, 2, ..., m$ and $\sum_{i=1}^{m} x_i = 0$.
2. To get principal axis by the diagonalization of covariance matrix $C = \frac{1}{m}\sum_{j=1}^{m} x_j x_j^T$, where C is positive definite and can be diagonalized with non-negative eigen values.
3. Solve $\lambda X = CX \;\; ; \lambda \geq 0, X \in \mathbb{R}^n \setminus \left\{0\right\}$ is a non-zero vector.

$$\therefore \;\; \lambda X = \frac{1}{m}\sum_{j=1}^{m} x_j x_j^T . X$$

$$\lambda X = \frac{1}{m}\sum_{j=1}^{m} \left\langle x_j . X\right\rangle x_j$$

The solutions of X with $\lambda \neq 0$ lie in the span of $x_1, x_2, ..., x_m$ and $\lambda X = CX$ is equivalent to $\lambda\left\langle x_i, X\right\rangle = \left\langle x_i, CX\right\rangle, \forall i = 1, 2, ..., m$.

To study PCA, we are interested in the principal components of variables or features, which are non-linearly related to the input variables. This can be done by the introduction of kernel in feature extraction.

9.1 Kernel Principal Component Analysis (k-PCA)

This technique is used to find non-linear PCA by taking into consideration eigen value problem.

Let us consider a non-linear feature space H mapped by $\Phi : \chi \rightarrow \text{H}, x \rightarrow \Phi\left(x\right)$

This feature space H is arbitrarily large and having infinite dimension.

Assuming that $\sum_{i=1}^{m} \Phi\left(x_i\right) = 0$

In H, the covariance matrix has the form $C = \frac{1}{m} \sum_{j=1}^{m} \Phi\left(x_j\right).\Phi\left(x_j\right)^T$.

If H has infinite dimensions, then $\Phi\left(x_j\right).\Phi\left(x_j\right)^T$ is a linear operator and mapping is $x \rightarrow \Phi\left(x_j\right)\left\langle \Phi\left(x_j\right)^T, x\right\rangle$

In order to find the eigen values and their corresponding eigen vectors, which satisfies $\lambda X = CX$, all the solutions vectors of X with $\lambda \neq 0$ lie in the span of $\Phi\left(x_1\right), \Phi\left(x_2\right), \ldots, \Phi\left(x_m\right)$.

This gives rise to two useful consequences as:

1. $\lambda\left\langle \Phi\left(x_n\right), X\right\rangle = \left\langle \Phi\left(x_n\right), CX\right\rangle, \ \forall n = 1, 2, \ldots, m$
2. $\exists \alpha_i \left(i = 1, 2, \ldots, m\right)$ such that $X = \sum_{i=1}^{m} \alpha_i \ \Phi\left(x_i\right)$ (9.1)

Using these consequences, we have

$$\lambda \sum_{i=1}^{m} \alpha_i \left\langle \Phi\left(x_n\right), \Phi\left(x_i\right)\right\rangle = \frac{1}{m} \sum_{i=1}^{m} \alpha_i \left\langle \Phi(x_n), \sum_{j=1}^{m} \Phi(x_j)\left\langle \Phi(x_j), \Phi(x_i)\right\rangle \right\rangle, \forall n = 1, 2, \ldots, m$$

In terms of gram matrix, $\left[K_{ij}\right]_{m \times m} = \left\langle \Phi\left(x_i\right), \Phi\left(x_j\right)\right\rangle$ (9.2)or $m\lambda\alpha = k\alpha$ (9.3)where, α is a column vector for non-zero eigen values.

Let $\lambda_1 \geq \lambda_2 \geq \ldots\ldots\ldots \geq \lambda_m$ be the eigen values of k and $\alpha^1, \alpha^2, ----\alpha^m$ be the corresponding eigen vectors, assuming that λ_p being the last non-zero eigen value.

Normalize $\alpha^1, \alpha^2, ----\alpha^p$ with the aim that corresponding vectors in H be normalized.i.e. $\left\langle X^n, X^n\right\rangle = 1, \quad \forall n = 1, 2, \ldots\ldots, p$

From (9.1) and (9.3), we get

$$1 = \sum_{i,j=1}^{m} \alpha_i^n \alpha_j^n \left\langle \Phi\left(x_i\right), \Phi\left(x_j\right)\right\rangle = \sum_{i,j=1}^{m} \alpha_i^n \alpha_j^n K_{ij} \tag{9.4}$$

$$1 = \left\langle \alpha^n, K\alpha^n\right\rangle = \lambda_n \left\langle \alpha^n, \alpha^n\right\rangle$$

For the extraction of principal component, we need to compute projection onto the eigen vectors X^n in feature space H.

Let $\Phi(x)$ be an image of a test point x in H, then

$$\langle X^n, \Phi(x) \rangle = \sum_{i=1}^{m} \alpha_i^n \langle \Phi(x_i), \Phi(x) \rangle \tag{9.5}$$

These are the non-linear principal components or features corresponding to Φ.

9.2 Kernel PCA (k-PCA) Algorithm

The algorithm used for the feature extraction and further applicable in decision making processes. This is explained in the Figure 2 and 3. Following are the steps as:

1. Compute Gram Matrix $K_{ij} = k(x_i, x_j)_{ij}$
2. Diagonalize K.
3. Normalize the eigen vector expansion coefficients α^n by requiring $\lambda_n \langle \alpha^n, \alpha^n \rangle = 1$.
4. To extract principal components from the feature space, corresponding to kernel k of a test point x as shown in Figure 3, compute projections onto the eigen vectors by $\langle X^n, \Phi(x) \rangle = \sum_{i=1}^{m} \alpha_i^n k(x_i, x), \forall n = 1, 2, \ldots\ldots, p$.

Note

For the sake of simplicity, we assume that observations are centered, which makes us easy to get the input space but difficult to implement in the feature space H. That is why, there is a little modification in the equation for kernel PCA.

Figure 2. Linear PCA as with classical PCA in input space

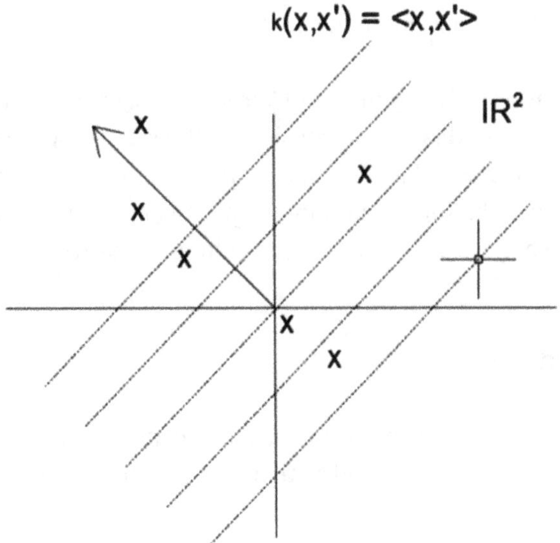

Figure 3. High-dimensional feature space H

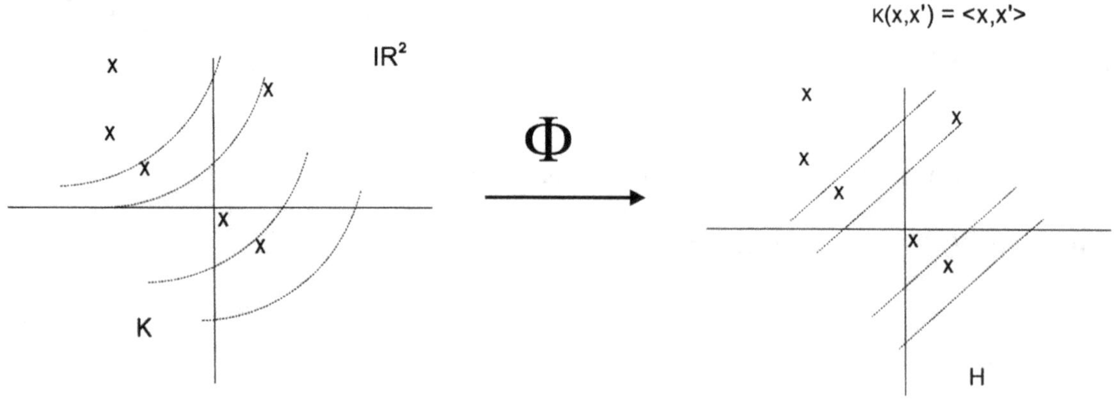

Therefore, diagonalize,

$$\widetilde{K_{ij}} = \left(K - I_m K - K\,1_m + 1_m K\,1_m\right)_{ij}$$

where

$$\left(1_m\right)_{ij} = \frac{1}{m} \qquad \forall i, j$$

Kernel PCA based on the centered matrix $\widetilde{K}$ can also be performed with the larger class of conditionally positive definite matrices.

Explanation of the Figure 3

Since feature space H is non-linearly related to input space Φ, the contour lines of constant projections onto the principal eigenvector are non-linear in input space. All the necessary computations are carried out by using kernel function k in input space $\mathbb{R}^2$.

Explanation of the Figure 4

Input vector is compared to a sample by means of kernel in first layer by choosing apriori (polynomial, Gaussian or sigmoid). In the second layer, we considered the sample space and taking the comparison of the values by considering kernels. The outputs are then combined by taking weights after solving an eigen vector problem. Since the function on input space is non-linear, therefore the function of the network can be found as the projection onto an eigen vector of a covariance matrix in high-dimensional feature space.

9.3 Properties of Kernel PCA

[Jolliffe, 1986, Diamantaras, 1996], In high-dimensional feature space, kernel PCA corresponds to standard PCA. Therefore, all mathematical and statistical properties of PCA corresponds to kernel PCA

Figure 4. Feature extractor constructed using kernel PCA

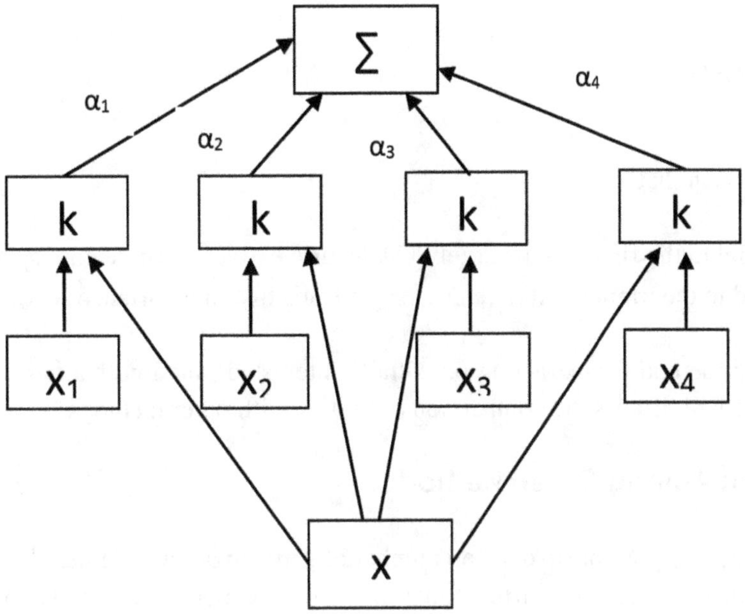

but only modification is that there is an involvement of function about a set of points $\Phi(x_i), i = 1, 2, ..., m$ in H rather than in $\mathbb{R}^n$.

9.3.1 Optimality Property of the Kernel

kernel PCA is the orthogonal basis transformation in H with the following properties (by sorted eigen vectors in decreasing order of eigen value size):

1. The first q principal components or projections on eigen vectors carry more variance than any other q orthogonal direction. $\forall q \in \{1, 2, ..., m\}$.
2. The mean squared approximation error in the observation in the feature space H by the first q principal components is minimal.
3. The principal components are uncorrelated.
4. The first principal components have maximal mutual information with respect to the inputs.

9.3.2 Connection Between k-PCA and SVM

[Scholkopf, 1999], the nth kernel PCA feature extractor, scaled by $\frac{1}{\lambda_n}\left(\forall n \in \{1, 2, ..., p\}\right)$ is optimal among all feature extractors of the form

$$f(x) = \sum_{i=1}^{m} \alpha_i k(x_i, x),$$

in the sense that it has minimal weight vector norm, i.e.

$$\|x\|^2 = \sum_{i,j=1}^{m} \alpha_i \alpha_j k\left(x_i, x_j\right),$$

subject to the condition that

1. It is orthogonal to the first $n-1$ kernel PCA feature extractors (in feature space)
2. When applied to the training set $x_1, x_2, \ldots, x_m$ it leads to a unit variance set of outputs.

kernel PCA is a method for extracting potentially interested function that has low capacity. In the coming section, we will discuss the comparison of k-PCA with other methods.

9.4 Comparison Among Other Methods

[Diamantaras, 1996], it is possible to develop number of generalizations of linear PCA to the non-linear case. By choosing an iterative algorithm to estimate principal components and make some of its non-linear parts to extract non-linear features. Using k-PCA, a non-linear generalization of PCA with a view that:

1. It performs PCA in feature spaces of arbitrarily large dimensionality.
2. If we use kernel $k\left(x, x'\right) = \left\langle x, x' \right\rangle$ we resolve original PCA algorithm.

The main advantage of kernel PCA is that non-linear optimization is not involved, linear algebra is involved as standard PCA. There is no need to specify the number of components that we wants to extract in advance. The comparisons of the methods with k-PCA are follows as:

9.4.1 Compared With Principal Curves [Hastie, 1989]

In k-PCA, hardly any interpretation is required in defining input space. For polynomial kernels, it has very clear interpretation in terms of higher-order features.

9.4.2 Compared With Neural Networks

[Oja, 1982], k-PCA has disadvantage if we process very large number of observations. It can only be possible to use sparse greedy methods to perform k-PCA approx. The sparse greedy method is not covered in this chapter. All these techniques provide non-linear feature extractors defined on the whole input space.

9.4.3 Compared With Multidimensional Scaling (MDS)

[Williams, 2001], non-linear feature extractors are evaluated on patterns irrespective of whether these are the elements of training set or not. But methods like locally linear embedding (LLE) and multi dimensionally scaling (MDS) are confined only to training set. The aim of the methods is only to provide a lower-dimensional representation of the training data. As a special case when we only extract features from the training data, k-PCA is closely connected to MDS.

Again, dimensionally reduction algorithm, LLE is closely related to k-PCA. One can obtain the solution of LLE by performing k-PCA on the Gram matrix computed from locally linear embedding kernel.

9.5 Frame Work for Feature Extraction

kernal PCA gives very promising results, but still some issues that needs to be addressed as:

1. The computational complexity of the standard version of k-PCA scales as $O\left(m^3\right)$ in the sample size m.
2. The resulting feature extractors are given as expansions in terms of the training patterns, but for each test point, the feature extractor requires m kernel evaluations.

Let us denote $X = \left\{x_1, x_2, ----, x_m\right\} \subset \chi$ be the set of patterns drawn independently and identically distributed from an underlying probability distribution $P\left(x\right)$. Our aim is to compute feature extractors that will satisfy certain criteria of simplicity and optimality (max. variance).

9.5.1 PCA

[Hotelling, 1933], Assuming that $\chi \subset \mathbb{R}^N$ the first principal component of a sample is given by the direction of projection with maximum variance.

For centered data,

$$\widetilde{X} = \left\{\widetilde{x}_i / \widetilde{x}_i = x_i - \frac{1}{m}\sum_{i=1}^{m} x_i, i = 1, 2, ---, m\right\} \tag{9.5.1}$$

and the first eigen vector v' is

$$v' = \arg\max_{\|v\|^2 \leq 1} \frac{1}{m}\sum_{i=1}^{m} \left|\left\langle v, \widetilde{x}_i \right\rangle\right|^2 \tag{9.5.2}$$

The successive eigenvectors $v^2, ---- v^N$ are chosen to be orthogonal, where each eigenvector v^i satisfies a property similar to (9.5.2) with respect to the remaining

$\left(N - i + 1\right)$- dimensional subspace.

The solution of this optimization problem is normally obtained by computing the largest principal component of the co-variance matrix of $\widetilde{X}$.

9.5.2 Kernel PCA

For centered data in feature space

$$\Phi\left(x_i\right) = \Phi\left(x_i\right) - \frac{1}{m}\sum_{i=1}^{m}\Phi\left(x_i\right)$$

Let us define $F_{\mathrm{H}} = \left\{ w/ w \in \mathrm{H}, \left\|w\right\|^2 \leq 1 \right\}$ (9.5.2.1)

be the set of candidate vectors to project on.

The first k-PCA eigen vector can be stated as: $v' = \underset{v \in F_{\mathrm{H}}}{\arg\max} \frac{1}{m}\sum_{i=1}^{m}\left\langle v, \Phi(x_i)\right\rangle^2$

$$= \underset{v \in F_{\mathrm{H}}}{\arg\max}\ var\left\{\left\langle v, \Phi\left(x_i\right)\right\rangle\right\} \tag{9.5.2.2}$$

10. APPLICATIONS OF MACHINE LEARNING IN THE IMPROVEMENT OF HEALTHCARE SYSTEMS

The cost of the treatment is increasing day by day and there is a need of intervention of some cost-effective technologies. Now a day, healthcare is a business and patients are treated as customer by healthcare institutions. They are taking into account the comfort of patients rather than the execution of the treatment, resulting increase in the cost of the service. Due to these interactions, it is feasible to introduce innovative methods for the treatment of diseases which not only provides quality healthcare solutions but also cost-effective. To achieve this goal, we discussed k-PCA, which is the non-linear generalization of PCA where non-linearity components in the data are taken into account when variance among the values is maximized. k-PCA helps in the improvement of performance of the existing systems.

The intensive collaboration between the healthcare practitioner and the machine learning scientist makes the healthcare system reliable, friendly, transparent and cost-effective for the users. Health care is the maintenance and restoration of health by the prevention and treatment of disease especially by trained and licensed professionals. Health care sector generated piles of data and is considered as a data goldmine, more data yields better decision making. [Mckinsey, 2013], the estimated annual revenue generated by machine learning in health care sector is $ 100 billion. The generated revenue is based on improved efficiency of clinical trials, better decision making, optimization techniques and the creation of new tools for physicians, consumers, regulators etc. Machine learning techniques effectively collects different types of data for better analysis and the treatment. Following are the applications of machine learning as:

10.1 Diagnosis of Diseases

Machine learning based kernel methods helps in the diagnosis of ailments and the identification of diseases. [MID, 2015], 800 medicines and vaccines are in trial to treat cancer. This is possible only by the collaboration between biologist and the data scientists to identify cancer and their treatments. Many research institutes like IBM Watson, Berg, Google's DeepMind Health etc. are engaged in developing diagnostics and their supplements. They are using kernel based machine learning techniques to achieve the overall goal. Moreover, diseases like depression are being treated by using predictive techniques.

10.2 Personalized Treatments

These are very effective and very much in practice, governed by supervised learning. This gives access to the physician to limited set of diagnosis based on the individual's information. It is considered as better disease assessment techniques, which prescribes effective treatments based on individual health by using predictive techniques. Over the coming decade, bio-medical devices and mobile apps will provide more health measurement and facilitate remote monitoring, which help treatment efficiency. This type of personalized attention to an individual has implication in health optimization and reduces the healthcare cost. Companies like IBM Watson is doing research in optimizing the treatment options based on patients medical information. They are using machine learning techniques to achieve personalized treatment plan.

10.3 Drug Discovery

Using machine learning in initial stage of drug discovery brings various facts of drug compounds to predict success rate of the drug based on biological factors. The type of research involves both supervised and unsupervised learning to identify patterns in data without predictions. Institutions like MIT clinical machine learning group is busy in the development of machine learning techniques to understand disease processes and design effective treatment plan of diseases. These techniques have the capability to reduce the time required to produce drugs and hence lowers costs.

10.4 Research in Clinical Trial

[Mckinsey, 2013], electronic medical records reduce data errors and enhance efficiency.

Clinical trials are very essential before the induction of drugs and the treatments. Machine learning has application in proving shape and structure to clinical trial research. Machine learning algorithms makes trails smaller, faster and less expensive, which are used to collect information of some specific population. These methods help in capturing real time data and monitor information getting through remote areas for increased safety.

10.5 Radiology

[Stat, 2016], in last two decades, radiologists gain its attention and their studies are more or like supervised learning. They studies thousands of related studies per minute and generate huge amount of data.

Machine learning algorithms gear up segmentation process and increase the accuracy in radiotherapy planning. An institute like Google's DeepMind Health is engaged in developing machine learning techniques which improve radiation related treatments.

10.6 Smart E-Health Records

Various machine learning technologies are used to classify the documents and transforming the desired information into digital form. MIT clinical machine learning group cited that there is a need for safe and robust machine learning techniques which understand natural language and generate it in medical settings.

10.7 Prediction of Epidemic Outbreak

Machine learning techniques are used to monitor and predict epidemic outbreaks over the globe on the basis of data collected from the sources like: satellites, web, real time updates and other reliable sources. For example, to predict malaria outbreaks by taking into consideration the data such as temperature, average rainfall, number of positive cases and other valid data points. These algorithms monitor the emerging diseases and providing real time reports.

11. CONCLUSION

In this chapter, we used machine learning algorithms for the purpose of easy diagnosis and treatments of diseases. These algorithms bring the diagnosis process and the treatments of ailments cost effective and transparent but can only be possible by the intensive collaboration between physicians and machine learning experts. k-PCA based decision making explained in the chapter demonstrates the applications of the algorithm in various fields of medical sciences. Moreover, the method is innovative and in practice for decision making purposes.

REFERENCES

Abrahamsen, P. (1992). *A review of Gaussian random fields and correlation functions.* Rapport 917, Norwegian Computing Center.

Aizerman, M. A., Braverman, E. M., & Rozonoer, L. I. (1964). Theoretical foundations of the potential function method in pattern recognition learning. *Automation and Remote Control, 25*, 821–837.

Aronszajn, N. (1950). Theory of reproducing kernels. *Transactions of the American Mathematical Society, 68*(3), 337–404. doi:10.1090/S0002-9947-1950-0051437-7

Ash, J., McCormack, J., Sittig, D., Wright, A., McMullen, C., & Bates, D. (2012). Standard practices for computerized clinical decision support in community hospitals: A national survey. *Journal of the American Medical Informatics Association, 19*(6), 980–987. doi:10.1136/amiajnl-2011-000705 PMID:22707744

Bartlett, P. L., & Scholkopf, B. (2001). *Some kernels for structured data. Technical report.* Biowulf Technologies.

Bashkirov, O. A., Braverman, E. M., & Muchnik, I. B. (1964). Theoretical foundations of the potential ′ function method in pattern recognition learning. *Automation and Remote Control, 25*, 629–631.

Berg, C., Christensen, J. P. R., & Ressel, P. (1984). *Harmonic Analysis on Semigroups.* New York: Springer-Verlag. doi:10.1007/978-1-4612-1128-0

Blumenthal, D. (2010). Launching HITECH. *The New England Journal of Medicine, 362*(5), 382–385. doi:10.1056/NEJMp0912825 PMID:20042745

Boser, B. E., Guyon, I. M., & Vapnik, V. (1992). A training algorithm for optimal margin classifiers. In D. Haussler (Ed.), *Proceedings of the 5th Annual ACM Workshop on Computational Learning Theory* (pp. 44–152). ACM Press. doi:10.1145/130385.130401

Burges, C. J. C. (1998). A tutorial on support vector machines for pattern recognition. *Data Mining and Knowledge Discovery, 2*(2), 121–167. doi:10.1023/A:1009715923555

Burges, C. J. C. (1999). Geometry and invariance in kernel based methods. In B. Scholkopf, C. J. C. Burges, & A. J. Smola (Eds.), *Advances in Kernel Methods — Support Vector Learning* (pp. 89–116). Cambridge, MA: MIT Press.

Burges, C. J. C., & Vapnik, V. (1995). *A new method for constructing artificial neural networks. Interim technical report, ONR contract N00014-94-c-0186.* AT&T Bell Laboratories.

Chaudhry, B., Wang, J., Wu, S., Maglione, M., Mojica, W., Roth, E., & Shekelle, P. et al. (2006). Systematic review: Impact of health information technology on quality, efficiency, and costs of medical care. *Annals of Internal Medicine, 144*(10), 742–752. doi:10.7326/0003-4819-144-10-200605160-00125 PMID:16702590

Cressie, N. A. C. (1993). *Statistics for Spatial Data.* New York: J. Wiley and Sons.

Cristianini, N., & Taylor, J. S. (2000). *An Introduction to Support Vector Machines.* Cambridge, UK: Cambridge University Press.

Diamantaras, K. I., & Kung, S. Y. (1996). *Principal Component Neural Networks.* New York: Wiley.

Girosi, F. (1998). An equivalence between sparse approximation and support vector machines. *Neural Computation, 10*(6), 1455–1480. doi:10.1162/089976698300017269 PMID:9698353

Guyon, I., Boser, B., & Vapnik, V. (1993). *Automatic capacity tuning of very large VC-dimension classifiers.* In S. J. Hanson, J. D. Cowan, & C. Lee Giles (Eds.), Advances in Neural Information Processing Systems (Vol. 5, pp. 147–155). San Mateo, CA: Morgan Kaufmann.

Hastie, T. J., & Stuetzle, W. (1989). Principal curves. *Journal of the American Statistical Association, 84*(406), 502–516. doi:10.1080/01621459.1989.10478797

Haussler, D. (1999). *Convolutional kernels on discrete structures*. Technical Report UCSC-CRL-99-10, Computer Science Department, University of California at Santa Cruz.

Hotelling, H. (1933). Analysis of a complex of statistical variables into principal components. *Journal of Educational Psychology, 24*, 417–441, 498–520.

Jaakkola, T. S., & Haussler, D. (1999). Probabilistic kernel regression models. *Proceedings of the 1999 Conference on AI and Statistics.*

Jolliffe, I. T. (1986). *Principal Component Analysis*. New York: Springer-Verlag. doi:10.1007/978-1-4757-1904-8

Kawamoto, K., Houlihan, C., Balas, E., & Lobach, D. (2005). Improving clinical practice using clinical decision support systems: A systematic review of trials to identify features critical to success. *BMJ (Clinical Research Ed.), 330*(7494), 765. doi:10.1136/bmj.38398.500764.8F PMID:15767266

MacKay, D. J. C. (1998). Introduction to Gaussian processes. In C. M. Bishop (Ed.), *Neural Networks and Machine Learning* (pp. 133–165). Berlin: Springer-Verlag.

Mitchell, T. (1997). *Machine Learning*. New York: McGraw-Hill.

Oja, E. (1982). A simplified neuron model as a principal component analyzer. *Journal of Mathematical Biology, 15*(3), 267–273. doi:10.1007/BF00275687 PMID:7153672

Page, D. (2015). *Predicting health events from electronic health records using machine learning. Talk by David Page at the Center for Predictive Computational Phenotyping*. University of Wisconsin.

Parthasarathy, K. R., & Schmidt, K. (1972). Positive definite kernels, continuous tensor products, and central limit theorems of probability theory. Springer-Verlag. doi:10.1007/BFb0058340

Radcliffe, N., & Surry, P. (1999). Differential response analysis: Modeling true response by isolating the effect of a single action. In Credit Scoring and Credit Control VI, Edinburgh, UK.

Roshanov, P., Fernandes, N., Wilczynski, J., Hemens, B., You, J., Handler, S., & Haynes, R. et al. (2013). Features of effective computerised clinical decision support systems: Meta-regression of randomised trials. *BMJ (Clinical Research Ed.)*, 346. PMID:23412440

Saitoh, S. (1988). *Theory of Reproducing Kernels and its Applications*. Harlow, UK: Longman Scientific & Technical.

Schoenberg, I. J. (1942). Positive definite functions on spheres. *Duke Mathematical Journal, 9*(1), 96–108. doi:10.1215/S0012-7094-42-00908-6

Scholkopf, B. (1997). *Support Vector Learning*. Munchen: R. Oldenbourg Verlag.

Scholkopf, B., & Smola, A. J. (1999). M uller, K.R. Kernel principal component analysis. In B. Scholkopf, C. J. C. Burges, & A. J. Smola (Eds.), *Advances in Kernel Methods - Support Vector Learning* (pp. 327–352). Cambridge, MA: MIT Press.

Schurmann, J. (1996). *Pattern Classification: a unified view of statistical and neural approaches*. New York: Wiley.

Stat News. (2016). Retrieved from https://www.statnews.com/2016/10/03/machine-learning-medicine-health/

Stitson, M., & Gammerman, A. (1999). Support vector regression with ANOVA decomposition kernels. In B. Scholkopf, C. J. C. Burges, & A. J. Smola (Eds.), *Advances in Kernel Methods — Support Vector Learning* (pp. 285–292). Cambridge, MA: Academic Press.

Vapnik, V. (1995). *The Nature of Statistical Learning Theory*. Springer. doi:10.1007/978-1-4757-2440-0

Vapnik, V. (1998). *Statistical Learning Theory*. Wiley.

Wahba, G. (1990). Spline Models for Observational Data. SIAM.

Williams, C. K. I. (2001). On a connection between kernel PCA and metric multi-dimensional scaling. In T. K. Leen, T. G. Dietterich, & V. Tresp (Eds.), Advances in Neural Information Processing Systems. MIT Press.

World Health Organization. (2015). *World Health Statistics 2015*. World Health Organization.

Compilation of References

Abaza, A., Harrison, M. A., Bourlai, T., & Ross, A. (2014). Design and evaluation of photometric image quality measures for effective face recognition. *IET Biometrics*, *3*(4), 314–324. doi:10.1049/iet-bmt.2014.0022

Abenstein, J. P., & Tompkins, W. J. (1982). A new data-reduction algorithm for real-time ECG analysis. *IEEE Transactions on Bio-Medical Engineering*, *BME-29*(1), 43–48. doi:10.1109/TBME.1982.324962 PMID:7076268

Abinaya, K. (2015). Data Mining with Big Data e-Health Service Using Map Reduce. *International Journal of Advanced Research in Computer and Communication Engineering, 4*(2).

Abrahamsen, P. (1992). *A review of Gaussian random fields and correlation functions.* Rapport 917, Norwegian Computing Center.

Adams, W. G., Fuhlbrigge, A. L., Miller, C. W., Panek, C. G., Gi, Y., & Loane, K. C. et al.. & Friedman, R. H. (2003). TLC-Asthma: an integrated information system for patient-centered monitoring, case management, and point-of-care decision support. In *AMIA Annual Symposium Proceedings* (Vol. 2003, p. 1). American Medical Informatics Association.

Agarwal, T. (n.d.). *Automatic Railway Gate Control System Alert via SMS.* Retrieved from https://www.elprocus.com/automatic-railway-gate-control-system-projects-using-microcontroller

Agarwal, P., & Searls, D. B. (2009, November). Can literature analysis identify innovation drivers in drug discovery? *Nature Reviews. Drug Discovery*, *8*(11), 865–878. doi:10.1038/nrd2973 PMID:19876041

Ågerfalk, P. J., & Fitzgerald, B. (2006). Introduction. *Communications of the ACM*, *49*(10), 26–34. doi:10.1145/1164394.1164416

Ahmad & Habibi. (2011). A Wimax Solution For Real-Time Video Surveillance In Public Transport. *International Journal of Computer Networks & Communications, 3*(2).

Ahmed, Björkman, Čaušsević, Fotouhi, & Linden. (n.d.). *An Overview on the Internet of Things for Health Monitoring Systems*. Retrieved from https://www.researchgate.net/publication/281062554

Aizerman, M. A., Braverman, E. M., & Rozonoer, L. I. (1964). Theoretical foundations of the potential function method in pattern recognition learning. *Automation and Remote Control*, *25*, 821–837.

Alam, M. R., Reaz, M. B. I., & Ali, M. A. M. (2012). A review of smart homes—Past, present, and future. *IEEE Transactions on Systems, Man and Cybernetics. Part C, Applications and Reviews*, *42*(6), 1190–1203. doi:10.1109/TSMCC.2012.2189204

Alappanavar, P., Shewale, K., Markad, Y., & Patil, N. (2016). *Intrusion Detection System for Networks Using K-Means ANN Algorithm.* Academic Press.

Alcaraz, J., Vales Alonso, J., & Garcia Haro, J. (2009). Control-based scheduling with QoS support for vehicle to infrastructure communications. *Wireless Communications*, *16*(6), 32–39. doi:10.1109/MWC.2009.5361176

Alexander, C. A., & Wang, L. (2017). Big data analytics in heart attack prediction. *The Journal of Nursing Care*, *6*(393). doi:10.4172/2167-1168.1000393

Alliance Cloud Security. (2013). *Top Ten Big Data Security and Privacy Challenges*. Alliance.

Al-Shaqi, R., Mourshed, M., & Rezgui, Y. (2016, May). Progress in ambient assisted systems for independent living by the elderly. *SpringerPlus*, *5*(1), 624. doi:10.1186/s40064-016-2272-8 PMID:27330890

Ambrose, A. F., Paul, G., & Hausdorff, J. M. (2013). Risk factors for falls among older adults: A review of the literature. *Maturitas*, *75*(1), 51–61. doi:10.1016/j.maturitas.2013.02.009 PMID:23523272

Aminikhanghahi, S., & Cook, D. (2017). A survey of methods for time series change point detection. *Knowledge and Information Systems*, *51*(2), 339–367. doi:10.1007/s10115-016-0987-z PMID:28603327

Anderson, K. M., Wilson, P. W. F., Odell, P. M., & Kannel, W. B. (1991). An updated coronary risk profile: A statement for health professionals. *Circulation*, *83*, 357–363. doi:10.1161/01.CIR.83.1.356

Anderson, R. A., Issel, L. M., & McDaniel, R. R. Jr. (2003). Nursing homes as complex adaptive systems: Relationship between management practice and resident outcomes. *Nursing Research*, *52*(1), 12–21. doi:10.1097/00006199-200301000-00003 PMID:12552171

Antman, E. M., Benjamin, E. J., Harrington, R. A., Houser, S. R., Peterson, E. D., Bauman, M. A., & Wayte, P. et al. (2015). Acquisition, analysis, and sharing of data in 2015 and beyond: A survey of the landscape. *Journal of the American Heart Association*, *4*(11), e002810. doi:10.1161/JAHA.115.002810 PMID:26541391

Aronszajn, N. (1950). Theory of reproducing kernels. *Transactions of the American Mathematical Society*, *68*(3), 337–404. doi:10.1090/S0002-9947-1950-0051437-7

Aryanto, K. Y. E., van Kernebeek, G., Berendsen, B., Oudkerk, M., & van Ooijen, P. M. A. (2016). Image de-identification methods for clinical research in the XDS environment. *Journal of Medical Systems*, *40*(4), 1–8. doi:10.1007/s10916-016-0431-7 PMID:26811074

Ash, J., McCormack, J., Sittig, D., Wright, A., McMullen, C., & Bates, D. (2012). Standard practices for computerized clinical decision support in community hospitals: A national survey. *Journal of the American Medical Informatics Association*, *19*(6), 980–987. doi:10.1136/amiajnl-2011-000705 PMID:22707744

Ashrafi, N., Kelleher, L., & Kuilboer, J.-P. (2014). The impact of business intelligence on healthcare delivery in the USA. *Interdisciplinary Journal of Information, Knowledge, and Management*, *9*, 117–130.

Ashton, K. (2009). That Internet of Things Thing: In the Real World Things Matter More than Ideas. *RFID Journal*. Retrieved from http://www.rfidjournal.com/articles/view?4986

AT&T Laboratories Cambridge. (2002). *The database of faces*. Retrieved from http://www.cl.cam.ac.uk/research/dtg/attarchive/facedatabase.html

Ataei, M., Shahsavany, H., & Mikaeil, R. (2013). Monte Carlo Analytic Hierarchy Process (MAHP) approach to selection of optimum mining method. *International Journal of Mining Science and Technology*, *23*(4), 573–578. doi:10.1016/j.ijmst.2013.07.017

Atallah, M. J., & Frikken, K. B. (2010). Securely outsourcing linear algebra computations. *Proceedings of the 5th ACM Symposium on Information, Computer and Communications Security - ASIACCS '10*, 48. https://doi.org/10.1145/1755688.1755695

Atallah, M. J., Pantazopoulos, K. N., Rice, J. R., & Spafford, E. E. (2002). Secure outsourcing of scientific computations. *Advances in Computers, 54*(C), 215–272. https://doi.org/10.1016/S0065-2458(01)80019-X

Au, A. W. S., Feng, C., Valaee, S., Reyes, S., Sorour, S., Markowitz, S. N., & Eizenman, M. et al. (2013). Indoor tracking and navigation using received signal strength and compressive sensing on a mobile device. *IEEE Transactions on Mobile Computing, 12*(10), 2050–2062. doi:10.1109/TMC.2012.175

Auffray, C. (2016). Making sense of big data in health research: Towards an EU action plan. *Genome Medicine, 8*(71), 1–13. doi:10.1186/s13073-016-0323-y PMID:26750923

Augusto, J., Kramer, D., Alegre, U., Covaci, A., & Santokhee, A. (2017). The user-centred intelligent environments development process as a guide to co-create smart technology for people with special needs. *Universal Access in the Information Society*, 1–16.

Azadeh, A., Saberi, M., Anvari, M., & Moghaddam, M. (2010). An integrated ANN-K-Means algorithm for improved performance assessment of electricity distribution units. *Journal of Scientific and Industrial Research, 69*, 672–679.

Baig, M. M., & Gholamhosseini, H. (2013). Smart health monitoring systems: An overview of design and modeling. *Journal of Medical Systems, 37*(2), 9898. doi:10.1007/s10916-012-9898-z PMID:23321968

Bajikar, S. (2002). Trusted platform module (tpm) based security on notebook pcs-white paper. Mobile Platforms Group Intel Corporation, 1–20.

Balubaid, M. A., & Basheikh, M. A. (2016). Using the analytic hierarchy process to prioritize alternative medicine: Selecting the most suitable medicine for patients with diabetes. *International Journal of Basic and Applied Sciences, 5*(1), 67. doi:10.14419/ijbas.v5i1.5607

Barlow, S. (2014). *Healthcare Data Warehouse Models Explained.* Retrieved June 20, 2016, https://www.healthcatalyst.com/best-healthcare-data-warehouse-model

Bartlett, P. L., & Scholkopf, B. (2001). *Some kernels for structured data. Technical report.* Biowulf Technologies.

Bashkirov, O. A., Braverman, E. M., & Muchnik, I. B. (1964). Theoretical foundations of the potential ´ function method in pattern recognition learning. *Automation and Remote Control, 25*, 629–631.

Becker, P. (2010). *Improving Healthcare: A Data Mining Approach.* Academic Press.

Belenkiy, M., Chase, M., Erway, C. C., Jannotti, J., Küpçü, A., & Lysyanskaya, A. (2008). Incentivizing outsourced computation. *Proceedings of the 3rd international workshop on Economics of networked systems*, 85–90. doi:10.1145/1403027.1403046

Bengio, Y., Courville, A., & Vincent, P. (2013). Representation learning: A review and new perspectives. *IEEE Transactions on Pattern Analysis and Machine Intelligence, 35*(8), 1798–1828. doi:10.1109/TPAMI.2013.50 PMID:23787338

Benioff. (2015). *Industrial Internet of Things: Unleashing the Potential of Connected Products and Services.* Academic Press.

Benjamin, D., & Atallah, M. J. (2008). Private and Cheating-Free Outsourcing of Algebraic Computations. *2008 Sixth Annual Conference on Privacy, Security and Trust*, 240–245. https://doi.org/10.1109/PST.2008.12

Berg, C., Christensen, J. P. R., & Ressel, P. (1984). *Harmonic Analysis on Semigroups.* New York: Springer-Verlag. doi:10.1007/978-1-4612-1128-0

Berry, J. A., & Linoff, G. (2004). *Data Mining Techniques: For Marketing, Sales, and Customer Relationship Management.* Wiley.

Bhattacharjee & Bera. (2014). Development of smart detachable wireless sensing system for environmental monitoring. *International Journal on Smart Sensing and Intelligent Systems*, *7*(3).

Big Data Value Association. (2016). *Big Data Technologies in Healthcare, Needs, opportunities and challenges*. TF/ Healthcare subgroup.

Big data. (2008). Retrieved from http://www.nature.com/news/specials/bigdata/ index.html

Bijandi, M., Maddah, M. G., & Mogharabi, V. (2014). *Using a combined method of hierarchical analysis and Monte Carlo simulation in order to identify and prioritize the target market selection criteria (Case study: Food distribution companies of Mashhad, Iran)*. Academic Press.

Blanton, M., Zhang, Y., & Frikken, K. B. (2013). Secure and verifiable outsourcing of large-scale biometric computations. *ACM Transactions on Information and System Security*, *16*(3), 1–33. doi:10.1145/2535523

Blumenthal, D. (2010). Launching HITECH. *The New England Journal of Medicine*, *362*(5), 382–385. doi:10.1056/ NEJMp0912825 PMID:20042745

Blythe, Rackliff, Holland, & Mageean. (2000). ITS applications in public transport: Improving the service to the transport system. *Article in Journal of Advance Transportation*. doi: 10.1002/atr.5670340302

Boguševičius, A., Maleckas, A., Pundzius, J., & Skaudickas, D. (2002). Prospective randomised trial of computer-aided diagnosis and contrast radiography in acute small bowel obstruction. *European Journal of Surgery*, *168*(2), 78–83. doi:10.1080/11024150252884287 PMID:12113275

Boser, B. E., Guyon, I. M., & Vapnik, V. (1992). A training algorithm for optimal margin classifiers. In D. Haussler (Ed.), *Proceedings of the 5th Annual ACM Workshop on Computational Learning Theory* (pp. 44–152). ACM Press. doi:10.1145/130385.130401

Bouchard, K., Bouchard, B., & Bouzouane, A. (2017). *Practical Guidelines to Build Smart Homes: Lessons Learned, Opportunistic Networking: Vehicular, D2D and Cognitive Radio Networks*. CRC Press, Taylor & Francis.

Bouchard, B. (2017). *Smart Technologies in Healthcare*. CRC Press, Taylor & Francis. doi:10.1201/9781315145686

Bouchard, B., Bouzouane, A., & Giroux, S. (2007, July). A Keyhole Plan Recognition Model for Alzheimers Patients. *Journal of Applied Artificial Intelligence, Taylor & Francis*, *22*(7), 623–658. doi:10.1080/08839510701492579

Bouchard, K., Gaboury, S., Bouchard, B., Bouzouane, A., & Giroux, S. (2016). Smart Homes in the Era of Big Data. In *Trends in Ambient Intelligent Systems* (pp. 117–137). Springer. doi:10.1007/978-3-319-30184-6_5

Boureau, Y. L., & Cun, Y. L. (2008). Sparse feature learning for deep belief networks. In Advances in neural information processing systems (pp. 1185-1192). Academic Press.

Bronstein, A. M., Bronstein, M. M., & Kimmel, R. (2007). Expression-invariant representations of faces. *IEEE Transactions on Image Processing*, *16*(1), 188–197. doi:10.1109/TIP.2006.884940 PMID:17283777

Burges, C. J. C. (1998). A tutorial on support vector machines for pattern recognition. *Data Mining and Knowledge Discovery*, *2*(2), 121–167. doi:10.1023/A:1009715923555

Burges, C. J. C. (1999). Geometry and invariance in kernel based methods. In B. Scholkopf, C. J. C. Burges, & A. J. Smola (Eds.), *Advances in Kernel Methods — Support Vector Learning* (pp. 89–116). Cambridge, MA: MIT Press.

Burges, C. J. C., & Vapnik, V. (1995). *A new method for constructing artificial neural networks. Interim technical report, ONR contract N00014-94-c-0186*. AT&T Bell Laboratories.

Burke, R. (2002). Hybrid recommender systems: Survey and experiments. *User Modeling and User-Adapted Interaction*, *12*(4), 331–370. doi:10.1023/A:1021240730564

Byrne, A., & Womack, J. P. (2012). *The Lean Turnaround: How Business Leaders Use Lean Principles to Create Value and Transform Their Company*. McGraw-Hill.

Cambria, E., & Hussain, A. (2015). *Sentic computing: a common-sense-based framework for concept-level sentiment analysis* (Vol. 1). Springer. doi:10.1007/978-3-319-23654-4

Can, A. (2013). *Benchmarking of data mining techniques as applied to power system analysis*. Department of Information Technology, Uppsala University.

Canadian Institute for Health Information (CIHI). (2011). *Les soins de santé au Canada 2011: Regard sur les personnes âgées et le vieillissement*. Author.

Canadian Mortage and Housing Coporation (CMHC). (2013). *Report, National Seniors' Housing Survey*. Author.

Canning, C. G. (2014). *Prevention of falls in Parkinson's disease: A review of fall risk factors and the role of physical interventions*. Future Medicine.

Cao, Z., & Liu, L. (2016). Comment on harnessing the Cloud for Securely Outsourcing Large-Scale Systems of Linear Equations.. *IEEE Transactions on Parallel and Distributed Systems*, *27*(5), 1551–1562. doi:10.1109/TPDS.2016.2531669

Carayon, P. (Ed.). (2012). *Handbook of Human Factors and Ergonomics in Health Care and Patient Safety*. CRC Press, Taylor & Francis.

Carayon, P., Schoofs, A. H., Karsh, B.-T., Gurses, A. P., Alvarado, C. J., & Smith, M. (2006). Flatley, Work system design for patient safety: The SEIPS model. *Quality & Safety in Health Care*, *15*(suppl_1), 50–58. doi:10.1136/qshc.2005.015842

Carberry, S. (2001). *Techniques for Plan Recognition, User Modeling and User Adapted-Interaction*. Academic Press.

Cederberg, S., & Widdows, D. (2003). Using LSA and noun coordination information to improve the precision and recall of automatic hyponymy extraction. *Proc of CoNLL'03*. doi:10.3115/1119176.1119191

Centers for Disease Control and Prevention. (2017). *Interactive atlas of heart disease and stroke*. Retrieved from the Centers for Disease Control and Prevention website: https://nccd.cdc.gov/dhdspatlas/

Chae, Y. M., Kim, H. S., Tark, K. C., Park, H. J., & Ho, S. H. (2003). Analysis of healthcare quality indicator using data mining and decision support system. *Expert Systems with Applications*, *24*(2), 167–172. doi:10.1016/S0957-4174(02)00139-2

Chamberlin, B. (n.d.). *Healthcare Internet of Things: 18 trends to watch in 2016*. IBM Center for Applied Insights. Retrieved from https://ibmcai.com/2016/03/01/healthcare-internet-of-things-18-trends-to-watch-in-2016/

Charalabidis, Y., Triantafillou, A., Karkaletsis, V., & Loukis, E. (2012). Public policy formulation through non moderated crowdsourcing in social media. In *International Conference on Electronic Participation* (pp. 156-169). Springer Berlin Heidelberg. doi:10.1007/978-3-642-33250-0_14

Chathurange, K. H. L., Rathnayaka, R. M. D. P. K., & Wimalasiri, T. S. N. (2015). Railway Warning and Control Systems. In *Proceedings of 8th International Research Conference*. KDU.

Chatzimilioudis, G. (2011). Crowdsourcing with Smartphones. *IEEE Internet Computing*.

Chaudhry, B., Wang, J., Wu, S., Maglione, M., Mojica, W., Roth, E., & Shekelle, P. et al. (2006). Systematic review: Impact of health information technology on quality, efficiency, and costs of medical care. *Annals of Internal Medicine*, *144*(10), 742–752. doi:10.7326/0003-4819-144-10-200605160-00125 PMID:16702590

Che, D., Safran, M., & Peng, Z. (2013). From Big Data to Big Data Mining: challenges, issues, and opportunities. In *Database Systems for Advanced Applications* (pp. 1–15). Berlin, Germany: Springer. doi:10.1007/978-3-642-40270-8_1

Chen, F., Xiang, T., Lei, X., & Chen, J. (2014). Highly Efficient Linear Regression Outsourcing to a Cloud. *IEEE Transactions on Cloud Computing*. https://doi.org/10.1109/TCC.2014.2378757

Chen, X., Li, J., & Ma, J. (2014). *New algorithms for secure outsourcing of modular exponentiations*. Academic Press.

Chen, D., Wang, X., Liu, W., Zeng, Y., & Chen, Z. (2016). Ebd extended analytic hierarchy process (Ahp) approach to evaluating the effectiveness of engineering projects. *Journal of Integrated Design and Process Science*, *19*(2), 49–70. doi:10.3233/jid-2015-0012

Chen, F., Xiang, T., Lei, X., & Chen, J. (2015). *Highly Efficient Linear Regression Outsourcing to a Cloud*. Academic Press.

Chen, F., Xiang, T., & Yang, Y. (2014). Privacy-preserving and verifiable protocols for scientific computation outsourcing to the cloud. *Journal of Parallel and Distributed Computing*, *74*(3), 2141–2151. doi:10.1016/j.jpdc.2013.11.007

Chen, X., Huang, X., Li, J., Ma, J., Lou, W., & Wong, D. S. (2015). *New Algorithms for Secure Outsourcing of Large-Scale Systems of Linear Equations*. Academic Press.

Christin, Reinhardt, Mogre, & Steinmetz. (n.d.). *Wireless Sensor Networks and the Internet of Things: Selected Challenges*. Retrieved from http://www.ti5.tu-harburg.de/events/fgsn09/proceedings/fgsn_031.pdf

Chuck, D., & Chang, J. M. (2010). Bandwidth Recycling in IEEE 802.16 Networks. *IEEE Transactions on Mobile Computing*, *9*(10), 1451–1465. doi:10.1109/TMC.2010.115

Chung, K. M., Kalai, Y., & Vadhan, S. (2010). Improved delegation of computation using fully homomorphic encryption. *Lecture Notes in Computer Science*, *6223*, 483–501. https://doi.org/10.1007/978-3-642-14623-7_26

Cisco, V. N. I. (2017). *The Zettabyte Era: Trends and Analysis*. White Paper. Cisco Public. Retrieved from http://www.cisco.com/c/en/us/solutions/collateral/service-provider/visual networking-index-vni/vni-hyperconnectivity-wp.html

Cohen, T., & Widdows, D. (2009). Empirical distributional semantics: Methods and biomedical applications. *Journal of Biomedical Informatics*, *42*(2), 390–405. doi:10.1016/j.jbi.2009.02.002 PMID:19232399

Colbaugh, R., & Glass, K. (2011). Agile sentiment analysis of social media content for security informatics applications. In *Intelligence and Security Informatics Conference (EISIC)* (pp. 327-331). IEEE. doi:10.1109/EISIC.2011.65

Cook, D., Crandall, A. S., Thomas, B. L., & Krishnan, N. C. (2013). CASAS: A smart home in a box. *Computer*, *46*(7), 62–69. doi:10.1109/MC.2012.328 PMID:24415794

Cook, D., Feuz, F., & Krishnan, N. (2013). Transfer learning for activity recognition: A survey. *Knowledge and Information Systems*, *36*(3), 537–556. doi:10.1007/s10115-013-0665-3 PMID:24039326

Cortes, C., & Vapnik, V. (1995). Support-vector networks. *Machine Learning*, *20*(3), 273–297. doi:10.1007/BF00994018

Cramer, R., & Damgård, I. (2001). Secure Distributed Linear Algebra in a Constant Number of Rounds. *Crypto*, *2139*, 119–136. https://doi.org/10.1007/3-540-44647-8_7

Cressie, N. A. C. (1993). *Statistics for Spatial Data*. New York: J. Wiley and Sons.

Cristianini, N., & Taylor, J. S. (2000). *An Introduction to Support Vector Machines*. Cambridge, UK: Cambridge University Press.

Cukier, K. (2010). *Data, data everywhere: a special report on managing information. Economist Newspaper.*

Curioni, Murtas, & Silari. (n.d.). *Internet of Sensors*. Politecnico di Milano. Retrieved from https://indico.cern.ch/event/470460/attachments/1303283/1948255/P10_TWD2016_Cur ioni.pdf

Dadkhah, A., Bayati, N., & Khodadadi, A. (2016). *An investigation of the impact of size and location of dg on system reliability by employing sequential Monte Carlo simulation*. Academic Press.

Dai, W. (2014). A mapreduce implementation of C4. 5 decision tree algorithm. *International Journal of Database Theory and Application*, 49-60. doi:10.1007/978-3-642-02196-1

Davies, R. (2015). *The Internet of Things Opportunities and challenges*. Retrieved from http://www.europarl.europa.eu/RegData/etudes/BRIE/2015/557012/EPRS_BRI(2015)557012_EN.pdf

de Miguel & Castro. (2001). *Requirements and guidelines for distributed laboratorios applications migration*. LONG Project IST-1999-20393, D3.1.

de Miguel, T. P., & Castro, E. M. (2012). *Programming guidelines on transition to IPv6*. LONG (Laboratories Over Next Generation networks) project, IST-1999-20393.

Dehghan, A., Kovacevic, A., Karystianis, G., Keane, J. A., & Nenadic, G. (2015). Combining knowledge and data-driven methods for de-identification of clinical narratives. *Journal of Biomedical Informatics*, *58*(1), S53–S59. doi:10.1016/j.jbi.2015.06.029 PMID:26210359

Deliens, T., Clarys, P., De Bourdeaudhuij, I., & Deforche, B. (2014). Determinants of eating behaviour in university students: A qualitative study using focus group discussions. *BMC Public Health*, *14*(1), 1. doi:10.1186/1471-2458-14-53 PMID:24438555

Demchenko, Ngo, & Membrey. (2013). *Big Security for Big Data: Addressing Security Challenges for the Big Data Infrastructure*. Academic Press.

Demiris, G., Hensel, B. K., Skubic, M., & Rantz, M. (2008). Senior residents perceived need of and preferences for smart home sensor technologies. *International Journal of Technology Assessment in Health Care*, *24*(1), 120–124. doi:10.1017/S0266462307080154 PMID:18218177

Deqiang, H., Jain, M., & Xiangyang, L. U. (2008). *Development of Onboard Metro Passenger Information System. Proceeding in ICWMMN*. doi:10.1049/cp:20081022

Diamantaras, K. I., & Kung, S. Y. (1996). *Principal Component Neural Networks*. New York: Wiley.

Dilts, D., Khamalah, J., & Plotkin, A. (1995). Using cluster analysis for medical resource decision making. *Medical Decision Making*, *15*(4), 333–347. doi:10.1177/0272989X9501500404 PMID:8544677

Di, P. H. (2011). *A novel fall prevention scheme for intelligent cane robot by using a motor driven universal joint. In Micro-NanoMechatronics and Human Science* (pp. 391–396). IEEE.

Djajadi. (2016). Ambient Environment quality monitoring Using IoT Sensor Network. Interworking Indonesia Journal, 8(1).

Dlodlo, N. (2012). Adopting the internet of things technologies in environmental management in South Africa. In *International Conference on Environment Science and Engineering* (vol. 3). IACSIT Press.

Douglas, M. M., Clifford, G. D., Reisner, A., Long, W. J., Moody, G. B., & Mark, R. G. (2005). De-identification algorithm for free-text nursing notes. *Proceedings of Computers in Cardiology, 05*, 331–334.

Doust, D., & Walsh, Z. (2011). *Data mining clustering: A healthcare application*. Academic Press.

Dragusin, M., Stanga, D., Gurau, D., & Ionescu, E. (2014). Radiation monitoring under emergency conditions. *Rom. Journal. Phys., 59*(9-10), 891–903.

Dreier, J., & Kerschbaum, F. (2011). *Practical Secure and Efficient Multiparty Linear Programming Based on Problem Transformation*. Retrieved from http://eprint.iacr.org/2011/108

Drowning in numbers - digital data will flood the planet - and help us understand it better. (n.d.). Retrieved from http://www.economist.com/blogs/daily chart/2011/11/bigdata-0

Du, W., & Atallah, M. J. (2001). Privacy-preserving cooperative scientific computations. *Proceedings of the Computer Security Foundations Workshop*, 273–282. https://doi.org/10.1109/CSFW.2001.930152

Du, W., Chen, S., & Han, Y. S. (2004). Privacy-Preserving Multivariate Statistical Analysis: Linear Regression and Classification. *Proceedings of the 4th SIAM International Conference on Data Mining*, 222–233. Retrieved from http://citeseerx.ist.psu.edu/viewdoc/summary?doi=10.1.1.2.423

Durairaj, M., & Ranjani, V. (2013). Data mining applications in healthcare sector: a study. *Int. J. Sci. Technol. Res., 2*(10).

Edwin, M. F. (n.d.). *Big Data Healthcare, An overview of the challenges in data intensive health care*. Discussion Paper. Academic Press.

Eiza, M. H., Randles, M., Johnson, P., Shone, N., Pang, J., & Bhih, A. (2015). Rail Internet of Things: An Architectural Platform and Assured Requirements Model. *Proceedings of 15th IEEE International Conference on Computer and Information Technology*. doi:10.1109/CIT/IUCC/DASC/PICOM.2015.52

El-Hasnony, I. M. (2015). Comparative study among data reduction techniques over classification accuracy. *International Journal of Computer Applications*, 8-15.

Emam, K. E., & Malin, B. (2015). Appendix B: concepts and methods for de-identifying clinical trial data. In *Sharing Clinical Trial Data: Maximizing Benefits, Minimizing Risk* (pp. 203–256). Institute of Medicine of the National Academies.

Eveborn, P., Flisberg, P., & Rönnqvist, M. (2006). Laps Care—an operational system for staff planning of home care. *European Journal of Operational Research, 171*(3), 962–976. doi:10.1016/j.ejor.2005.01.011

Ezechina, Okwara, & Ugboaja. (2015). The Internet of Things (Iot): A Scalable Approach to Connecting Everything. *The International Journal of Engineering and Science, 4*(1), 9-12.

Fact sheet. (2012). *Big data across the federal government*. Retrieved from http:// www.whitehouse.gov/sites/default/files/microsites/ostp/big data fact sheet 3 29 2012.pdf

Fan, H., Cao, Z., Jiang, Y., Yin, Q., & Doudou, C. (2014). *Learning deep face representation*. arXiv:1403.2802

Fatima. (2015). Internet of things: A Survey on Architecture, Applications, Security, Enabling Technologies, Advantages & Disadvantages. *International Journal of Advanced Research in Computer and Communication Engineering, 4*(12).

Feldman, R. (2013). Techniques and applications for sentiment analysis. *Communications of the ACM, 56*(4), 82–89. doi:10.1145/2436256.2436274

Ferreira, N., Meireles, T., & Fonseca, J. A. (2009). An RSU coordination scheme for WAVE safety services support. *Proceedings of the IEEE Conference on Emerging Technologies & Factory Automation*, 1-4. doi:10.1109/ETFA.2009.5347231

Few, S. (2006). *Information Dashboard Design: The Effective Visual Communication of Data*. O'Reilly.

Financial Express Online. (2016). Now, smart cities to have redeveloped 'smart' railway stations; 5 things to know. *Financial Express*. Retrieved from http://www.financialexpress.com/economy/indian-railways-smart-cities-railway-station-redevelopment-mou-urban-developmen t-suresh-prabhu-venkaiah-naidu/424492/

Fisher, E. S., Wennberg, D. E., Stukel, T. A., Gottlieb, D. J., Lucas, F. L., & Pinder, E. L. (2003). The implications of regional variations in Medicare spending. Part 1: The content, quality, and accessibility of care. *Annals of Internal Medicine*, *138*(4), 273–287. doi:10.7326/0003-4819-138-4-200302180-00006 PMID:12585825

Fokum, D. T., & Victor, S. (2010). A Survey on Methods for Broadband Internet Access on Trains. IEEE Communications Surveys & Tutorials, 12(2).

Fortin-Simard, D., Bilodeau, J. S., Bouchard, K., Gaboury, S., Bouchard, B., & Bouzouane, A. (2015). Exploiting passive RFID technology for activity recognition in smart homes. *IEEE Intelligent Systems*, *30*(4), 7–15. doi:10.1109/MIS.2015.18

Fortnow, L., & Lund, C. (1993, May). Interactive proof systems and alternating time—space complexity. *Theoretical Computer Science*, *113*(1), 55–73. doi:10.1016/0304-3975(93)90210-K

Friedman, J. (2001). The elements of statistical learning (Vol. 1). New York: Springer.

Gaikwad, S. M., Joshi, R. R., & Kulkarni, A. J. (2017). Cohort Intelligence and Genetic Algorithm Along with Modified Analytical Hierarchy Process to Recommend an Ice cream to Diabetic Patient. In *Proceedings of the International Conference on Data Engineering and Communication Technology* (pp. 279-288). Springer Singapore. doi:10.1007/978-981-10-1675-2_29

Gaikwad, S. M., Joshi, R. R., & Mulay, P. (2016). System Dynamics Modeling for Analyzing Recovery Rate of Diabetic Patients by Mapping Sugar Content in Ice cream and Sugar Intake for the Day. In *Proceedings of the Second International Conference on Computer and Communication Technologies* (pp. 743-749). Springer India. doi:10.1007/978-81-322-2517-1_71

Gaikwad, S. M., Joshi, R. R., & Kulkarni, A. J. (2015, December). Cohort Intelligence and Genetic Algorithm along with AHP to recommend an Ice cream to a Diabetic Patient. In *International Conference on Swarm, Evolutionary, and Memetic Computing* (pp. 40-49). Springer International Publishing.

Gaikwad, S. M., Joshi, R. R., & Mulay, P. (2015). Analytical Network Process (ANP) to Recommend an Ice cream to a Diabetic Patient. *International Journal of Computers and Applications*, *121*(12).

Gaikwad, S. M., Joshi, R., & Gaikwad, S. M. (2016, March). Modified analytical hierarchy process to recommend an ice cream to a diabetic patient. In *Proceedings of the Second International Conference on Information and Communication Technology for Competitive Strategies* (p. 138). ACM. doi:10.1145/2905055.2905198

Gaikwad, S. M., Mulay, P., & Joshi, R. R. (2015). Analytical Hierarchy Process to Recommend an Ice cream to a Diabetic Patient Based on Sugar Content in it. *Procedia Computer Science*, *50*, 64–72. doi:10.1016/j.procs.2015.04.062

Ganasegeran, K., Al-Dubai, S. A., Qureshi, A. M., Al-Abed, A. A. A., Rizal, A. M., & Aljunid, S. M. (2012). Social and psychological factors affecting eating habits among university students in a Malaysian medical school: A cross-sectional study. *Nutrition Journal*, *11*(1), 1. doi:10.1186/1475-2891-11-48 PMID:22809556

Gantz, J., & Reinsel, D. (2011). Extracting value from chaos. *IDC iView*, 1–12.

Garfinkel, S. L. (2015). *De-identification of personal information. National Institute of Standards and Technology Internal Report 8053*. Department of Commerce. doi:10.6028/NIST.IR.8053

Gennaro, R., Gentry, C., & Parno, B. (2010). Non-interactive verifiable computing: Outsourcing computation to untrusted workers. *Lecture Notes in Computer Science, 6223*, 465–482. https://doi.org/10.1007/978-3-642-14623-7_25

Gentry, C. (2009). *A Fully Homomorphic Encryption Scheme* (PhD thesis). https://doi.org/10.1145/1536414.1536440

Gentry, C. (2010). Computing arbitrary functions of encrypted data. *Communications of the ACM*, *53*(3), 97. doi:10.1145/1666420.1666444

Ghosh & Nath. (2015). Big Data Security Issues and Challenges. *International Journal of Innovative Research in Advanced Engineering, 2*, 15-20.

Gilligan. (2002). *Basic Socket Interface Extensions for IPv6*. Obsoletes RFC 2553.

Girosi, F. (1998). An equivalence between sparse approximation and support vector machines. *Neural Computation*, *10*(6), 1455–1480. doi:10.1162/089976698300017269 PMID:9698353

Giroux, S., & Pigot, H. (2013). Smart homes for people suffering from cognitive disorders. *Computer Science and Ambient Intelligence*, 225-262.

Glenisson, P., Antal, P., Mathys, J., Moreau, Y., & Moor, B. D. (2003). Evaluation Of The Vector Space Representation In Text-Based Gene Clustering. *Proc Pacific Symposium of Biocomputing*, 391–402.

Glorot, X., Bordes, A., & Bengio, Y. (2011, June). Deep sparse rectifier neural networks. In *Proceedings of the Fourteenth International Conference on Artificial Intelligence and Statistics* (pp. 315-323). Academic Press.

Goldreich, O., Micali, S. W. A., Goldreich, O., Micali, S., & Wigderson, A. (1987). How To Play Any Mental Game, or A Completeness Theorem for Protocols with Honest Majority. *Proceedings of 19th Annual ACM Symposium on Theory of Computing*. https://doi.org/10.1145/28395.28420

Goldwasser, S., Kalai, Y. T., & Rothblum, G. N. (2008). Delegating Computation: Interactive Proofs for Muggles. *Stoc, 62*(4), 113–122. https://doi.org/http://doi.acm.org/10.1145/1374376.1374396

Goldwasser, S., Micali, S., & Rackoff, C. (1989). The Knowledge Complexity of Interactive Proof Systems. *SIAM Journal on Computing*, *18*(1), 186–208. doi:10.1137/0218012

Gonçalves, P., Araújo, M., Benevenuto, F., & Cha, M. (2013). Comparing and combining sentiment analysis methods. In *Proceedings of the first ACM conference on Online social networks* (pp. 27-38). ACM. doi:10.1145/2512938.2512951

Grant, T. J. (2014). *Measuring sit-to-stand timing variability over time using under mattress pressure sensor technology. In Medical Measurements and Applications*. IEEE.

Granville, V. (2014). *16 analytic disciplines compared to data science*. Retrieved June 20, 2016, http://www.datasciencecentral.com/profiles/blogs/17-analytic-disciplines-compared

Groves, P., Kayyali, B., Knott, D., & Kuiken, S. V. (2016). *The big data revolution in healthcare: Accelerating value and innovation*. Academic Press.

Groves, P., Kayyali, B., Knott, D., & Van Kuiken, S. (2013). The 'big data' revolution in healthcare. *The McKinsey Quarterly*, *2*, 3.

Guidi, G., Miniati, R., Mazzola, M., & Iadanza, E. (2016). Case study: IBM Watson Analytics cloud platform as analytics-as-a-service system for heart failure early detection. *Future Internet*, *8*(32), 1–16. doi:10.3390/fi8030032

Guimaraes, V. R. (2013). *A smartphone-based fall risk assessment tool: Measuring one leg standing, sit to stand and falls efficacy scale. In e-Health Networking, Applications & Services*. IEEE.

Gutierrez, D. (2013). *Data Science 101: Probability and Monte Carlo Methods*. Retrieved July 05, 2016, http://insidebigdata.com/2013/12/26/data-science-101-probability-monte-carlo-methods/

Guyon, I., Boser, B., & Vapnik, V. (1993). *Automatic capacity tuning of very large VC-dimension classifiers.* In S. J. Hanson, J. D. Cowan, & C. Lee Giles (Eds.), Advances in Neural Information Processing Systems (Vol. 5, pp. 147–155). San Mateo, CA: Morgan Kaufmann.

Hamilton, B. (2012). *Big Data is the Future of Healthcare*. Cognizant 20-20 Insights.

Hao, M., Rohrdantz, C., Janetzko, H., Dayal, U., Keim, D. A., Haug, L.-E., & Hsu, M.-C. (2011). Visual sentiment analysis on twitter data streams. In *Visual Analytics Science and Technology (VAST)* (pp. 277-278). IEEE. doi:10.1109/VAST.2011.6102472

Harsh, K.P., & Seshadri, R. (n.d.). *Big data security and privacy issues in healthcare*. Academic Press.

Hastie, T. J., & Stuetzle, W. (1989). Principal curves. *Journal of the American Statistical Association, 84*(406), 502–516. doi:10.1080/01621459.1989.10478797

Haussler, D. (1999). *Convolutional kernels on discrete structures*. Technical Report UCSC-CRL-99-10, Computer Science Department, University of California at Santa Cruz.

Haykin, S. (1999). *Neural Networks: A Comprehensive Foundation*. Pearson education.

He, W., Goodkind, D., & Kowal, P. (2016). *An Aging World: International Population Report*. National Institute on Aging (NIA).

Health Care. (n.d.). Retrieved July 01, 2016, http://www.shimko1to1.com/health-care/

Helal, S., Mann, W., El-Zabadani, H., King, J., Kaddoura, Y., & Jansen, E. (2005). The gator tech smart house: A programmable pervasive space. *Computer, 38*(3), 50–60. doi:10.1109/MC.2005.107

Hersh, W. (2009). *Information retrieval: a health and biomedical perspective* (3rd ed.). New York: Springer Verlag. doi:10.1007/978-0-387-78703-9

HIPAA. (1996). *Health Insurance Portability and Accountability Act of 1996. 104th United State Congress.*

Hirata, Y. M. (2006). *Motion control of intelligent passive-type walker for fall-prevention function based on estimation of user state. In Robotics and Automation* (pp. 3498–3503). IEEE.

Hodge, V. J., OKeefe, S., Weeks, M., & Moulds, A. (2015). Wireless Sensor Networks For Condition Monitoring In The Railway Industry: A Survey. *IEEE Transactions on Intelligent Transportation Systems, 16*(3), 1088–1106. doi:10.1109/TITS.2014.2366512

Hogenboom, A., Bal, D., Frasincar, F., Bal, M., de Jong, F., & Kaymak, U. (2013). Exploiting emoticons in sentiment analysis. In *Proceedings of the 28th Annual ACM Symposium on Applied Computing* (pp. 703-710). ACM. doi:10.1145/2480362.2480498

Homann, M., Banova, V., Oelbermann, P., Wittges, H., & Krcmar, H. (2014). Towards User Interface Components for Dashboard Applications on Smartphones. In G. Memmi & U. Blanke (Eds.), *Mobile Computing, Applications, and Services. MobiCASE 2013. Lecture Notes of the Institute for Computer Sciences, Social Informatics and Telecommunications Engineering* (Vol. 130, pp. 19–32). Springer. doi:10.1007/978-3-319-05452-0_2

Hong, Y., Vaidya, J., & Lu, H. (2012). Secure and efficient distributed linear programming. *Journal of Computer Security, 20*(5), 583–634. doi:10.3233/JCS-2012-0452

Horta, E. T. (2013). *Real time falls prevention and detection with biofeedback monitoring solution for mobile environments. In e-Health Networking, Applications & Services*. IEEE.

Horwitz-Bennett, B. (2014). *Staff Support: Designing Optimal Healthcare Work Environments*. Healthcare Design Magazine.

Hotelling, H. (1933). Analysis of a complex of statistical variables into principal components. *Journal of Educational Psychology, 24*, 417–441, 498–520.

Hough, A. (2012). *Ice cream as 'addictive as drugs' says new study*. Retrieved June 22, 2016, http://www.telegraph.co.uk/news/science/science-news/9118768/Ice-cream-as-addictive-as-drugs-says-new-study.html

Hsu, P. F., Lin, E. P., & Tsai, C. W. (2016). Optimal Selection of Business Managers for Integrated Marketing Communications Companies Using AHP and GRA. *International Journal of Customer Relationship Marketing and Management, 7*(2), 16–29. doi:10.4018/IJCRMM.2016040102

Hsu, T. H., & Pan, F. F. (2009). Application of Monte Carlo AHP in ranking dental quality attributes. *Expert Systems with Applications, 36*(2), 2310–2316. doi:10.1016/j.eswa.2007.12.023

Huang, Dong, Duan, & Li. (n.d.). Similarity Measure Between Patient Symptoms for Clinical Pathway Analysis: Problem, Method, and Applications. *IEEE Journal of Biomedical and Health Informatics, 18*(1), 4-14.

Hunter, J. G., & Cason, K. L. (n.d.). *Healthy Eating Habits for Children*. Retrieved from http://www.clemson.edu/extension/hgic/food/pdf/hgic4109.pdf

Huston, G. (2010). *IPv4 Address Report*. Tech. Rep. Available: http://www.potaroo.net/tools/ipv4

Hu, X., & Tang, C. (2015). Secure outsourced computation of the characteristic polynomial and eigenvalues of matrix. *Journal of Cloud Computing, 4*(1), 4–9. https://doi.org/10.1186/s13677-015-0033-9

I. S. I. at University of Southern California. (1981). *Internet Protocol, DARPA Internet Program, Protocol Specification*. Author.

IEEE Secretary. (2007). Wireless LAN Medium Access Control (MAC) and Physical Layer (PHY) Specifications. IEEE Std. 802.11.

IETF RFC 791. (2011). *Internet Usage Statistics*. Miniwatts Marketing Group, Tech. Rep. Available: http://www.internetworldstats.com

Inanloo, M., Ashouri, M., Gheibi, S., & Hemmatyar, A. A. (2012, October). A new approach for multi-source data prediction in Wireless Sensor Networks: Collaborative filtering. In *Wireless Communications & Signal Processing (WCSP), 2012 International Conference on* (pp. 1-6). IEEE.

Informatica. (2012). *Healthcare data management: expanding insight, increasing efficiency, improving care*. Informatica Corporation.

International Markets Bureau. (n.d.). *The Global Flavour Industry*. Retrieved from https://www.gov.mb.ca/agriculture/market-prices-and-statistics/food-and-value-added-agriculture-statistics/pubs/ma_global_flavours_industry_en.pdf

Jaakkola, T. S., & Haussler, D. (1999). Probabilistic kernel regression models. *Proceedings of the 1999 Conference on AI and Statistics*.

Jain, A. K., & Li, S. Z. (2011). Handbook of face recognition. New York: Springer.

Jain, A. K., Flynn, P., & Ross, A. A. (2007). *Handbook of biometrics*. Secaucus.

Jiang, P., Xia, H., He, Z., & Wang, Z. (2009). Design of a Water Environment Monitoring System Based on Wireless Sensor Networks. *Sensors (Basel, Switzerland)*, *9*(9), 6411–6434. doi:10.3390/s90806411 PMID:22454592

Jing, L., Chen, B., Zhang, B., Li, P., & Zheng, J. (2012). Monte Carlo simulation–aided analytic hierarchy process approach: Case study of assessing preferred non-point-source pollution control best management practices. *Journal of Environmental Engineering*, *139*(5), 618–626. doi:10.1061/(ASCE)EE.1943-7870.0000673

Jin, R., Goswami, A., & Agrawal, G. (2006). Fast and exact out-of-core and distributed K-Means clustering. *Knowledge and Information Systems*, *10*(1), 17–40. doi:10.1007/s10115-005-0210-0

Joanne, M., & Demand, M. (n.d.). *Advantages & Disadvantages of Ice cream to Human Health.* Retrieved from http://healthyeating.sfgate.com/advantages-disadvantages-ice-cream-human-health-2858.html

Jolliffe, I. T. (1986). *Principal Component Analysis*. New York: Springer-Verlag. doi:10.1007/978-1-4757-1904-8

Jones, S., Hara, S., & Augusto, J. C. (2015). eFRIEND: An ethical framework for intelligent environments development. *Ethics and Information Technology*, *17*(1), 11–25. doi:10.1007/s10676-014-9358-1

Joshi, R. R., Kadam, K. D., Shelke-Bembde, M., & Deshmukh-Joshi, V. (2015). PBR: Perspective Based Ranking of Selected State IT Policy Documents in India using AHP. *International Journal of Applied Engineering Research*, *10*(20), 41353–41356.

Kakulapati, V. (2011). Improved Web Search Engine by New Similarity Measures. *Proc of TREC'11*. doi:10.1007/978-3-642-22726-4_30

Kanungo, T., Mount, D. M., Netanyahu, N. S., Piatko, C. D., Silverman, R., & Wu, A. Y. (2002). An efficient K-Means clustering algorithm: Analysis and implementation. *IEEE Transactions on Pattern Analysis and Machine Intelligence*, *24*(7), 881–892. doi:10.1109/TPAMI.2002.1017616

Kaur & Singh. (2016). A Survey Report on Internet of Things Applications. *International Journal of Computer Science Trends and Technology*, *4*(2).

Kawamoto, K., Houlihan, C., Balas, E., & Lobach, D. (2005). Improving clinical practice using clinical decision support systems: A systematic review of trials to identify features critical to success. *BMJ (Clinical Research Ed.)*, *330*(7494), 765. doi:10.1136/bmj.38398.500764.8F PMID:15767266

Kharya, S. (2012). Using data mining techniques for diagnosis and prognosis of cancer disease. *International Journal of Computer Science, Engineering and Information Technology, 2*(2).

Kientz, J. A., Patel, S. N., Jones, B., Price, E. D., Mynatt, E. D., & Abowd, G. D. (2008). The georgia tech aware home. In *CHI'08 extended abstracts on Human factors in computing systems* (pp. 3675–3680). ACM.

Kiltz, E., Mohassel, P., Weinreb, E., & Franklin, M. K. (2007). Secure Linear Algebra Using Linearly Recurrent Sequences. *Theory of Cryptography, 4th Theory of Cryptography Conference Proceedings, 4392*, 291–310. https://doi.org/10.1007/978-3-540-70936-7_16

Koh, H. C., & Tan, G. (2011). Data mining applications in healthcare. *Journal of Healthcare Information Management*, *19*(2), 65. PMID:15869215

Konasani, V., Biswas, M., & Koleth, P.K. (2012). *Healthcare Fraud Management using Big Data Analytics*. A White-paper by Trendwise Analytics.

Kou, G., Ergu, D., Peng, Y., & Shi, Y. (2012). *Data Processing for the AHP/ANP* (Vol. 1). Springer Science & Business Media.

Krizhevsky, A., Sutskever, I., & Hinton, G. E. (2012). Imagenet classification with deep convolutional neural networks. In Advances in neural information processing systems (pp. 1097-1105). Academic Press.

Krumholz, H. M. (2008). Outcomes research: Generating evidence for best practice and policies. *Circulation, 118*(3), 309–318. doi:10.1161/CIRCULATIONAHA.107.690917 PMID:18625906

Kulkarni, A., Tokekar, V., & Kulkarni, P. (2015). Discovering context of labeled text documents using context similarity coefficient. Procedia Computer Science, 49C(9), 118-127.

Kulkarni, P. A., & Mulay, P. (2013). Evolve systems using incremental clustering approach. *Evolving Systems*, *4*(2), 71–85. doi:10.1007/s12530-012-9068-z

Kumar, R. (2015). *IoT, Internet of Things and Indian Railway*. Retrieved from http://www.blog.indianrailways.gov.in / internet-of-things-iot-and-indian-railways/

Kumar. (2012). A Framework for Integration and Standardization of Data from Heterogeneous Sources. *American Journal of Database Theory and Application*. DOI: 10.5923/j.database.20120101.01

Laddha, A. R., Joshi, R. R., & Mulay, P. (2016). Enriching process of ice cream recommendation using combinatorial ranking of AHP and Monte Carlo AHP. *Journal of Theoretical & Applied Information Technology*, *85*(3), 298.

Lampropulos, J. F., Gupta, A., Kulkarni, V. T., Mody, P., Chen, R., Bikdeli, B., & Dharmarajan, K. (2013). Most important outcomes research papers on variation in cardiovascular disease. *Circulation: Cardiovascular Quality and Outcomes*, *6*(2), e9–e16. doi:10.1161/CIRCOUTCOMES.113.000185 PMID:23481532

Lapointe, J., Verreault, A., Bouchard, B., Bouchard, J., Potvin, A., & Bouzouane, A. (2013). How to maximize the effectiveness of prompts in assistive technologies according to the particular cognitive profile of people with alzheimer. *International Journal of Smart Home*, *7*(5), 19–38. doi:10.14257/ijsh.2013.7.5.03

Laud, P., & Pankova, A. (n.d.). *Transformation-Based Outsourcing of Linear Equation Systems over Real Numbers*. Retrieved from http://eprint.iacr.org/2015/322

Lee, Tewolde, & Kwon. (2014). Design and Implementation of Vehicle Tracking System UsingGPS/GSM/GPRS Technology and Smart Phone Application. *IEEE World Forum on Internet of Things (WF-IoT)*.

Lee, J., Maslove, D. M., & Dubin, J. A. (2015). Personalized mortality prediction driven by electronic medical data and a patient similarity metric. *PLoS ONE*, *10*(5), e0127428. doi:10.1371/journal.pone.0127428 PMID:25978419

Lee, W. S. (2001). *Real time data mining-based intrusion detection. In Information Survivability Conference & Exposition* (pp. 89–100). IEEE.

Lei, X., Liao, X., Huang, T., Li, H., & Hu, C. (2013). Outsourcing Large Matrix Inversion Computation to A Public Cloud. *IEEE Transactions on Cloud Computing, 1*(1), 1–1. https://doi.org/10.1109/TCC.2013.7

Lei, X., Liao, X., Huang, T., & Heriniaina, F. (2014). Achieving security, robust cheating resistance, and high-efficiency for outsourcing large matrix multiplication computation to a malicious cloud. *Information Sciences*, *280*, 205–217. doi:10.1016/j.ins.2014.05.014

Lei, X., Liao, X., Member, S., Huang, T., & Li, H. (2015). Cloud Computing Service. *The Case of Large Matrix Determinant Computation*, *8*(5), 688–700.

Lemuye, E. (2011). *HIV Status Predictive Modeling Using Data Mining Technology* (Doctoral dissertation). AAU.

Li, D., Park, H. W., Batbaatar, E., Piao, Y., & Ryu, K. H. (2016). Design of health care system for disease detection and prediction on Hadoop using DM techniques. In *Proceedings of the 2nd International Conference on Health Informatics and Medical Systems* (pp. 124-129). Las Vegas, NV: WORLDCOMP.

Liao, M., Li, Y., Kianifard, F., Obi, E., & Arcona, S. (2016). Cluster analysis and its application to healthcare claims data: A study of end-stage renal disease patients who initiated hemodialysis. *BMC Nephrology*, *17*(1), 25. doi:10.1186/s12882-016-0238-2 PMID:26936756

Li, L., Cheng, W.-Y., Glicksberg, B. S., Gottesman, O., Tamler, R., Chen, R., & Dudley, J. T. et al. (2015). Identification of type2 diabetes sub groups through topological analysis of patient similarity. *Science Translational Medicine*, *7*(311), 311ra174. doi:10.1126/scitranslmed.aaa9364 PMID:26511511

Lin, K., & Chen, M. S. (2010). Privacy-preserving outsourcing support vector machines with random transformation. *Proceedings of the 16th ACM SIGKDD International Conference on Knowledge Discovery and Data Mining*, 363–372. https://doi.org/10.1145/1835804.1835852

Lin, C. C., Chiu, M. J., Hsiao, C. C., Lee, R. G., & Tsai, Y. S. (2006). Wireless health care service system for elderly with dementia. *IEEE Transactions on Information Technology in Biomedicine*, *10*(4), 696–704. doi:10.1109/TITB.2006.874196 PMID:17044403

Lindell, Y., & Pinkas, B. (2009). Secure Multiparty Computation for Privacy-preserving Data Mining. *Journal of Privacy and Confidentiality*, *1*(1), 59–98.

Linden, G., Smith, B., & York, J. (2003). Amazon. com recommendations: Item-to-item collaborative filtering. *IEEE Internet Computing*, *7*(1), 76–80. doi:10.1109/MIC.2003.1167344

Liu, W., & Park, E. K. (2014). Big Data as an e-Health Service. *International Conference on Computing, Networking and Communications*, 982-988.

Li, Y., Wu, C., Guo, L., Lee, C. H., & Guo, Y. (2014). Wiki-Health: a big data platform for health sensor data management. In A. Moumtzoglou & A. Kastania (Eds.), *Cloud Computing Applications for Quality Health Care Delivery* (pp. 59–77). Hershey, PA: IGI Global. doi:10.4018/978-1-4666-6118-9.ch004

Loghmanpour, N. A., Kormos, R. L., Kanwar, M. K., Teuteberg, J. J., Murali, S., & Antaki, J. F. (2016). A Bayesian model to predict right ventricular failure following left ventricular assist device therapy. *JACC: Heart Failure*, *4*(9), 722–725. doi:10.1016/j.jchf.2016.04.004 PMID:27289403

Lohr, S. (2012). The age of big data. *New York Times*, p. 11.

Lopes, J. B.-A. (2010). *Traffic and mobility data collection for real-time applications. Intelligent Transportation Systems* (pp. 216–223). IEEE.

López-Alt, A., Tromer, E., & Vaikuntanathan, V. (2012). On-the-fly multiparty computation on the cloud via multikey fully homomorphic encryption. *Proceedings of the 44th Symposium on Theory of Computing - STOC '12*, 1219. https://doi.org/10.1145/2213977.2214086

MacKay, D. J. C. (1998). Introduction to Gaussian processes. In C. M. Bishop (Ed.), *Neural Networks and Machine Learning* (pp. 133–165). Berlin: Springer-Verlag.

Majumder, A. J. (2013). iPrevention: Towards a novel real-time smartphone-based fall prevention system. *Symposium on Applied Computing* (pp. 513-518). ACM. doi:10.1145/2480362.2480462

Majumder, A. J. (2013). *SmartPrediction: A real-time smartphone-based fall risk prediction and prevention system. In Research in Adaptive and Convergent Systems*. ACM. doi:10.1145/2513228.2513267

Mäkelä, K., Belt, S., Greenblatt, D., & Häkkilä, J. (2007). Mobile interaction with visual and RFID tags: a field study on user perceptions. In *Proceedings of the SIGCHI conference on Human factors in computing systems* (pp. 991-994). ACM. doi:10.1145/1240624.1240774

Mandwel, A. A., & Anjum, A. (2013). Detection of Brain Tumor Using K-Means Clustering. *International Journal of Science and Research, 5*(6).

Maniya, H., Hasan, M. I., & Patel, K. P. (2011). Comparative study of Naïve Bayes Classifier and KNN for Tuberculosis. *International Conference on Web Services Computing (ICWSC).*

Manyika, J., Chui, M., Brown, B., Bughin, J., Dobbs, R., Roxburgh, C., & Byers, A.H. (2011). *Big data: The next frontier for innovation, competition, and productivity*. Report McKinsey Global Institute.

Marie, J., & Media, D. *Advantages & Disadvantages of Ice cream to Human Health.* Retrieved June 28, 2016, http://healthyeating.sfgate.com/advantages-disadvantages-ice-cream-human-health-2858.html

Matsumoto. (2014). Development of On-board Passenger Information Display. Hitachi Review, 63(10).

Mattern & Floerkemeier. (n.d.). *From the Internet of Computers to the Internet of Things*. Academic Press.

McCarney, R. W., Warner, J., Iliffe, S., van Haselen, R., Griffin, M., & Fisher, P. (2007). The Hawthorne Effect: A randomised, controlled trial. *BMC Medical Research Methodology, 7*(1), 30. doi:10.1186/1471-2288-7-30 PMID:17608932

McLachlan, G. J. (1992). Cluster analysis and related techniques in medical research. *Statistical Methods in Medical Research, 1*(1), 27–48. doi:10.1177/096228029200100103 PMID:1341650

Mell, P., & Grance, T. (2011). The NIST Definition of Cloud Computing Recommendations of the National Institute of Standards and Technology. *National Institute of Standards and Technology, Information Technology Laboratory, 145*, 7. https://doi.org/10.1136/emj.2010.096966

Miceli. (2013). *Energy Management and Smart Grids Energies*. Academic Press.

Mihailidis, A., Boger, J., & Kautz, H. (2011). *Technology and Aging, Assistive Technology Research Series* (Vol. 21). IOS Press.

Mingle, D. (n.d.). *4 big reasons why healthcare needs data science*. Retrieved July 10, 2016, http://www.cio.com/article/3001216/analytics/4-big-reasons-why-healthcare-needs-data-science.html

Mirzabeiki. (n.d.). *An Overview of the Freight Intelligent Transportation Systems*. Division of Logistics and Transportation, Chalmers University of Technology. Retrieved from http://www.bth.se/tek/intelligent_gods.nsf/bilagor/Mirzabeiki,2010,ITS%20World%20Busan_pdf/$file/Mirzabeiki,2010,ITS%20World%20Busan.pdf

Mitchell, M. (1996). *An Introduction to Genetic Algorithms*. Cambridge, MA: MIT Press.

Mitchell, T. (1997). *Machine Learning*. New York: McGraw-Hill.

Moatamed, B., Shahmohammadi, F., Ramezani, R., Naeim, A., & Sarrafzadeh, M. (2016). Low-cost indoor health monitoring system. In *Wearable and Implantable Body Sensor Networks (BSN), 2016 IEEE 13th International Conference on* (pp. 159-164). IEEE.

Mohammad, S. M. (2016). Challenges in sentiment analysis. In A Practical Guide to Sentiment Analysis. Springer.

Mohammeda & Ahmedb. (2017). Internet of Things Applications, Challenges and Related Future Technologies. *WSN, 67*(2), 126-148.

Mohanty, S., Jagadeesh, M., & Srivatsa, H. (2013). *Big Data Imperatives*. Apress Publications. doi:10.1007/978-1-4302-4873-6

Mohassel, P. (2011). Efficient and Secure Delegation of Linear Algebra. *IACR Cryptology ePrint Archive*, 1–33. Retrieved from http://eprint.iacr.org/2011/605.pdf

Mohassel, P., & Weinreb, E. (2008). Efficient secure linear algebra in the presence of covert or computationally unbounded adversaries. *Lecture Notes in Computer Science, 5157*, 481–496. https://doi.org/10.1007/978-3-540-85174-5_27

Mohassel, R. R. (2014). A survey on Advanced Metering Infrastructure. *International Journal of Electrical Power & Energy Systems, 63*, 473–484. doi:10.1016/j.ijepes.2014.06.025

Momani, A. M., & Ahmed, A. A. (2011). Material handling equipment selection using hybrid Monte Carlo simulation and analytic hierarchy process. *World Academy of Science, Engineering and Technology, 59*, 953–958.

Monrose, F., Wyckoff, P., & Rubin, A. (1999). Distributed execution with remote audit. *Ndss*. Retrieved from http://www.isoc.org/isoc/conferences/ndss/99/proceedings/papers/monrose.pdf

Motwani, M. (2017). Machine learning for prediction of all-cause mortality in patients with suspected coronary artery disease: A 5-year multicentre prospective registry analysis. *European Heart Journal, 38*, 500–507. doi:10.1093/eurheartj/ehw188 PMID:27252451

Moura & Serrao. (n.d.). *Security and Privacy Issues of Big Data*. Academic Press.

Mubashir, M. S., Shao, L., & Seed, L. (2013). A survey on fall detection: Principles and approaches. *Neurocomputing, 100*, 144–152. doi:10.1016/j.neucom.2011.09.037

Mudur, G. (2015). *App to pick right ice cream- Engineers propose tool to match tastes with health needs*, Retrieved June 29, 2016, http://www.telegraphindia.com/1150517/jsp/frontpage/story_20548.jsp#.V45o3qIzzIU

Muir, S. W., Berg, K., Chesworth, B., & Speechley, M. (2008). Use of the Berg Balance Scale for predicting multiple falls in community-dwelling elderly people: A prospective study. *Physical Therapy, 88*(4), 449–459. doi:10.2522/ptj.20070251 PMID:18218822

Mukherji, A. (n.d.). *Indian Healthcare system: Challenges and Opportunities*. Retrieved from http://tejas.iimb.ac.in/interviews/41.php

Mulay, P., & Kulkarni, P. A. (2013). Knowledge augmentation via incremental clustering: New technology for effective knowledge management. *International Journal of Business Information Systems, 12*(1), 68–87. doi:10.1504/IJBIS.2013.050660

Munaye. (2016). Big data: Security issues, challenges and future scope. *International Journal of Computer Engineering & Technology, 4*(7), 12-24.

Murray, Minevich, & Abdoullaev. (2011). Being smart about smart cities. *KM World*.

Nagaraj, R. (2016). Health care analysis for process deviation using alpha-fitness algorithm in process mining. *Journal of Theoretical & Applied Information Technology, 88*(3).

National Guideline Clearinghouse. (2013). *Guideline summary: 2013 AHA/ACC guideline on lifestyle management to reduce cardiovascular risk: a report of the American College of Cardiology/American Heart Association Task Force on Practice Guidelines*. Rockville, MD: Agency for Healthcare Research and Quality (AHRQ). Available: https://www.guideline.gov

National Rural Health Mission (NRHM). (n.d.). Retrieved from http://nrhm.gov.in/

Naveed, N., Gottron, T., Kunegis, J., & Alhadi, A. C. (2011). Bad news travel fast: A content-based analysis of interestingness on twitter. In *Proceedings of the 3rd International Web Science Conference* (p. 8). ACM. doi:10.1145/2527031.2527052

Niewolny, D. (n.d.). *How the Internet of Things Is Revolutionizing Healthcare*. Retrieved from https://cache.freescale.com/files/corporate/doc/white_paper/IOTREVHEALCARWP.pdf

Nimbalkar, S. P. (2016). Real-Time Data Pre-processing Technique in Web Usage Mining. *International Journal of Innovative Research in Computer.*

Niño, M., & Illarramendi, A. (2015). Understanding big data: Antecedents, origin and later development. *DYNA New Technologies*, *2*, 1–8. doi:10.6036/NT7835

Nissim, K., & Weinreb, E. (2006). Communication efficient secure linear algebra. *Lecture Notes in Computer Science, 3876*, 522–541. https://doi.org/10.1007/11681878_27

Nordmark, E. (2000). *Stateless IP/ICMP Translator (SIIT)*. RFC 2765.

Nuaimi. (2015). Applications of big data to smart cities. *Journal of Internet Services and Applications.*

Oderanti, F. O. (2012). *Commercialisation of Assisted Living Technologies and Services: A Framework for Sustainable Business Models*. Cardiff, UK: BAM.

Oja, E. (1982). A simplified neuron model as a principal component analyzer. *Journal of Mathematical Biology*, *15*(3), 267–273. doi:10.1007/BF00275687 PMID:7153672

O'Reilly, T., Loukides, M., Steele, J., & Hill, C. (2012). *How data science is transforming health care*. O'Reilly Media, Inc.

Ostankov, A., Röhrbein, F., & Waltinger, U. (2014). LinkedHealthAnswers: towards linked data-driven question answering for the healthcare domain. In *Proceedings of the Ninth International Conference on Language Resources and Evaluation* (pp. 2613-2620). Reykjavik, Iceland: ELRA.

Otis, M. J. (2012). *Toward an augmented shoe for preventing falls related to physical conditions of the soil. In Systems, Man, and Cybernetics (SMC)* (pp. 3281–3285). IEEE.

Page, D. (2015). *Predicting health events from electronic health records using machine learning. Talk by David Page at the Center for Predictive Computational Phenotyping*. University of Wisconsin.

Papadaki, A., Hondros, G., Scott, J. A., & Kapsokefalou, M. (2007). Eating habits of university students living at, or away from home in Greece. *Appetite*, *49*(1), 169–176. doi:10.1016/j.appet.2007.01.008 PMID:17368642

Parthasarathy, K. R., & Schmidt, K. (1972). Positive definite kernels, continuous tensor products, and central limit theorems of probability theory. Springer-Verlag. doi:10.1007/BFb0058340

Patel, S., & Patel, H. (2016). Survey of data mining techniques used in healthcare domain. *International Journal of Information*, *6*(1/2).

Patsadu, O., Nukoolkit, C., & Watanapa, B. (2012). Human gesture recognition using Kinect camera. *International Joint Conference on Computer Science and Software Engineering (JCSSE)* (pp. 28-32). IEEE.

Paul, R., & Hoque, A. S. M. L. (2010, July). Clustering medical data to predict the likelihood of diseases. In *Digital Information Management (ICDIM), 2010 Fifth International Conference on* (pp. 44-49). IEEE. doi:10.1109/ICDIM.2010.5664638

Perk, J. et al.. (2012). European guidelines on cardiovascular disease prevention in clinical practice. *European Heart Journal*, *33*(13), 1635–1701. doi:10.1093/eurheartj/ehs092

Peter, A. D. (2014). Big Data Analytics and Hadoop in Developing Indias Healthcare Services. *International Journal of Computers and Applications*, *89*(16), 44–50. doi:10.5120/15719-4622

Ponemon Institute. (2016). *Sixth annual benchmark study on privacy & security of healthcare data*. Ponemon Institute LLC.

Prabowo & Thelwall. (2009). Sentiment analysis: A combined approach. *Journal of Informetrics, 3*(2), 143-157. doi.org/10.1016/j.joi.2009.01.003

Preeti, M., Rahul, J., Aditya, A., Alisha, G., & Deepankar, G. (2017). *Threshold based clustering algorithm analyzes diabetic mellitus*. Academic Press.

Priyavadana, V., Sivashankari, A., & Senthil Kumar, R. (2015). A comparative study of data mining applications in diagnosing diseases. *International Research Journal of Engineering and Technology, 2*(7).

Qureshi, F., & Terzopoulos, D. (2008). Smart Camera Networks in Virtual Reality. *Proceedings of the IEEE*, *96*(10), 1640–1656. doi:10.1109/JPROC.2008.928932

Rabiner, L. (1990). A Tutorial on Hidden Markov Models and Selected Applications in Speech Recognition. *Proceeding of the IEEE, 77*(2).

Radcliffe, N., & Surry, P. (1999). Differential response analysis: Modeling true response by isolating the effect of a single action. In Credit Scoring and Credit Control VI, Edinburgh, UK.

Rafferty, J., Nugent, C. D., Liu, J., & Chen, L. (2017). From activity recognition to intention recognition for assisted living within smart homes. *IEEE Transactions on Human-Machine Systems*, *47*(3), 368–379. doi:10.1109/THMS.2016.2641388

Ram, J., & Comesa, P. (n.d.). *Secure Direct and Iterative Protocols for Solving Systems of Linear Equations. Academic Press.*

Ramos, C. (2008). Ambient Intelligence: The Next Step for AI. *IEEE Intelligent Systems*, *23*(2), 15–18. doi:10.1109/MIS.2008.19

Ranjan, J. (2007). Applications of data mining techniques in pharmaceutical industry. *Journal of Theoretical and Applied Information Technology*, *3*(4), 61–67.

Raychaudhuri, S. (2008, December). *Introduction to monte carlo simulation. In 2008 Winter Simulation Conference* (pp. 91–100). IEEE. doi:10.1109/WSC.2008.4736059

Revelant, J. (2014). *4 shocking ways sugar affects your kid's health*. Retrieved from http://www.foxnews.com/health/2014/08/17/4-shocking-ways-sugar-affects-your-kids-health.html

Ricquebourg, V., Menga, D., Durand, D., Marhic, B., Delahoche, L., & Loge, C. (2006). The smart home concept: our immediate future. In *1st IEEE International Conference on E-Learning in Industrial Electronics* (pp. 23-28). IEEE. doi:10.1109/ICELIE.2006.347206

Rogers, G., & Joyner, E. (1997, March). Mining your data for health care quality improvement. *SAS User Group International Conference*, 641-647.

Romesburg, H. C. (1984). *Cluster analysis for researchers*. Belmont: Lifetime Learning Publications.

Rosen, J. A. (n.d.). *Data science solutions for healthcare*. Retrieved from https://www.leidos.com/sites/default/files/Leidos%20WP%20-%20Data%20Science%20Solutions%20for%20Health%201.15.pdf

Rosenthal, S., Nakov, P., Kiritchenko, S., Mohammad, S. M., Ritter, A., & Stoyanov, V. (2015). Semeval-2015 task 10: Sentiment analysis in twitter. In *Proceedings of the 9th international workshop on semantic evaluation (SemEval 2015)* (pp. 451-463). doi:10.18653/v1/S15-2078

Roshanov, P., Fernandes, N., Wilczynski, J., Hemens, B., You, J., Handler, S., & Haynes, R. et al. (2013). Features of effective computerised clinical decision support systems: Meta-regression of randomised trials. *BMJ (Clinical Research Ed.)*, 346. PMID:23412440

Roy, P., Bouchard, B., Bouzouane, A., & Giroux, S. (2013). *Ambient Activity Recognition in Smart Environments for Cognitive Assistance. International Journal of Robotics Applications and Technologies.*

Rumsfeld, J. S., Joynt, K. E., & Maddox, T. M. (2016). Big data analytics to improve cardiovascular care: Promise and challenges. *Nature Reviews. Cardiology*, *13*(6), 250–359. doi:10.1038/nrcardio.2016.42 PMID:27009423

Russell, S., & Norvig, P. (2009). Artificial Intelligence: A modern approach (3rd ed.). Academic Press.

Saad, Y. (2001). Parallel iterative methods for sparse linear systems. *Studies in Computational Mathematics, 8*(C), 423–440. https://doi.org/10.1016/S1570-579X(01)80025-2

Saaty, T. L. (2008). Decision making with the analytic hierarchy process. *International Journal of Services Sciences, 1*(1), 83-98.

Sahoo, Chiang, & Wu. (2014). SVANET: A Smart Vehicular *Ad Hoc* Network for Efficient Data Transmission with Wireless Sensors. *Positioning and Tracking Sensors and Technologies in Road Transport, 14*(12), 22230-22260. Retrieved from https://www.ncbi.nlm.nih.gov/pmc/articles/PMC4299011/

Saitoh, S. (1988). *Theory of Reproducing Kernels and its Applications*. Harlow, UK: Longman Scientific & Technical.

Salleh, S. (2013). *When Multiattribute Decision Analysis Needs Monte Carlo*. Retrieved from http://www.lumina.com/blog/when-multiattribute-decision-analysis-needs-monte-carlo

Sapna, S., Tamilarasi, A., & Pravin Kumar, M. (2012). Implementation of Genetic Algorithm in Predicting Diabetes. *International Journal of Computer Science Issues, 9*(1).

Saranya, C. M., & Nitha, K. P. (2015). Analysis of Security methods in Internet of Things. *International Journal on Recent and Innovation Trends in Computing and Communication, 3*(4).

Sartipi, K., Najafi, M., & Kazemzadeh, R. S. (2008). *Data and mined-knowledge interoperability in eHealth systems.* INTECH Open Access Publisher. doi:10.5772/6413

Schafer, J. B., Frankowski, D., Herlocker, J., & Sen, S. (2007). Collaborative filtering recommender systems. In *The adaptive web* (pp. 291–324). Springer Berlin Heidelberg.

Schatten, M., & Kakulapati, V. (2010). Reasoning about Social Semantic Web Applications using String Similarity and Frame Logic. *Proceedings of Central European Conference on Information and Intelligent System.* Doi:10.13140/2.1.4489.2163

Schmitt, C., Shoffner, M., Owen, P., Wang, X., Lamm, B., & Barker, M. J. (2013). Security and Privacy in the era of Big Data. *RENCI, 1.*

Schoenberg, I. J. (1942). Positive definite functions on spheres. *Duke Mathematical Journal, 9*(1), 96–108. doi:10.1215/S0012-7094-42-00908-6

Scholkopf, B. (1997). *Support Vector Learning*. Munchen: R. Oldenbourg Verlag.

Scholkopf, B., & Smola, A. J. (1999). M uller, K.R. Kernel principal component analysis. In B. Scholkopf, C. J. C. Burges, & A. J. Smola (Eds.), *Advances in Kernel Methods - Support Vector Learning* (pp. 327–352). Cambridge, MA: MIT Press.

Schurmann, J. (1996). *Pattern Classification: a unified view of statistical and neural approaches*. New York: Wiley.

Schwendimann, R. B., Bühler, H., De Geest, S., & Milisen, K. (2006). Falls and consequent injuries in hospitalized patients: Effects of an interdisciplinary falls prevention program. *BMC Health Services Research*, *6*(1), 69. doi:10.1186/1472-6963-6-69 PMID:16759386

Scruggs, S. B., Watson, K., Su, A. I., Hermjakob, H., Yates, J. R. III, Lindsey, M. L., & Ping, P. (2015). Harnessing the heart of big data. *Circulation Research*, *116*(7), 1115–1119. doi:10.1161/CIRCRESAHA.115.306013 PMID:25814682

Seel, T., Raisch, J., & Schauer, T. (2014). IMU-based joint angle measurement for gait analysis. *Sensors (Basel, Switzerland)*, *14*(4), 6891–6909. doi:10.3390/s140406891 PMID:24743160

Seetha Lakshmi, G., & Isakki, P. (2017). A Comparative Study of Data Mining Classification Technique Using HIV/AIDS and STD data. *International Journal of Innovative Research in Computer and Communication Engineering*, *5*(1).

Seshadri, A., Luk, M., Shi, E., Perrig, A., Van Doorn, L., & Khosla, P. (2005). Pioneer: Verifying integrity and guaranteeing execution of code on legacy platforms. In *Proceedings of ACM Symposium on Operating Systems Principles (SOSP)* (Vol. 173). doi:10.1145/1095810.1095812

Sharma, A., & Gupta, P. C. (2012). Predicting the number of blood donors through their age and blood group by using data mining tool. *International Journal of Communication and Computer Technologies*, *1*(6), 6-10.

Sharmila, K., & Vethamanickam, S. A. (2015). Application of mapreduce in diabetic dataset using hadoop platform. *International Journal of Applied Engineering Research.*, *10*(60), 15–20.

Shin et al. (2002). *Application Aspects of IPv6 Transition*. Academic Press.

Shiraz, M., Gani, A., Khokhar, R. H., & Buyya, R. (2013). A review on distributed application processing frameworks in smart mobile devices for mobile cloud computing. *IEEE Communications Surveys and Tutorials*, *15*(3), 1294–1313. doi:10.1109/SURV.2012.111412.00045

Shirudkar & Motwani. (2015). Big-Data Security. *International Journal of Advanced Research in Computer Science and Software Engineering*, 1100-1109.

Shortliffe, E. H., Davis, R., Axline, S. G., Buchanan, B. G., Green, C. C., & Cohen, S. N. (1975). Computer-based consultations in clinical therapeutics: Explanation and rule acquisition capabilities of the MYCIN system. *Computers and Biomedical Research, an International Journal*, *8*(4), 303–320. doi:10.1016/0010-4809(75)90009-9 PMID:1157471

Shumway-Cook, A. B. S. (2000). Predicting the probability for falls in community-dwelling older adults using the Timed Up & Go Test. *Physical Therapy*, 896–903. PMID:10960937

Siddique, H. (n.d.). *Sugar should be no more than 5% of daily calories, say nutrition experts*. Retrieved from https://www.theguardian.com/society/2015/jul/17/cut-recommended-daily-allowance-sugar-5-percent-daily-calories-report

Singh, A., Yadav, A., & Rana, A. (2013, April). K-means with Three different Distance Metrics. *International Journal of Computers and Applications*, *67*(10).

Smart Grid enabling energy efficiency and low-carbon transition. (n.d.). Retrieved from https://www.gov.uk/government/uploads/system/uploads/attachment_data/file/321852/Policy_Factsheet_-_Smart_Grid_Final__BCG_.pdf

Smith, S. W., & Weingart, S. (1999). Building a high-performance, programmable secure coprocessor. *Computer Networks*, *31*(8), 831–860. doi:10.1016/S1389-1286(98)00019-X

Smullyan, R. M. (1995). *First-Order Logic*. Dover Publications.

Special online collection: dealing with big data. (2011). Retrieved from http:// www.sciencemag.org/site/special/data/

Spring, G., Cook, D., Fritz, R., & Schmitter-Edgecombe, M. (2016). Detecting Health and Behavior Change by Analyzing Smart Home Sensor Data. *IEEE International Conference on Smart Computing*.

Srinivas, K., Rani, B. K., & Govrdhan, A. (2010). Applications of data mining techniques in healthcare and prediction of heart attacks. *International Journal on Computer Science and Engineering*, *2*(02), 250–255.

Srisuresh & Egevang. (2001). *Traditional IP Network Address Translator (Traditional NAT)*. RFC 3022.

Staranowicz, A. B. (2013). Evaluating the accuracy of a mobile Kinect-based gait-monitoring system for fall prediction. In *International Conference on Pervasive Technologies Related to Assistive*. ACM.

Stat News. (2016). Retrieved from https://www.statnews.com/2016/10/03/machine-learning-medicine-health/

StatCrunch. (2012). *Ice cream Survey Report*. Retrieved June 10, 2016, http://www.statcrunch.com/5.0/viewreport.php?reportid=25427

Statistics Canada. (2011). Canada Year Book 2011 Catalogue no. 11-402-X. Author.

Statistics Canada. (n.d.). *2016 Census*. Statistics Canada Catalogue no. 98-316-X2016001. Author.

Stitson, M., & Gammerman, A. (1999). Support vector regression with ANOVA decomposition kernels. In B. Scholkopf, C. J. C. Burges, & A. J. Smola (Eds.), *Advances in Kernel Methods — Support Vector Learning* (pp. 285–292). Cambridge, MA: Academic Press.

Stonová, M. (2014). Unstructured data in healthcare. *International Journal on Biomedicine and Healthcare*, *2*(1), 34–36.

Subaira, A.S., Gayathri, R., & Sindhujaa, N. (n.d.). Security Issues and Challenges in Big Data Analysis. *International Journal of Advanced Research in Computer Science and Software Engineering, 6*, 530-536.

Subramaniam, S., Dhillon, J. S., Ahmad, M. S., Teoh, C., Hassan, N. H., Ismail, Z., & Ranjan, K. S. (2016). Integrating health behavioural change theories in the design of prediabetes self-care applications: A systematic literature review. *Journal of Theoretical and Applied Information Technology*, *88*(2).

Suhas, G., Rahul, J., & Preeti, M. (2015). Cluster mapping with the help of new proposed algorithm and MCF algorithm to recommend an ice cream to the diabetic patient. *International Journal of Applied Engineering Research, 10*(8), 21259-21266.

Suhonen, J. (2013). *Experiences and Future Plans for WSN-enabled Service Development in Home Environment*. Realin white paper.

Suresh, S., & Sruthi, P. V. (2015). A review on smart home technology. *IEEE International Conference on Green Engineering and Technologies (IC-GET)*, 1-8.

Susmitha, P., & Sowmyabala, G. (2014). Design and Implementation of Weather Monitoring and Controlling System. *International Journal of Computers and Applications*, *97*(3).

Taigman, Y., Yang, M., Ranzato, M. A., & Wolf, L. (2014). Deepface: Closing the gap to human-level performance in face verification. In *Proceedings of the IEEE conference on computer vision and pattern recognition* (pp. 1701-1708). doi:10.1109/CVPR.2014.220

Talasila, Curtmola, & Borcea. (n.d.). *Mobile Crowd Sensing*. New Jersey Institute of Technology. Retrieved from https://web.njit.edu/~mt57/publications/Chapter4.pdf

Tamblyn, R., Huang, A., Perreault, R., Jacques, A., Roy, D., & Hanley, J. et al. Laprise, R. (2003). The medical office of the 21st century (MOXXI): Effectiveness of computerized decision-making support in reducing inappropriate prescribing in primary care. *Canadian Medical Association Journal, 169*(6), 549-556. PMID:12975221

Tanner, , Schreiber, M., Low, J. G. H., Ong, A., Tolfvenstam, T., Lai, Y. L., & Ooi, E. E. et al. (2008, March). Decision Tree Algorithms Predict the Diagnosis and Outcome of Dengue Fever in the Early Phase of Illness. *PLoS Neglected Tropical Diseases*, *2*(3), e196. doi:10.1371/journal.pntd.0000196 PMID:18335069

The Office of the National Coordinator for Health Information Technology. (2015). *Guide to privacy and security of electronic health information*. HHS.

Tomar, D., & Agarwal, S. (2013). A survey on Data Mining approaches for Healthcare. *International Journal of Bio-Science and Bio-Technology*, *5*(5), 241–266. doi:10.14257/ijbsbt.2013.5.5.25

Toor. (2008). Vehicle Ad Hoc Networks: Applications and Related Technical issues. *IEEE Communications Surveys & Tutorials, 10*(3), 74-88.

Tsirtsis & Srisuresh. (2000). *Network Address Translation – Protocol Translation (NAT-PT)*. RFC 2766.

Tsoi, K. K. F., Chan, F. C. H., Hirai, H. W., Leung, G. K. S., Kuo, Y. H., Tai, S., & Meng, H. (2017). Data visualization on global trends on cancer incidence an application of IBM Watson Analytics. In *Proceedings of the 50th Hawaii International Conference on System Sciences* (pp. 3283-3288). Waikoloa, HI: UH Mānoa Shidler College of Business. doi:10.24251/HICSS.2017.397

Tsuchiya, Higuchi, & Atarashi. (2000). *Dual Stack Hosts using the Bump-In-The-Stack technique (BIS)*. RFC 2767.

Tweets by @regionalvoice. (2014). *Open data in health+care- a blueprint*. Retrieved June23, 2016, http://www.regionalvoices.org/node/230

United Nations. (2015). *World Population Ageing. Dep. of Economic and Social Affairs*. Population Division.

ur Rehman, M. H. (2016). Big data reduction methods: a survey. *Data Science and Engineering*, 265-284. doi:10.1145/2504335.2504396

Vaishali, G., & Kalaivani, V. (2016). Big data analysis for heart disease detection system using map reduce technique. In *Proceedings of the 2016 International Conference on Computing Technologies and Intelligent Data Engineering* (pp. 1-6). Kovilpatti, India: IEEE. doi:10.1109/ICCTIDE.2016.7725360

Van Der Aalst, W. (2012, July 1). Process mining: Overview and opportunities. *ACM Transactions on Management Information Systems*, *3*(2), 7. doi:10.1145/2229156.2229157

Van Dijk, M., Gentry, C., Halevi, S., & Vaikuntanathan, V. (2010). Fully homomorphic encryption over the integers. *Advances in Cryptology–EUROCRYPT '10*, 24–43. https://doi.org/10.1007/978-3-642-38348-9_20

VanderMey, A. (2014). *Do we still scream for ice cream?* Retrieved June 10, 2016,http://fortune.com/2014/07/24/ice-cream-sales/

Vapnik, V. (1995). *The Nature of Statistical Learning Theory*. Springer. doi:10.1007/978-1-4757-2440-0

Vapnik, V. (1998). *Statistical Learning Theory*. Wiley.

Vellas, B. J., Wayne, S. J., Romero, L., Baumgartner, R. N., Rubenstein, L. Z., & Garry, P. J. (1997). One-leg balance is an important predictor of injurious falls in older persons. *Journal of the American Geriatrics Society*, *45*(6), 735–738. doi:10.1111/j.1532-5415.1997.tb01479.x PMID:9180669

Vermesan & Fries. (2014). *Internet of Things-From Research and Innovation to Market Deployment*. River Publisher Series in Communication.

Verstichel, S. (2006). On the Design of a Train Communication Management Platform. *Symposium on Communications and Vehicular Technology*, 29–34. doi:10.1109/SCVT.2006.334366

Wahba, G. (1990). Spline Models for Observational Data. SIAM.

Wang, C., Ren, K., Wang, J., & Urs, K. M. (2011). Harnessing the Cloud for Securely Solving Large-Scale Systems of Linear Equations. *2011 31st International Conference on Distributed Computing Systems, 24*(6), 549–558. https://doi.org/10.1109/icdcs.2011.41

Wang, C., Ren, K., & Wang, J. (2011). Secure and practical outsourcing of linear programming in cloud computing. *Proceedings - IEEE INFOCOM*, 820–828. https://doi.org/10.1109/INFCOM.2011.5935305

Wang, C., Ren, K., Wang, J., & Wang, Q. (2013). Harnessing the Cloud for Securely Outsourcing Large-Scale Systems of Linear Equations. *IEEE Transactions on Parallel and Distributed Systems, 24*(6), 1172–1181. doi:10.1109/TPDS.2012.206

Wang, H., Wang, W., Yang, J., & Yu, P. S. (2002). Clustering by Pattern Similarity in Large Data Sets. *Proceeding SIGMOD '02,* 394-405. doi:10.1145/564691.564737

Wazid & Goudar. (2013). *Big Data: Issues, Challenges, Tools and Good Practices*. Institute of Electrical and Electronics Engineers.

Weiss, A. S., Shimkin, I., Giladi, N., & Hausdorff, J. M. (2010). Automated detection of near falls: Algorithm development and preliminary results. *BMC Research Notes, 3*(1), 62. doi:10.1186/1756-0500-3-62 PMID:20205708

Whitworth, E., & Biddle, R. (2007). The social nature of agile teams. In Agile conference (AGILE), 2007 (pp. 26-36). IEEE. doi:10.1109/AGILE.2007.60

Wickramasinghe, N., Bali, R. K., Gibbons, M. C., Choi, J. H., & Schaffer, J. L. (2009). A systematic approach: Optimization of healthcare operations with knowledge management. *Journal of Healthcare Information Management, 23*(3), 44–50. PMID:19663164

Williams, C. K. I. (2001). On a connection between kernel PCA and metric multi-dimensional scaling. In T. K. Leen, T. G. Dietterich, & V. Tresp (Eds.), Advances in Neural Information Processing Systems. MIT Press.

Witten, H., Frank, E., & Hall, M. (2011). *Data Mining: Practical Machine Learning Tools and Techniques* (3rd ed.). Morgan Kaufmann.

World Health Organization. (2015). *World Health Statistics 2015*. World Health Organization.

World Health Organization. (2016). *HEARTS: Technical package for cardiovascular disease management in primary health care*. Geneva, Switzerland: World Health Organization.

Worldometers. (2014). *Real time world statistics*. Retrieved from http://www.worldometers.info/world-population/

Wu, Cui, & Wu, Liu, & Metz. (n.d.). Transition from IPv4 to IPv6: A State-of-the-Art Survey. *IEEE Communications Surveys and Tutorials*.

Xie, J., Xu, L., & Chen, E. (2012). Image denoising and inpainting with deep neural networks. In Advances in Neural Information Processing Systems (pp. 341-349). Academic Press.

Yang, X. (2010). *Engineering Optimization: An Introduction with Metaheuristic Applications*. Wiley. doi:10.1002/9780470640425

Yao, A. C. (1982). Protocols for secure computations. *23rd Annual Symposium on Foundations of Computer Science (Sfcs 1982)*, 1–5. https://doi.org/10.1109/SFCS.1982.38

Yao, A. C.-C. (1986). How to generate and exchange secrets. *27th Annual Symposium on Foundations of Computer Science (Sfcs 1986)*, (1), 162–167. https://doi.org/10.1109/SFCS.1986.25

Yaraghi, N., Tabesh, P., Guan, P., & Zhuang, J. (2015). Comparison of AHP and monte carlo AHP under different levels of uncertainty. *IEEE Transactions on Engineering Management*, *62*(1), 122–132. doi:10.1109/TEM.2014.2360082

Yee, B. (1994). *Using secure coprocessors*. Citeseer.

Yi, J., Nasukawa, T., Bunescu, R., & Niblack, W. (2003). Sentiment analyzer: Extracting sentiments about a given topic using natural language processing techniques. In *Data Mining, 2003. ICDM 2003. Third IEEE International Conference on* (pp. 427-434). IEEE. doi:10.1109/ICDM.2003.1250949

Yuki, N. (2011). *Following digital breadcrumbs to big data gold*. Retrieved from http://www.npr.org/2011/11/29/142521910/thedigitalbreadcrumbsthat-lead-to-big-data

Yuki, N. (2011). *The searchfor analysts to make sense ofbig data*. Retrieved from http://www.npr.org/2011/11/30/142893065/the-searchforanalyststo-make-sense-of-big-data

Zakrzewska, D. M.-L. (2009). *Methods and Supporting Technologies for Data Analysis*. Springer.

Zhang, S., Huang, Z., Sun, Y., & Guo, K. (2016). A Fuzzy Integrated Multi-Criteria Decision Approach to Select Green Logistics Provider for Sustainable Supply Chain. *Transylvanian Review, 24*(4).

Zhang, Y., & Blanton, M. (2014). *Efficient Secure and Verifiable Outsourcing of Matrix Multiplications*. https://doi.org/10.1007/978-3-319-13257-0_10

Zhang, Y., Liu, H., Su, X., Jiang, P., & Wei, D. (2015). Remote mobile health monitoring system based on smart phone and browser/server structure. *Journal of Healthcare Engineering, 6*(4), 717-738.

Zhang, P. (2014). Towards personalized medicine: Leveraging patient similarity and drug similarity analytics. *AMIAJt. Summits Transl. Sci. Proc.*, *2014*, 132–136. PMID:25717413

Zhang, Y., & Li, W. (2012, March). AHP Construct Mining Component strategy applied for data mining process. In *2012 IEEE International Conference on Information Science and Technology* (pp. 591-595). IEEE. doi:10.1109/ICIST.2012.6221714

Zhao, W., Ma, H., & He, Q. (2009). Parallel K-means clustering based on mapreduce. *Springer-Verlag Berlin Heidelberg.*, *5931*, 674–679.

Zhou, L., Li, C., & Member, S. (2016). *Outsourcing Eigen-Decomposition and Singular Value Decomposition of Large Matrix to a Public Cloud*. Academic Press.

Zhu, Z., Luo, P., Wang, X., & Tang, X. (2013). Deep learning identity-preserving face space. In *Proceedings of the IEEE International Conference on Computer Vision* (pp. 113-120). Academic Press.

Zwicker, M., Seitz, J., & Wickramasinghe, N. (2012). Identifying Critical Issues for Developing Successful E-Health Solutions. *Proceedings of the Pacific Asia Conference on Information Systems (PACIS)*. Retrieved from http://aisel.aisnet.org/pacis2012/33

About the Editors

Brojo Kishore Mishra (Ph.D. in Computer Science) is working as an Associate Professor in the Department of Information Technology at C. V. Raman College of Engineering (Autonomous), Bhubaneswar. He has been selected as State Student Coordinator (Odisha) and Regional Student Coordinator (CSI Region – IV) of Computer Society of India in 2015-16 and 2016-17 respectively. Now he has been elected as National Nomination Committee Member (2017-18) for Computer Society of India. Similarly he has been selected as IEEE Day Ambassador for Kolkata Section of IEEE Region – 10 for the year 2015, 2016 and 2017. He was the Jury Coordination Committee Member of All IEEE Young Engineers' Humanitarian Challenge (AIYEHUM 2015) project competition organized by IEEE Region 10 (Asia pacific). Currently he is guiding 05 Ph.D Scholar registered under the BPUT (A State Government Technical University). His present areas of research are Opinion Mining and Sentimental Analysis, Machine Learning, Data Science. He has already published more than 40 research papers in internationally reputed journals and referred conferences, 6 book chapters, has edited 1 book, and is acting as a member of the editorial board/associate editor / Guest editor of various International journals. He served in the capacity of Keynote Speaker, Plenary Speaker, Program Chair, Proceeding chair, Publicity chair, Special session chairperson and as member of programme committees of many international conferences also. He was associated with a CSI funded research project as a Principal Investigator. He is a life member of ISTE, CSI, and member of IEEE, IAENG, UACEE, and ACCS.

Raghvendra Kumar, Ph.D., has been working as Assistant Professor in Computer Science and Engineering Department at L.N.C.T Group of College Jabalpur, M.P. India. He received B. Tech. in Computer Science and Engineering from SRM University Chennai (Tamil Nadu), India, M. Tech. in Computer Science and Engineering from KIIT University, Bhubaneswar, (Odisha) India and Ph.D. in Computer Science and Engineering from Jodhpur National University, Jodhpur (Rajasthan), India. He has published 86 research papers in international/national journal and conferences including IEEE, Springer and ACM as well as serve as session chair, Co-chair, Technical program Committee members in many international and national conferences and serve as guest editors in many special issues from reputed journals (Indexed By: Scopus, ESCI). He also received best paper award in IEEE Conference 2013 and Young Achiever Award-2016 by IEAE Association for his research work in the field of distributed database. His researches areas are Computer Networks, Data Mining, cloud computing and Secure Multiparty Computations, Theory of Computer Science and Design of Algorithms. He authored 12 computer science books in field of Data Mining, Robotics, Graph Theory, and Turing Machine by IGI Global Publication, USA, IOS Press Netherland, Springer, Lambert Publication, Scholar Press, Kataria Publication, Narosa, Edupedia Publication, S. Chand Publication and Laxmi Publication.

Index

G

H

I

K

L

M

N

O

P

R

S

T

U

V

W

Purchase Print, E-Book, or Print + E-Book

IGI Global books can now be purchased from three unique pricing formats: Print Only, E-Book Only, or Print + E-Book. Shipping fees apply.

www.igi-global.com

Recommended Reference Books

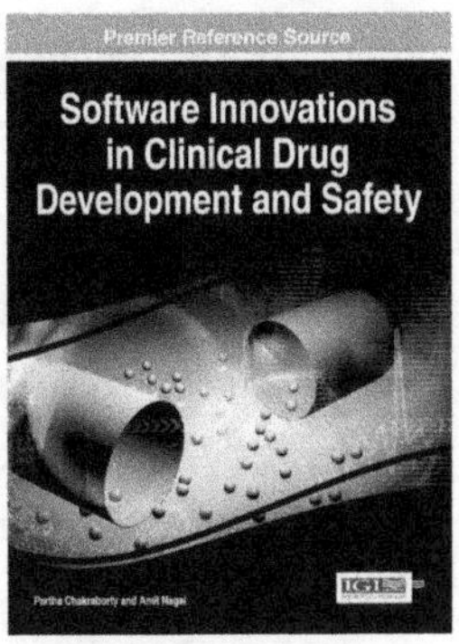

ISBN: 978-1-4666-8726-4
© 2016; 305 pp.
List Price: $225

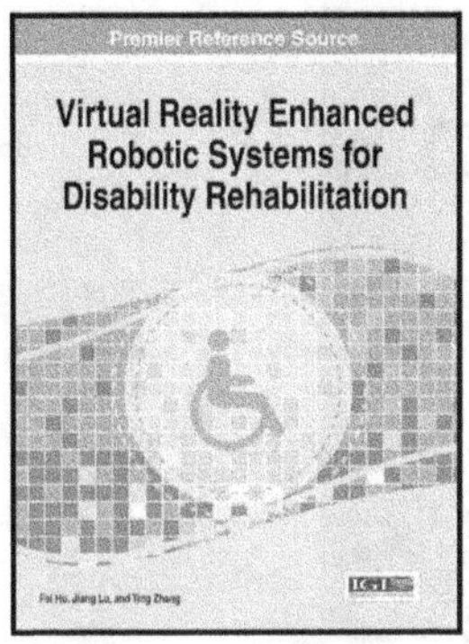

ISBN: 978-1-4666-9740-9
© 2016; 383 pp.
List Price: $210

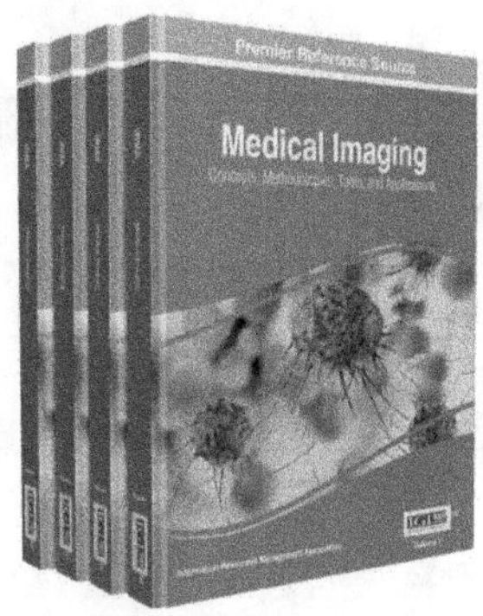

ISBN: 978-1-5225-0571-6
© 2017; 2,081 pp.
List Price: $2,150

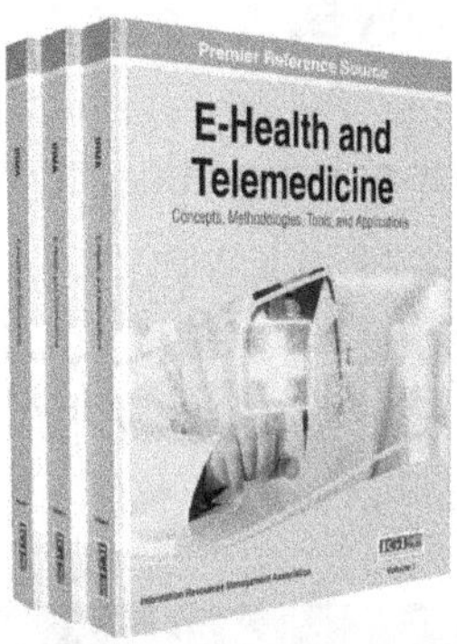

ISBN: 978-1-4666-8756-1
© 2016; 1,759 pp.
List Price: $2,435

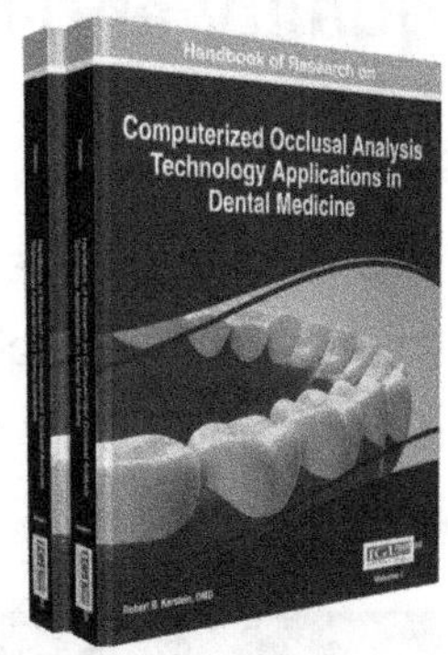

ISBN: 978-1-4666-6587-3
© 2015; 973 pp.
List Price: $475

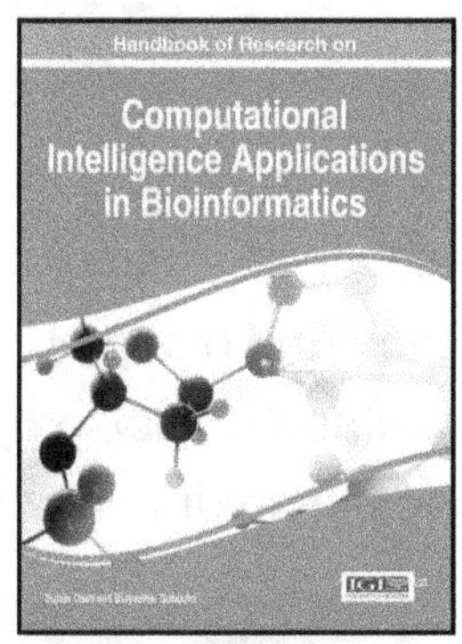

ISBN: 978-1-5225-0427-6
© 2016; 514 pp.
List Price: $230

Looking for free content, product updates, news, and special offers?
Join IGI Global's mailing list today and start enjoying exclusive perks sent only to IGI Global members.
Add your name to the list at **www.igi-global.com/newsletters.**

Publishing Information Science and Technology Research Since 1988

IGI Global
DISSEMINATOR OF KNOWLEDGE

www.igi-global.com Sign up at www.igi-global.com/newsletters facebook.com/igiglobal twitter.com/igiglobal

Stay Current on the Latest Emerging Research Developments

Become an IGI Global Reviewer for Authored Book Projects

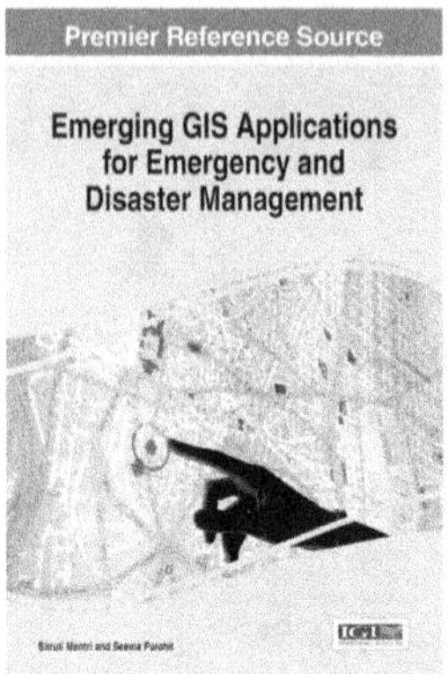

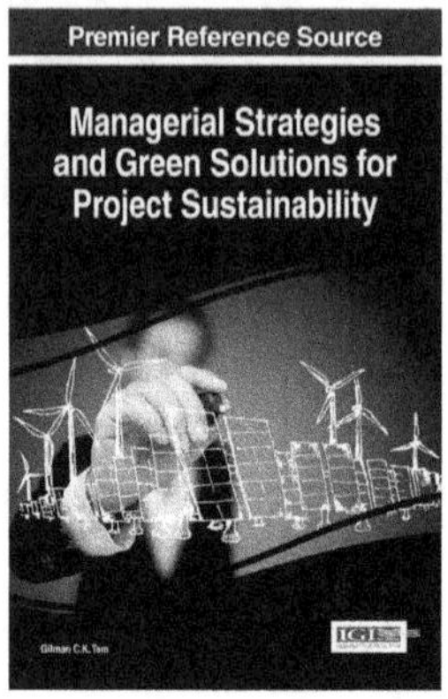

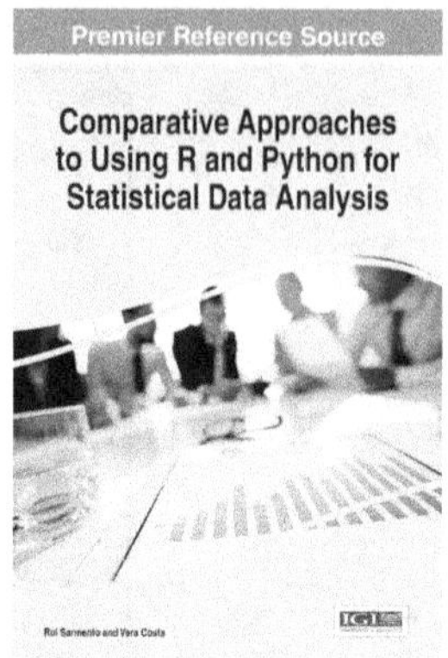

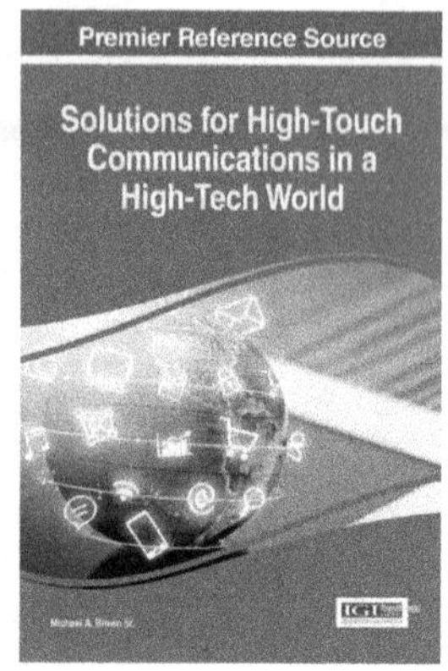

The overall success of an authored book project is dependent on quality and timely reviews.

In this competitive age of scholarly publishing, constructive and timely feedback significantly decreases the turnaround time of manuscripts from submission to acceptance, allowing the publication and discovery of progressive research at a much more expeditious rate. Several IGI Global authored book projects are currently seeking highly qualified experts in the field to fill vacancies on their respective editorial review boards:

Applications may be sent to:
development@igi-global.com

Applicants must have a doctorate (or an equivalent degree) as well as publishing and reviewing experience. Reviewers are asked to write reviews in a timely, collegial, and constructive manner. All reviewers will begin their role on an ad-hoc basis for a period of one year, and upon successful completion of this term can be considered for full editorial review board status, with the potential for a subsequent promotion to Associate Editor.

If you have a colleague that may be interested in this opportunity, we encourage you to share this information with them.

www.igi-global.com

InfoSci®-Books

A Database for Information Science and Technology Research

Maximize Your Library's Book Collection!

Invest in IGI Global's InfoSci®-Books database and gain access to hundreds of reference books at a fraction of their individual list price.

The InfoSci®-Books database offers unlimited simultaneous users the ability to precisely return search results through more than 80,000 full-text chapters from nearly 3,900 reference books in the following academic research areas:

Business & Management Information Science & Technology • Computer Science & Information Technology
Educational Science & Technology • Engineering Science & Technology • Environmental Science & Technology
Government Science & Technology • Library Information Science & Technology • Media & Communication Science & Technology
Medical, Healthcare & Life Science & Technology • Security & Forensic Science & Technology • Social Sciences & Online Behavior

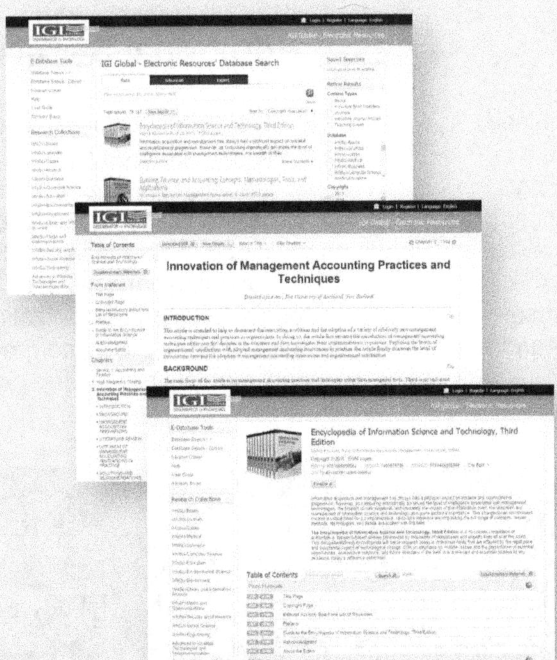

Peer-Reviewed Content:

- Cutting-edge research
- No embargoes
- Scholarly and professional
- Interdisciplinary

Award-Winning Platform:

- Unlimited simultaneous users
- Full-text in XML and PDF
- Advanced search engine
- No DRM

Librarian-Friendly:

- Free MARC records
- Discovery services
- COUNTER4/SUSHI compliant
- Training available

To find out more or request a free trial, visit: www.igi-global.com/eresources

IGI Global DISSEMINATOR OF KNOWLEDGE

www.igi-global.com

IGI Global
DISSEMINATOR OF KNOWLEDGE
www.igi-global.com

IGI Global Proudly Partners with

eContent Pro International

Enhance Your Manuscript with eContent Pro's Professional and Academic **Copy Editing Service**

Expert Copy Editing

eContent Pro copy editors, with over 70 years of combined experience, will provide complete and comprehensive care for your document by resolving all issues with spelling, punctuation, grammar, terminology, jargon, semantics, syntax, consistency, flow, and more. In addition, they will format your document to the style you specify (APA, Chicago, etc.). All edits will be performed using Microsoft Word's Track Changes feature, which allows for fast and simple review and management of edits.

Additional Services

eContent Pro also offers fast and affordable proofreading to enhance the readability of your document, professional translation in over 100 languages, and international marketing services to help businesses and organizations localize their content and grow into new markets around the globe.

IGI Global Authors Save 25% on eContent Pro's Services!

Scan the QR Code to Receive Your 25% Discount

The 25% discount is applied directly to your eContent Pro shopping cart when placing an order through IGI Global's referral link. Use the QR code to access this referral link. eContent Pro has the right to end or modify any promotion at any time.

Email: customerservice@econtentpro.com

econtentpro.com

Information Resources Management Association

Advancing the Concepts & Practices of Information Resources Management in Modern Organizations

Become an IRMA Member

Members of the **Information Resources Management Association (IRMA)** understand the importance of community within their field of study. The Information Resources Management Association is an ideal venue through which professionals, students, and academicians can convene and share the latest industry innovations and scholarly research that is changing the field of information science and technology. Become a member today and enjoy the benefits of membership as well as the opportunity to collaborate and network with fellow experts in the field.

IRMA Membership Benefits:

- **One FREE Journal Subscription**
- **30% Off Additional Journal Subscriptions**
- **20% Off Book Purchases**
- Updates on the latest events and research on Information Resources Management through the IRMA-L listserv.
- Updates on new open access and downloadable content added to Research IRM.
- A copy of the Information Technology Management Newsletter twice a year.
- A certificate of membership.

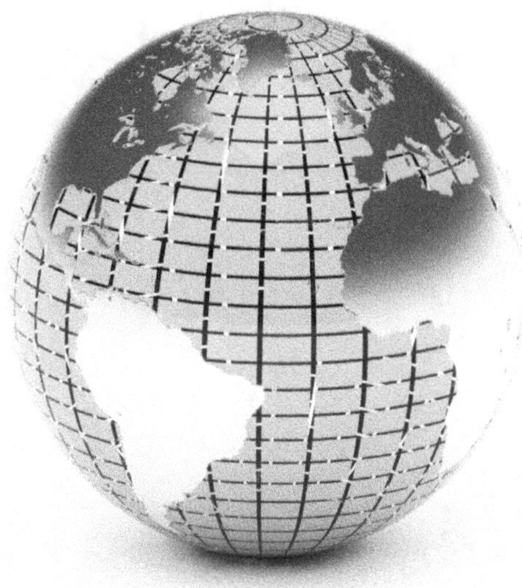

IRMA Membership $195

Scan code or visit **irma-international.org** and begin by selecting your free journal subscription.

Membership is good for one full year.

www.irma-international.org

www.ingramcontent.com/pod-product-compliance
Lightning Source LLC
LaVergne TN
LVHW060423300926
849162LV00006B/1506